GLOWING PRAISE FROM
LEADING CHILDBIRTH EXPERTS

"This is a superb book. Though it's called "official," it isn't written in bureaucratic language and isn't heaped with instructions. It's humane, funny, tender, down-to-earth and joyful. Essential reading for all pregnant women who seek autonomy in childbirth."

—Sheila Kitzinger, author of *The Complete Book of Pregnancy and Childbirth*

"*The Official Lamaze Guide: Giving Birth with Confidence* is the first book that every pregnant woman should read before she makes any decisions about her maternity care. This book is a breath of fresh air. By following these explanations and recommendations women will gain the best chance of having a normal, natural, healthy, and empowering birth."

—Marshall Klaus, MD, and Phyllis Klaus, MFT, CSW, authors of *The Doula Book*, *Your Amazing Newborn*, and *Bonding*

"This book is a wonderful resource that provides information, knowledge, and skills to expectant parents who want to play a central role in their children's births."

—Penny Simkin, coauthor of *Pregnancy, Childbirth, and the Newborn*

"At last there is a resource that emphasizes normal birth and increases parents' confidence. The honest information and reassuring tone of the authors truly get to the heart of women's fears and allow them to explore those fears in a safe way. The book contains life skills such as communication and negotiation and tells the simple story of birth in a manner that left me in awe. I wish I had been able to share this book with expectant families during my first seventeen years of teaching and being a doula."

—Ann Grauer, LCCE, CD(DONA), PCD(DONA), Past President of DONA International

"*The Official Lamaze Guide: Giving Birth with Confidence* is a no-nonsense handbook for laboring without medical interventions. The authors point out that Lamaze is no longer a method but a philosophy: Birth is normal and women can handle it."

—Melissa Chianta, *Mothering* magazine

"*The Official Lamaze Guide: Giving Birth with Confidence* is one of the rare books today containing an unapologetically woman-centered view of birth.... The authors strongly advocate natural birth.... They emphasize that women's bodies are beautifully designed to grow, birth, and nurture babies. *The Official Lamaze Guide*...should be in every [pregnant mother's] hands."

—Jane Pincus, BA, MAT, MFA, *Birth: Issues in Perinatal Care*

"Warm and wise, honest yet reassuring, chock full of information, and based on the latest and best research—any pregnant woman who wants a normal birth should put this book on her A list."

—Henci Goer, author of *The Thinking Woman's Guide to a Better Birth*

No. 1 pick on About.com Top 10 Pregnancy Books:
    "This book is an instant classic! With great advice, humor, and birth stories, Lothian and DeVries share the truth about birth and how to make it a wonderful time in your life. The factual information is provided in a practical way, including how to pick a place of birth, talk to your doctor or midwife, and most importantly how to trust your body."

—Robin Elise Weiss, LCCE, About.com

"*The Official Lamaze Guide* is a source of information that women *need* to have and a message that women need to hear. I think it accomplishes its purpose skillfully and has the potential to be a transformative influence. I hope women read it, absorb it, and begin to celebrate birth!"

—Molly Remer, MSW, CCCE

The Official Lamaze® Guide

Judith Lothian RN, PhD, LCCE, FACCE &
Charlotte DeVries of Lamaze International

Ⓜ Meadowbrook Press
Distributed by Simon & Schuster
New York

Library of Congress Cataloging-in-Publication Data

Lothian, Judith.
  Official Lamaze guide : giving birth with confidence / by Judith Lothian and Charlotte DeVries.
  — [New ed.]
  p. cm.
  ISBN 978-0-88166-566-6 (Meadowbrook Press) — ISBN 978-1-4391-7979-6 (Simon & Schuster)
  1. Childbirth—Popular works. 2. Natural childbirth—Popular works. 3. Labor (Obstetrics)—
Popular works. I. DeVries, Charlotte. II. Lamaze International. III. Title.
  RG525.L63 2011
  618.4—dc22
  2010023626

Editors: Christine Zuchora-Walske, Angela Wiechmann, and Megan McGinnis
Creative Director: Tamara JM Peterson
Production Manager: Paul Woods
Cover Photo: © Larry Williams/Corbis
Interior Photos: © BananaStock, Ltd; © Brand X Pictures; © Comstock, Inc; © Getty Images;
       © Marilyn Nolt (noltphotos@mail.com).
Index: Beverlee Day

Text © 2005, 2010 by Judith Lothian and Charlotte DeVries

Published by Meadowbrook Press, 5451 Smetana Drive, Minnetonka, MN 55343

www.meadowbrookpress.com

BOOK TRADE DISTRIBUTION by Simon and Schuster, a division of Simon and Schuster, Inc.
1230 Avenue of the Americas, New York, NY 10020

15 14   10 9 8 7 6 5 4 3

Printed in the United States of America

DEDICATION

To my seven granddaughters: Nora, Mary Brigid, Margaret,
Catherine, and Claire Gibbons, and Margaret and Ellen Lothian.
When it is time to birth their babies, I am hoping they will not
need to read this book. They will know from their wise,
confident mothers about birth and will trust, simply
and easily, their own power to give birth.

—J. L.

To Raymond, Anna, Rocky, and Jesse,
who have midwifed me as friend, partner, and mother,
and to lovely Mae, who made me a grandmother.

—C. D.

Acknowledgments

Making books, like making babies, takes more than one person. We would like to thank the collective of friends, colleagues, and family members who played important roles in bringing this book to light. Special thanks to Steven Polansky for steerage; to Linda Harmon and the Lamaze International board of directors for their continued hard work on behalf of mothers and babies; to Christine Zuchora-Walske for her patience and keen editing, to Megan McGinnis for her editing of this second edition, and to the other good folks at Meadowbrook Press; to Barbara Bonner and Will Healy for their support in so many ways; to the Institute for Advanced Study in Princeton, New Jersey, where we connected in beautiful surroundings to work on this project; to colleagues and students at the Seton Hall University College of Nursing; to the many women who have written about and modeled natural childbirth with practical knowledge and wisdom; and to Jim and Ray for their loving support and their confidence in our confidence in birth.

PREFACE

Why Another Birth Book?

In the previous edition of *The Official Lamaze Guide: Giving Birth with Confidence*, we noted that stepping into a bookstore revealed hundreds of birth books on the shelves. Some claimed to be the "complete guide" or the "better way" to have a baby. Some were filled with illustrations of developing babies, charts listing possible complications, and intricate biological details. Some were technical and scientific; others were warm and even funny.

When we reviewed all those birth books, we found that instead of encouraging women, the bestsellers cataloged what to fear when you're expecting. It was no surprise that their readers often ended up alarmed, afraid, and eager to choose medical interventions like epidurals and cesareans.

As we prepared to write this new edition of our book, we discovered that things have not changed much. Today, as in 2005, very few pregnancy books deliver the simple message that we think pregnant women need to hear most: *Birth is a natural part of life*. We conceived this book nearly a decade ago from our deep conviction that women know how to give birth—and that women need to rediscover this very important, basic truth.

Throughout history, the wisdom of birthing has belonged to the family and community. The majority of the world's women have given birth among people they know, in a familiar and comfortable place. Birth has been considered a family event, not a medical one—until recently. In our modern, technology-centered culture, birth has moved from the home to the hospital, from the care of friends and family to the oversight of medical professionals, where touch and patience often give way to tests and timekeeping.

We believe deeply that birth is a process you can trust, just as millions of women before you have. This belief isn't sentimental; it's based on our thorough understanding of the physiologic birth process and research that confirms interfering in that process is harmful, unless there's clear evidence that interference provides benefit.

Unlike many other pregnancy and birth books—and, surprisingly, much of standard obstetric care—this book is evidence-based. We often refer to *The Cochrane Library* (a collection of careful studies and systematic reviews of current research) and *A Guide to Effective*

Care in Pregnancy and Childbirth (a summary of *The Cochrane Library*'s maternity research findings with recommendations for practice). In this edition, the research has been updated. As you read this book, you'll see that research continues to support the excellence of nature's design for birth.

Simply said, it's safer and healthier for you and for your baby to allow the natural process of labor and birth unfold in the way that nature intended. In this new edition, we highlight over and over again that the best way to ensure a safe and healthy birth is to not interfere in the natural process without a serious medical indication.

Lamaze: It's Not Just about Breathing

Lamaze has been around for a long time. In the 1950s Fernand Lamaze, a French obstetrician, developed a method of breathing and relaxation that helped women manage childbirth pain. The Lamaze that people have come to know is women puffing and panting their way through labor.

But Lamaze isn't just about breathing techniques. In the years since 1960, when the Lamaze organization began, we've learned many lessons from research and women's experiences giving birth naturally. Lamaze classes provide opportunities to understand the process of birth, gain confidence in your ability to give birth simply, and have the safest, healthiest birth possible. Lamaze provides women with the latest, best information about birth and breastfeeding, and it helps women make sense of that information by simplifying maternity care decisions. In this edition, we share Lamaze's belief that it takes an entire pregnancy to prepare for birth and motherhood, not just six weeks of formal classes at the end of pregnancy.

In 1960, many women wanted more control of their pregnancy and birth experiences than women typically had at that time. These women wanted their husbands with them during labor and birth; a say in who would attend to their needs; safer, more humane treatment; and more comfortable surroundings for this important life event. Thanks to the efforts of these informed, vocal women who knew things could be better, midwives reemerged as caregivers, labor and birthing rooms became more homelike, and hospitals eliminated some unnecessary routine procedures, like enemas and perineal shaving.

Recently, the birth pendulum has taken an alarming swing backward. Our high-tech healthcare system is designed to look for trouble, and as a result, it labels more and more pregnancies and births as "complicated" or "high-risk." By the end of pregnancy, few women trust their bodies enough to believe they can give birth without drugs and machines. Today we see epidurals used almost routinely, labor induced (started artificially) at epidemic rates, women still confined to their beds in labor and on their backs during birth (the worst position for birthing a baby), and record-breaking numbers of cesarean surgeries performed.

Since the previous edition of this book was published, things have gotten even worse. The cesarean rate has continued to rise. Now almost one third of women in the United States give birth by cesarean. There has been a shocking rise in the maternal mortality rate. More babies are being admitted to the neonatal intensive care unit (NICU), and there has been an alarming increase in postpartum depression and post traumatic stress disorder related to childbirth. *Evidence-Based Care: What It Is and What It Can Achieve*,[1] published jointly by Childbirth Connection, the Reforming States Group, and the Milbank Memorial Fund, outlines problems with the current maternity care system and identifies the evidence-based care that will make birth safer and healthier for mothers and babies.

In spite of what women may hear—from their doctors, their hospitals, the media, or the books they read—women *do* know how to give birth simply. And doctors, hospitals, and technology have not made birth safer for mothers or babies. We hope this book will help you understand that pregnancy is not a disease requiring medical heroics, and that you, like all women, are well equipped to give birth.

Although the name *Lamaze* will seldom appear in these pages, it's inspired by the plain wisdom of the Lamaze belief that birth is simply and beautifully designed, and that interfering in that process without a medical reason increases risk to mothers and babies.

This book is a simple guide for the journey to motherhood. It's written clearly in plain English. It's not an encyclopedia of everything that anyone could possibly know about pregnancy, birth, and breastfeeding. It's not an endless list of obscure and unlikely complications. It's not a textbook laced with clinical terms that ends with a quiz. It's not a guide to medical birth but a guide to safe and healthy birth. It encourages you to lay down the heavy burden of what-ifs that can squash confidence. It invites you to replace fear with knowledge, and to build confidence in your ability to give birth on that foundation of knowledge.

In the pages that follow, we'll walk beside you on the path to motherhood. We'll invite you into conversations with other women who've faced the many choices you now face. We'll challenge you to consider which options are right for you and whether standard American obstetric care is actually conducive to safe, healthy, uncomplicated birth. When you look beyond the menu of options typically offered to expectant mothers, you'll find that birthing a baby is a much simpler event than you may have thought.

We believe that you have the right and the responsibility to get full and accurate information, and to choose what's best for you and your baby based on that information. We believe that the best start for mothers and babies is a safe and healthy pregnancy and birth. We believe the facts speak loudly that the safest and healthiest way to give birth is to avoid unnecessary medical interventions. This book will provide evidence that supports this belief and will show you how to give birth in the safest and healthiest way.

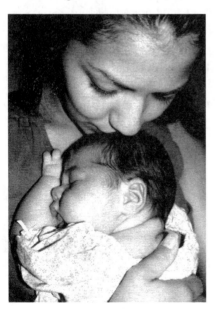

You are not an accident.
Even at the moment of your conception,
out of many possibilities,
only certain cells combined,
survived, grew to be you.
You are unique, created for a purpose.
Go confidently into the days ahead.

Contents

HAVING A SAFE, HEALTHY BIRTH

*We are just one generation away from the days when a
girl grew up on a farm watching the sheep and pigs give birth.
Anyone who saw that year after year knew that giving birth
was a natural process, a process that could be trusted.*
—Ina May Gaskin

The mission of Lamaze International and this book is to promote, support, and protect safe and healthy birth. We—like midwife Ina May Gaskin and the millions of other women who have witnessed and experienced simple, natural birth—believe that a woman's body is beautifully designed to grow, birth, and nurture a baby. To work properly, this elegant design requires patience and trust. For most women, the safest birth is one that unfolds naturally, free of unnecessary interventions. (See Chapter 7.)

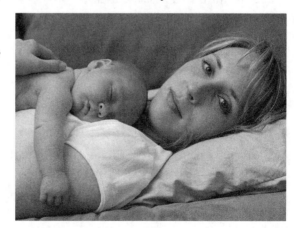

PORTRAIT OF BIRTH TODAY

Many women are surprised to learn that pregnancy, birth, and breast-feeding happen quite simply for most mothers and babies. But it's true. A woman conceives, and as she moves through her life—often without even thinking about pregnancy—a miracle happens. Cells divide, a tiny heart starts beating, brain and nerves grow. Nature orchestrates a baby's second-to-second development. It also orchestrates the release of hormones that help the mother's body adapt; that trigger labor and birth at just the right time; that help her cope with the pain and work of labor; that prepare her emotionally and physically to feed and care for her baby; and that ensure that her baby is alert and ready to nurse and meet the world.

Women don't need to read books to grow babies. Women shouldn't need to read books or take classes to give birth either. (But these days, a good book or class can be helpful in achieving a safe and healthy birth. For more on childbirth education, see pages 99–104.) We are designed perfectly for both jobs, with very few exceptions.

Let's be clear. Some labors and births do require intervention. Some women with very long, difficult labors benefit from medication. The few women who don't go into labor by forty-two weeks may need their labors jump-started. Some babies experience distress that mandates immediate intervention. Some pregnant women have preexisting health problems, like diabetes or heart disease, that require treatment affecting labor and birth. But medicalized births should be a very small percentage of all births.

An evolving body of research repeatedly shows the danger of interfering without a valid reason in the natural processes of pregnancy, birth, and breastfeeding. Any intervention, no matter how simple it

> "Someone once told me that having a baby is our way of assisting God in a miracle. I couldn't have said it better myself. My birth experience was important to me because I knew that I had a very specific and important job to do at that moment: to bring my baby into the world as healthy as possible. Every contraction, every breath, every push was bringing me closer to the end result: giving birth to my son. The moment he was born, I realized what a miracle he was, what a miracle conception and birth are to us as parents and to humankind. I felt a kinship with every woman throughout history who has given birth. This is what my body was made to do."
>
> —April

seems, may disrupt hormone release and create problems that, in turn, must be managed with more interventions. (For more on this "cascade of interventions," see Chapter 4.) In light of such evidence, the World Health Organization (WHO), a leader in the international public health effort to promote safe birth, says that maternity care should aim to achieve a healthy mother and child with the *least* intervention as possible.[1]

"With my second pregnancy I wanted a normal birth, a process where I would be left alone, to let things take their natural course.... In some profound way, which surprised me, I felt dehumanized by the cesarean I had with my first baby. I felt I had missed out on something, been robbed of something central to being me, in order to make things simpler for somebody else. As I gave birth to my second daughter, despite the pain, I was aware of something eternal in a woman giving birth, surrounded and helped by other women who had given birth themselves. I felt a connection to *life* that I did not feel the first time."
—Indira

In the United States, reality falls far short of this goal.[2] Most births in the U.S. today are interrupted by procedures designed to start, maintain, and finish labor according to an arbitrary schedule. Few women experience their pregnant bodies unfolding and opening in their own time, in their own way.

Nearly half of all expectant mothers in the U.S. receive drugs to begin labor, more than half receive drugs to speed up labor, and more than 76 percent receive drugs to dull labor pain. In contrast, pain management strategies that women describe as very helpful, like birth balls and showers and tubs, are rarely available at hospital births.[3] According to the National Center for Health Statistics, more than 90 percent of laboring women have their babies' heart rates tracked continuously by electronic fetal monitors (EFMs),[4] even though no research has shown that routine EFM use keeps babies safer.[5]

Despite all these "helpful" interventions, the U.S. cesarean rate is at an all-time high: Almost one third percent of American babies are born surgically.[6] This far exceeds the 6-percent rate considered reasonable by the WHO.[7] Although cesarean surgery is safer today than in the past, it still carries significant short-term risks for babies, and both short- and long-term risks for mothers.[8]

We're just beginning to understand the impact of birth practices on breastfeeding, but already it's clear that intervention-intensive labors and routine separation of babies and mothers interfere with nature's plan for babies' easy transition to life outside the womb. (See Healthy Birth Practice #6 on page 129.) Yet despite a wealth of research and history that prove "babies were born to be breastfed"[9] and show the many negative effects on mothers and babies who don't breastfeed,[10] formula feeding continues to be the norm in our society. Women are bombarded with advertising—and other cultural images and messages—that imply formula feeding is just as good as breastfeeding.

PRACTICES THAT PROMOTE SAFE, HEALTHY BIRTH

Research reveals not only the dangers of interfering in the natural process of birth, but also six simple strategies for keeping birth safe and healthy. The WHO identifies four practices, and Lamaze adds two more (marked with asterisks: *).

1. Let labor begin on its own.
2. Walk, move around, and change positions throughout labor.*
3. Bring a loved one, friend, or doula for continuous support.
4. Avoid interventions that aren't medically necessary.*
5. Avoid giving birth on your back and follow your body's urges to push.
6. Keep mother and baby together—it's best for mother, baby, and breastfeeding.

We explain these practices in detail and give you evidence to support their importance in Chapter 8. (Also see Appendix A.)

WHY DO SO FEW WOMEN GIVE BIRTH NATURALLY?

If the facts speak so loudly in favor of birth that unfolds naturally, why don't more women choose and experience it? We believe that because this way of birth is uncommon in the U.S., many women either don't know it's an option or don't understand that it's the safest and healthiest way to give birth for them and their babies. If women don't understand the importance of letting birth and breastfeeding happen as nature intended, they can't make truly informed choices.

Here's another way to think about informed choice: Let's say you like the taste of cod and live in a little Midwestern town, where you've grown up content with frozen cod, the only kind your local grocer stocks. But then one summer you take a seaside vacation, and for the first time you taste fresh cod! You discover that the options offered by your grocer back home are very limited. Now you know that eating fresh cod is an entirely different experience from eating frozen cod. When you return home, you persistently ask your grocer for more options in the seafood section, and eventually they become available.

Our current birth culture is like that little grocery store. Our society sets an array of choices before us, leading us to think, "These are my options. They must be the best available." But there are other options besides what "everyone else" is doing, what your hospital or doctor says is "standard" or "best," and what you've read in magazines or seen on TV.

This book introduces you to those other options. As you read on, you'll learn about the physiology of labor and birth and how to keep your labor and birth as safe and healthy as possible.

There's another reason that so few women give birth simply and naturally in the United States. Standard U.S. maternity care can sabotage nature's best plans. Birth practices like the routine use of electronic fetal monitoring (EFM) and restrictions on eating, drinking, and movement make it difficult for even the most committed woman to give birth simply and easily.

Playing in the background and haunting women's thoughts is fear for the safety of themselves and their babies. Most women have heard all their lives that doctors, hospitals, and technology make birth safe for mothers and babies. Women rarely hear that that no one can make birth—or life, for that matter—completely safe. What we do know is that the more we interfere in the natural process of labor and birth, the less safe mothers and babies are.

What you learn about birth and standard maternity care will give you a

> In spite of the evidence, U.S. maternity care continues to make it difficult for women to give birth the way nature intended. In 2006, the *Listening to Mothers II* survey learned that among nearly 1,600 new mothers across the U.S., 41 percent had labor induced, 76 percent did not move freely during labor, 93 percent had electronic fetal monitoring, 80 percent had intravenous lines, 92 percent gave birth on their backs or slightly propped up, and almost 50 percent of their babies spent the first hours after birth with hospital staff.[11]

strong foundation to make the best possible decisions for you and your baby. This knowledge will also build your confidence and help you let go of your fears. It'll help you know that you can trust your body's design as you join the circle of women who have powerfully and simply birthed their babies.

WHY YOU SHOULD BOTHER
TO LEARN MORE

Your upcoming birth experience is about much more than getting your baby out of your belly and into your arms. How your birth unfolds will profoundly affect your life, regardless of whether you think it will. It's an event you'll never forget.

Research shows that the day a woman gives birth is not "just another day," and that decades later, women clearly recall positive and negative aspects of their birth experiences.[12] Women's satisfaction with their births has little to do with the length, difficulty, or painfulness of their labors and more to do with their personal expectations, their involvement in decision making, and how they were treated by their caregivers.[13] Even women who are content to let others make decisions (including birth decisions) for them are more satisfied with their births if they're more involved in making birth decisions.[14]

Your memories of birth can influence your confidence and self-image in the future. Childbirth educator Penny Simkin says, "The potential for positive impact is great, but it takes planning, advance preparation, and safe, respectful nurturing. I'd urge women to take their upcoming childbirth very seriously. It matters too much to turn the experience of a lifetime over to someone else."[15]

Your baby's birth is a life-changing event, and it is *your* experience—not the hospital's, not the doctor's—to remember and cherish. If you seize the opportunity to prepare for and expect a positive birth experience, you'll most likely find that giving birth increases your confidence and strengthens your self-image—which will make you a more capable woman in all aspects of your life. If, instead, you hand over this important event to the direction of others, you'll do nothing to build your self-esteem.

You can make many choices to guide your pregnancy and birth down the path you prefer. You can choose how to care for yourself during pregnancy, where to have your baby, who will help you give birth, how to labor, how to give birth, how to meet your newborn, and how to feed and care for your baby. But even if your pregnancy, labor, and birth don't go as you'd hoped, your positive attitude, your care of your body, and your careful learning, planning, and choosing will build you up.

> "I was at a birth recently where the mother was very afraid of needles and pain. As she methodically moved through the stages of birth, she became more and more empowered to believe in her own body and her ability to bring into the world a beautiful, healthy baby boy. Her self-identity will never be the same."
>
> —Vicki

A snapshot of the dramatic changes during the last century will help you understand why current U.S. maternity care makes birth more difficult and less safe for us than it was for our great-grandmothers. Turn the page to learn more. We think the information will inspire you to think about birth in a new way.

Chapter 2

THE HISTORY OF BIRTH: BACK TO THE FUTURE

Stories have to be told or they die, and when they die,
we can't remember who we are or why we're here.
—Sue Monk Kidd

THE HISTORY OF BIRTH IS FULL OF STORIES

Many historians and anthropologists have chronicled the global story of birth throughout the ages. Despite the cultural flourishes associated with time and place, it's remarkable how universal the experience of pregnancy and birth is—how much a pregnant North American woman shares with a pregnant Asian woman today, how physically and spiritually similar pregnancy was for a Kenyan woman in the late 1900s and a Victorian Englishwoman. No matter where or when it happens, pregnancy brings with it special clothing and foods,

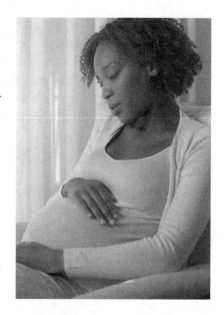

changes in relationships, growth in maturity and inner strength, and a gathering of helpers who share their wisdom and profoundly touch both mother's and baby's lives.

In the South Pacific island nation of Fiji, a whole community takes responsibility for the pregnancy of one of its women; everybody participates somehow in household preparation, labor, delivery, and postpartum care, providing support and encouragement to the growing family. In the Netherlands, a family and midwife get to know each other as they prepare the home for birth together. In Mexico, a midwife does simple exercises with an expectant mother to encourage her and help her get ready for labor. In New York, a pregnant woman gathers a simple wardrobe for her newborn, laundering and folding tiny socks and sleepers as she longs for the day she'll meet her little one face to face.

Birth: Then and Now

Allison's Story

As little girls, my sister and I hung on our grandmother's every word when she spoke of her birth in 1910. She and three of her siblings had been born on the kitchen table at the family's Brooklyn home. (Her eldest brother had been born in the hospital, which was a sign of wealth and status at the time. Apparently, the family had scraped together money to be able to afford that birth.)

Laboring and giving birth at home sounded so simple for my great-grandmother: No need to rush anywhere or pack anything, just be home and comfortable. Women in the family and building would come in and out to help during and after the birth, which sounded so nice to me. It all sounded joyous and stress-free, despite my grandmother's belief that her mother had difficult births.

Often when my grandmother shared these stories, we were gathered around our own antique oak kitchen table. I always wondered if any baby had been born on it. Could the place where I ate my breakfast be so sacred?

When I was pregnant with my first baby, I knew I'd use a midwife. A good friend had used a midwife for her child's birth, and her great birth story and account of pre- and postnatal care convinced me to find a midwife. My husband and I assumed we'd have the best of both worlds by opting for a midwifery practice that attended births at our local hospital. The prenatal visits and birth were amazing, but the hospital practices and attitudes were so foreign to us. Our loving and knowledgeable midwives had protected us in a wonderful bubble of confidence and support, which popped after we were transferred to the postpartum unit. Although we were able to advocate our wishes for ourselves, the experience was definitely one I didn't want to have again.

During labor and birth, I kept thinking about my great-grandmother, whom I never knew in person. She was, in my mind, a strong and powerful woman and mother, and she inspired me as I labored. I almost felt that she was with me, and I drew from her power—if she could birth four babies in her kitchen, I sure could birth mine! In the days following my daughter Jane's birth, I reflected on my great experience and tried to imagine what it would have been like to birth her at home. I had so many questions about home birth, but I knew that my next baby would be born at home.

My intuition was right, and I had a beautiful home water birth with my son Gavin. I again found a loving and knowledgeable midwife, and again felt the power and wisdom of my great-grandmother. As I labored, I chuckled to myself, thinking how lovely this labor was. It was still hard work, but I was in my comfortable home and surrounded by people who cared about me.

My home was only three New York City blocks from the hospital of my first birth, but it was miles and miles away in so many other ways! I thought of the women laboring at the hospital and felt guilty for the experience I was having; I knew what awaited them there. Gavin and I were treated with the highest standard of care imaginable. I tear up when I think of my gentle and loving midwife welcoming my baby boy. She asked for his permission before weighing and measuring him, which took place after as much skin-to-skin contact with me as we both needed.

Jane had also been treated beautifully by the midwife who attended her birth, but the hospital staff was focused on timing, charting, and moving things along. It wasn't an awful experience, but this one at home was so incredibly better, I was in awe. At home, birth was the normal work of bringing my baby into the world. The joy and elation that followed were the highlights. For my hospital birth, labor and birth seemed like the cliffhanger, and my daughter's arrival seemed like something to be acknowledged for just a moment before the list of other things had to be done.

For my third birth, I of course planned to be at home again, in the water, and surrounded by loving and knowledgeable people. I'm so thankful that this was how we welcomed our daughter Nora just seven months ago. It was another amazing experience. In many ways, birth in my family has come full circle. My girlhood fascination with my great-grandmother's births will always be there, but now I have firsthand experience to share. I almost feel as though I'm in on a secret of the past.

Of course, some of the practices I encountered were likely different from those my great-grandmother experienced, but the important points were intact: excellent care, health and safety for mother and baby, loving support, confidence, joy, and normalcy. It always makes me smile to think about how normal home birth feels. It sort of slips into the day or night and just happens like anything else. What a dichotomy! Birth is the biggest and most important thing I've ever done, yet the most normal. It's life, right? We just keep moving forward and getting done what we must.

Judith's Postscript

I was honored to be at the birth of Nora, and as I found my way home that night, I passed that hospital three blocks away. Women giving birth there that night would have been strapped to electronic fetal monitoring, given intravenous lines, restricted to bed, and not allowed to eat or drink. Their babies would have been whisked to the nursery almost immediately after birth. Woman just like Allison would have had a 40 percent change of having a cesarean. Allison is right: Her home was just three blocks away from the hospital, but it was miles farther in so many other ways!

FROM NATURAL TO MEDICAL

So much of what we hear and see about birth these days suggests that women are lacking, that what we bring to birth isn't enough, that we need technological help to get our babies born. Listen to a few medical stories about birth, and you'll probably wonder how women were able to have babies in past centuries.

But if you investigate the history of birth more closely, you'll see that once upon a time, as Allison's story illustrates on page 10, birth was (and still can be) a much simpler process. Ironically, as birth technology has become more sophisticated, complication and intervention rates have increased. The result is that while medical interventions, when used appropriately, make birth today safer for some mothers and babies than it was in 1910, those same interventions make birth *less* safe when they're used inappropriately.

Medical doctors led childbirth's relocation from the home to the hospital. Doctors are trained to view the world as a place where people need curing and fixing, as indeed many do. But if something isn't broken, it doesn't need to be fixed. Pregnancy is not a disease, yet many doctors treat it that way. When obstetricians imposed the "disease model" on birth, they redefined a very natural, normal event as risky business.

Until the 1900s, most women gave birth at home with a midwife's help. In the 1910s and 1920s, medical education was improving and doctors were becoming more organized as a profession. As doctors unified, they helped develop laws that enhanced and protected their own power—especially in running hospitals. The prestige of medical science grew, and upper-class women began to seek the care of doctors (who were usually male). People began to view midwives as backward, suitable only for lower-class women who couldn't afford to have doctors at their births.[1]

> Many people today still view birth as a medical event fraught with danger. "What if something goes wrong?" they ask. "Look how many mothers and babies died in the old days!" they exclaim.
>
> Midwife Ina May Gaskin is quick to differ: "Our bodies *must* work pretty well, or there wouldn't be so many humans on the planet."[8] Of the more than 2,300 babies born at the Farm, Gaskin's midwifery center in Tennessee, 96 percent were delivered without medical assistance.
>
> Indeed, there's no research that shows medical birth is safer for women and babies. Actually, research reveals more risks for mother and baby when the birth team "expects trouble" and where medical intervention is routine.[9]

The medical establishment fostered prejudice against midwives' intelligence, abilities, training, and skill. Many midwives were immigrants and didn't speak English fluently. Many were poor, many were black, and most were women. They weren't equipped to challenge the campaign being waged against them, and so began a long debate among doctors, government agencies, and midwifery supporters. This argument—which never even started in most of the rest of the world—continues today in the U.S.

So what resulted when birth shifted from homes and midwives to hospitals and doctors? It's hard to compare hospital and home birth statistics fairly, but the death rates of mothers and babies during this period can tell us a few important things.

The period when childbirth shifted from home to hospital did see some positive effects for mothers and babies. The maternal and infant death rates in the United States were high around 1900—as high as today's rates in developing countries. Over the next forty years, as the overall standard of living improved thanks to better water treatment, housing, and sanitation, the health of mothers and babies followed suit. During that same period, medical advances—specifically, the introduction of antibiotics and blood transfusions in the early 1940s— contributed to further dramatic declines in perinatal death rates.[2]

However, medical science had negative effects on mothers and babies during this time, too. To hasten delivery, doctors used procedures and instruments that often harmed mother and baby. Studies show that in the United States, obstetric interference in hospitals was associated with a large increase in baby deaths from birth injuries.[3] Hospitals also harbored germs and allowed practices that led to childbed fever in mothers. A 1925 national study concluded that "untrained midwives approach and trained midwives surpass the record of physicians in normal deliveries."[4]

Even though reports confirmed that midwives were better assistants at normal births, the medical campaign worked. Male doctors became the preferred birth attendants as middle- and lower-class women followed the example of the upper class. Statistics show the grim result: In the 1920s, more mothers and babies died in hospitals than at home births attended by midwives.[5] This is information that most women do not know.

Gradually, childbirth came to be seen as an affliction that required medical help, and the womanly art of midwifery gave way to the powerful politics of medicine. By the mid-1930s, most births were happening in hospitals. Despite evidence that told a very different story, doctors convinced women that midwives were dirty, illiterate, and incompetent and declared themselves the only competent baby deliverers. From here on, the home was deemed an unfit place for birth, although to this day there is no research that supports this claim.[6] Women birthing in the hospital, unlike at home, now "required" outside help and such "improvements" as twilight sleep (morphine and scopolamine injection), which heavily drugged a laboring woman and erased her memory of birth. Just as importantly, the combination of heavy medication and the nearly routine use of forceps for delivery put babies at risk.

Childbirth's move from home to hospital improved the lives of doctors. In a hospital, one doctor could care for many women at once. Doctors no longer had to travel to mothers' homes and work at inconvenient hours in unfamiliar territory.

This change did not, however, improve the lives of women. It swept away respect for the abilities of both birthing women and midwives. It dried up the flow of empowering birth stories.[7] As a result of twilight sleep, women had no memories of their births to treasure and pass along.

If you could step into a 1950s American hospital, you'd see women left to labor alone—often drugged and confined to bed—then moved to loud, bright delivery rooms and strapped onto sterile tables, lying on their backs with their feet pressed high overhead in metal stirrups. Gowned and masked doctors and nurses directed these births and typically forbade mothers to have family present and to hold or sometimes even see their babies right after birth. Home birth was becoming a distant memory.

> "I was knocked out as soon as I got to the hospital. I didn't remember anything until the next day. My husband said I kept asking him if the baby was born and what it was. I was in a fog."
>
> —Doris

By the 1960s, medicalized birth was so common in the United States that most women didn't know there was any other kind. They routinely labored without support, were given enemas, had their genitals shaved and disinfected, and gave birth on their backs, draped with sterile sheets to prevent them from touching (and possibly infecting) their newborns. Hospital staff whisked the babies away, washed and clothed them, wrapped them in sterile receiving blankets, and put them on display in nurseries far from their mothers. Formula feeding at scheduled times became the norm. Women were told that this was good, modern medical practice. We now know that these practices harmed both mothers and babies. The documentary *The Business of Being Born* presents a vivid picture of this era in U.S. maternity care. (See Recommended Resources.)

MOTHERS SPEAK OUT

Luckily, some women didn't accept the medical view of birth, and they spoke out. It began as just a murmur, but as more and more women demanded an active role in birth, their voices grew too strong to ignore. They insisted on—and got—childbirth education and breastfeeding information and support. Their steady work rekindled midwifery and natural childbirth.

In the late 1950s, Marjorie Karmel wrote *Thank You, Dr. Lamaze* after birthing her baby in Paris with Fernand Lamaze at her side. (She'd been inspired to try Lamaze's natural childbirth method after reading Grantly Dick-Read's *Childbirth without Fear*.) When she met Elisabeth Bing in New York City soon afterward, the two women set about teaching as many women as possible to approach childbirth without fear and to learn how to work with their bodies in labor and birth. In 1960, Karmel and Bing established Lamaze International (then called the American Society for Psychoprophylaxis in Obstetrics, or ASPO), one of the most important childbirth organizations in the country.

Like so many other social changes in the U.S., the natural childbirth movement gained strength as a consumer movement. More and more women and men convinced their doctors and nurses that women

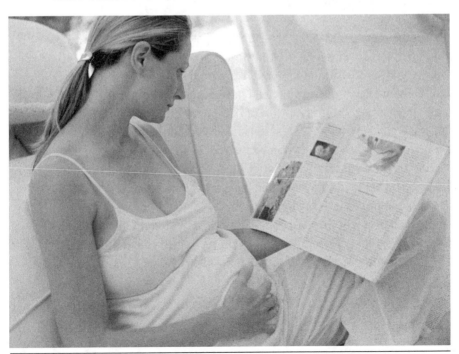

would have better births and healthier babies if they were better educated and better prepared for birth. Medication use could be reduced, and women could be awake, in control, and supported by those around them in what could be a more rewarding, less traumatic event for everyone.

More challenges to medicalized birth came in the 1960s. Across the Atlantic, British anthropologist Sheila Kitzinger burst onto the scene with her book *The Experience of Childbirth* in 1962, suggesting that labor pain shouldn't be drugged away, but rather embraced as "pain with a purpose" in the perfect design of birth. American obstetrician Robert Bradley's 1965 book *Husband-Coached Childbirth* stressed the importance of women having their companions present during labor and delivery. In 1967, Elisabeth Bing's *Six Practical Lessons for an Easier Childbirth* became a guide for thousands of women who wanted to prepare actively for birth.

The birth revolution continued in the next decade. The Boston Women's Health Book Collective (a women's health education and advocacy group) published its historic book *Our Bodies, Ourselves* in 1970. This book told women that they had the power to bring about change in women's health and suggested that the medical approach to normal life events like birth might not be effective or healthy. Soon more writers woke up and spoke up with books like Doris Haire's *The Cultural Warping of Childbirth* (1972), Suzanne Arms' *Immaculate Deception* (1975), and Ina May Gaskin's *Spiritual Midwifery* (1975).

As like-minded women around the country sought out one another and made birth choices not offered in hospitals at the time, they angered the medical community by challenging its long-standing authority. Elisabeth Bing recalls, "The fight for recognition of the idea of family-centered maternity care, in which fathers and children become part of the birth experience, was a slow and hard fight. Acceptance did not come overnight. I remember well how I was told that surely this was all a fad, that women would soon forget, and that ideas as strange as encouraging a woman to be awake and aware while giving birth were beyond all rational thinking."[10]

Governments and healthcare systems were slow to react. But the evidence supporting a move toward more natural birth was so strong that even bureaucrats and members of the very profession being criticized were compelled to respond. In 1975, Uruguayan obstetrician Roberto Caldeyro-Barcia, who later served as president of the International Federation of Gynecology and Obstetrics, advocated getting laboring women off their backs and out of stirrups and allowing women to labor in their own chosen positions.[11] In the late 1970s, U.S. congressional hearings called for reducing the alarmingly high cesarean rate and for improving prenatal care around the country. During the same decade, French obstetrician Michel Odent's research led him to promote the use of showers and baths for comfort during natural birth.[12] In the late 1980s, the Carnegie Foundation for the Advancement of Teaching made midwife recruitment and education recommendations that highlighted the importance of and growing demand for midwife care.[13] In 1992, the United Kingdom's House of Commons finally admitted that research showed the home to be as safe as a hospital for birth and that, in fact, home birth *should* be a publicly supported option.[14]

Meanwhile, across the North Sea, women in the Netherlands have enjoyed watching the international birth pendulum swing back and forth. The Dutch government has supported midwife-assisted home birth for decades. A third of Dutch births happen at home, and nearly half of Dutch women have their babies with midwives in attendance. The Netherlands consistently ranks among the top countries in the world for successful birth outcomes, along with Japan, Iceland, Sweden, and Finland.[15]

Obstetrics under the Microscope

The Cochrane Group Is Born

In 1979 Archie Cochrane, then director of a prestigious epidemiology research unit in the UK, identified obstetrics as the medical specialty with the worst record for using randomized, controlled trials (the gold standard in research) to evaluate the effectiveness of patient care. Three obstetrician-epidemiologists took on the challenge of changing that: Murray Enkin from Canada, Iain Chalmers from the UK, and Marc Keirse from the Netherlands.

The efforts of Enkin, Chalmers, and Keirse produced *The Cochrane Library*[16] (a collection of careful studies and systematic reviews of current research) and *A Guide to Effective Care in Pregnancy and Childbirth*[17] (a summary of *The Cochrane Library*'s maternity research findings with recommendations for practice). Currently more than nine thousand controlled trials from almost four hundred medical journals, in eighteen languages from eighty-five countries, are registered in *The Cochrane Library*, which is available electronically and is constantly updated. Its research team includes doctors, midwives, nurses, public health experts, and statisticians who find and evaluate the world's best research and then make recommendations for practice.

A Guide to Effective Care in Pregnancy and Childbirth (full text available at http://www.childbirthconnection.org) classifies maternity care practices as:

- beneficial
- probably beneficial
- both risky and potentially beneficial
- of unknown effectiveness
- probably not beneficial
- probably ineffective or harmful[18]

The most important thing we learn from the work of *The Cochrane Library* is that interfering without a serious medical indication in the process of labor and birth disrupts the process, causing unintended consequences that increase risk for mother and baby. Over and over again, the research confirms the danger inherent in disrupting the normal, natural process of labor and birth. The research also confirms the value of medical interventions when used appropriately.

Thanks to *The Cochrane Library*, caregivers and women now have easy access to high-quality research and can provide evidence-based care to women and their babies. As a result, births should be safer. Nonetheless, for many reasons, most U.S. obstetricians still don't consistently base their practices on best evidence.[19]

The Role of Technology

Why, when research continually supports natural birth as the safest and healthiest way to give birth and shows the danger of routine birth interventions, does birth remain stuck in the realm of medicine? There's no doubt that technology *can* improve our lives, but it doesn't *always* do so. Any device, drug, or procedure can cause either good or bad results. Using technology just because we can often leads to unintended consequences. This is what has happened in obstetrics.

Modern medical technology, used routinely in an effort to increase safety, changes how birth is meant to proceed and actually increases risks for mothers and babies. Here are just some of the routine interventions that often divert mothers from natural birth and increase risk when not used appropriately:

- **Prenatal tests** are often misinterpreted, causing unnecessary stress, loss of confidence, and sometimes misinformed decisions. (See page 81.)
- **Drugs** can begin a woman's labor on the spot, even though her body and her baby may not be ready for birth. They intensify labor, which may necessitate other drugs to help manage her pain if contractions get too intense. Babies are born too soon and require special care. (See page 141.)
- An **epidural** removes a mother's labor pain, but also scrambles her body's signals and disrupts the natural course of labor. The medication used in epidurals also affects her baby. (See page 154.)
- **Electronic fetal monitoring (EFM)** records a baby's response to labor. External EFM, the most common type, is held against a mother's abdomen with a belt. The belt is connected to a large machine that limits the mother's ability to move around. Research shows that medical staff interpret EFM information inconsistently. (Some research shows that the confinement required for EFM actually causes the problems EFM records.) If the information is misread, staff may intervene further, disrupting the normal flow of labor and birth even more.

EFM certainly *seems* like a good idea. A machine that measures and records a baby's response to contractions provides scientific data about a particular woman's labor. Logic says—and many people assume—that EFM improves birth outcomes.

Actually, three decades of research shows that EFM *doesn't* improve birth outcomes. When EFM is used during labor, no fewer babies die and no fewer have problems at birth. However, more women have cesareans when EFM is used.[20] If EFM doesn't help babies and puts mothers at higher risk of surgical intervention, it is *not* safer care.

In 1988, a Harvard Medical School report described EFM as a "failed technology" but also predicted that doctors wouldn't stop using it because they fear being sued.[21] Fear of malpractice litigation is pervasive in obstetrics. Doctors too often make patient care decisions based on their fear of a lawsuit rather than on evidence-based standards of practice established by their profession.

- **A scheduled cesarean** is faster and more convenient for a doctor and mother than allowing the mother to labor when and for as long as her body might need to. But a cesarean is surgery, and like all surgery, it carries risks for mother and baby that most women don't realize. (See page 156 and 269.)

- **Newborn care procedures and equipment**, such as tests, shots, and warmers (isolettes), separate mothers and babies. But we know that a mother's warm arms provide the perfect setting for her newborn baby's first hours, and separating mothers and babies increases risk for both of them. (See page 129.)

Albert Einstein looked at the state of the world late in his career and said, "It has become appallingly obvious that our technology has exceeded our humanity." We think Einstein is right. As we increasingly pursue and rely on birth technology—that force we've come to trust as faster, safer, better—we not only forget what normal birth is, we also forget how to respond to birth with humanity and patience.

Much of modern birth technology has not improved birth outcomes in the United States. Forty-one countries have lower infant mortality rates than the U.S.[22] The countries with the lowest infant and maternal death rates share, among other practices, a reliance on midwives for primary care at most births.[23] Research suggests that doctors may not be the best birth attendants,[24] and history shows that until the early 1900s they never attended complication-free births.

Obstetricians are trained to diagnose and treat disease and complications in pregnancy and childbirth. They do this extremely well. Medical advances like the development of antibiotics, the diagnosis and treatment of pregnancy-induced hypertension, and the use of blood transfusions have done a lot to reduce maternal death and disease rates.

But doctors are not trained to understand and trust the natural process of birth. They're trained to expect trouble and to manage birth rather than let it move at its own pace. An obstetrician's expertise at fixing problems may make him or her less cautious about disrupting the natural process than a midwife would be. Many obstetricians fear litigation more than intervention. American lawyers and jurors tend to equate good medicine with interventions and technology rather than evidence-based standards of practice. Obstetricians are stuck between a rock and a hard place.

As a result, we perpetuate a system of intervention-intensive birth that too often puts mothers and babies at risk. Childbirth educator and author Penny Simkin warns, "I think we're fiddling with a process that is showing us more and more that it really shouldn't be fiddled with, except where there is clear indication that something is wrong."[25]

Support for Natural Birth Today

Midwives

According to both the American College of Nurse-Midwives (ACNM) and the Midwives Alliance of North America (MANA), a midwife recognizes pregnancy and birth as normal processes and believes the education and empowerment of pregnant women are just as important as good prenatal care.[26]

Midwifery training focuses on understanding and protecting what is normal and natural in pregnancy and birth, while obstetric training focuses on understanding and looking for complications. Holding a midwifery textbook in one hand and an obstetrics textbook in the other illustrates the different outlooks of the two professions: The obstetrics text is much heavier, since it's full of descriptions of rare complications.

One midwife says, "There's a lot of pressure on midwives, particularly if you're hospital-based, to become like hospital residents, to see as many patients as possible and keep pushing people through." But that's not what midwife care is about. Doctor visits average eight or nine minutes per patient.[27] A midwife will tell you that her routine prenatal visit takes up to thirty minutes. The medical part of this visit—checking blood pressure, listening to the baby's heartbeat, and measuring the mother's belly—takes only about four minutes. The rest of the time is for building relationship, trust, and confidence—for getting to know a woman, answering questions, alleviating fears.

Unfortunately, time isn't the only aspect of midwifery that's being threatened by developments in medicine. The very future of midwifery is at risk. Midwifery centers across the country are being forced to close because their malpractice insurance is getting too costly (though midwives are rarely sued) and because obstetricians are refusing to offer backup support to midwives (a legal requirement in most states)—partly because of *their* huge malpractice costs.

Just as parents needed to organize into a consumer movement to improve childbirth in past decades, midwives have realized the need to speak and work together to change harmful legislation and discriminatory practices. As more women choose midwives as caregivers and share their empowering birth stories, the demand for midwives continues to grow in the United States. Midwifery programs around the country continue to train new midwives each year, despite the political pressures working against them.

Citizens for Midwifery is a grass-roots organization dedicated to spreading the word about the midwifery model of care. Their website, http://cfmidwifery.org, is an excellent resource for basic research on midwifery and out-of-hospital birth, and on legislation related to midwifery and out-of-hospital birth nationally and in individual states.

> "In every country where I have seen real progress in maternity care, it was women's groups working together with midwives that made the difference."
> —Marsden Wagner, MD, MS

Lamaze International and Other Birth Advocacy Groups

For fifty years **Lamaze International** has been a strong advocate for safe, healthy birth. It continues to develop and support initiatives that provide credible, relevant, and useful information about safe, healthy birth for both professionals and childbearing families.[28] Lamaze's six evidence-based Healthy Birth Practices, adapted from the work of the World Health Organization (WHO), help women have the safest, healthiest birth possible. (See Chapter 8 and Appendix A.) In addition to training and certifying childbirth educators, Lamaze International has a strong internet presence (http://www.lamaze.org), providing evidence-based information for professionals and parents, including blogs, forums, videos, and a weekly pregnancy e-newsletter.

The list of other North American organizations advocating for natural birth is ever-growing. In 1994, Lamaze International hosted a gathering of individuals representing more than fifty of these organizations to discuss how to improve care for birthing women and their babies. This meeting gave birth to the **Coalition for Improving Maternity Services (CIMS)**, a group that works to improve birth outcomes while reducing the cost of maternity care.[29] CIMS has developed a Mother-Friendly Childbirth Initiative (MCFI) that hospitals, birth centers, and home birth services can implement to offer the best possible care for both mothers and babies.

The MCFI is based on the following principles. (For the full text of the MCFI, see Appendix B.)

- Birth is a normal, natural, and healthy process.
- Women are empowered when they receive sensitive, respectful care.
- When women are accurately informed of their options in birth, they will make good choices.
- Routine tests, procedures, drugs, and restrictions on laboring and birthing women should be avoided.
- The interests of mothers and babies should come first in maternity care.
- Any maternity care practice should be backed by evidence that it is best for mother and baby.

CIMS works to educate pregnant women as well as professionals and, unsurprisingly, the group supports the work of midwives because of their long history of promoting, protecting, and supporting normal birth.

Working alongside CIMS in supporting and promoting natural, safe, healthy birth are dozens of more specialized groups of nurses, midwives, childbirth educators, and doulas (professionals who support birthing women and their families). Here are just a few:

- **DONA International** believes in the highest quality of emotional, physical, and educational support for women and their families during and after childbirth. DONA has trained about three thousand doulas in evidence-based programs that teach the importance of continuous support for childbearing women. Doula Christina McGhee explains the value of her work: "I strongly believe that the support of another woman through pregnancy, labor, and postpartum has a profound impact on the health and happiness of the mother, the baby, and the family unit."[30]
- **Childbirth Connection** (formerly Maternity Center Association) has been dedicated to improving maternity care since 1918.[31] Among many other firsts, the organization opened the first school of nurse-midwifery in the United States in 1931 and established the nation's first freestanding birth center in 1975. Childbirth Connection continues to be a strong voice in birth research and advocacy. Its website, http://www.childbirthconnection.org, offers free downloads of many documents that help mothers make informed decisions, such as the Cochrane Collaboration's *A Guide to Effective Care in Pregnancy and Childbirth* and

Listening to Mothers I (2002) and *II* (2006) and *New Mothers Speak Out* (2008), the only national surveys of U.S. women's childbearing and postpartum experiences. These are invaluable resources for both parents and professionals, and we refer to both over and over again in this book.

In 2008, Childbirth Connection in partnership with the Reforming States Group and the Milbank Memorial Foundation published *Evidence Based Care: What It Is and What It Can Achieve* (also known as the Milbank Report).[32] This report is a thorough analysis of the current maternity care system. Since the publication of the Milbank Report, Childbirth Connection has worked with national leaders representing medicine, nursing, childbirth education, doulas, midwives, insurance companies, government agencies—everyone who's involved in maternity care. The collaborative work of this group resulted in two direction-setting papers, "2020 Vision for a High Quality, High Value Maternity Care System," which describes an optimal maternity care system, and the "Blueprint for Action: Steps Toward a High Quality, High Value Maternity Care System," which charts the pathway for moving toward the vision. (The full reports of these papers are available at the organization's website.) Through these initiatives, Childbirth Connection continues to provide leadership in creating change in the maternity care system in order to protect the safety and health of mothers and babies.

Across the country, Childbirth Connection and other birth networks are providing education and support to childbearing women, and advocating locally and nationally to protect women's rights and choices related to birth. Visit http://www.birthnetwork.org to find other birth networks.

- **Choices in Childbirth** was founded in New York City in 2003 by a handful of doulas and childbirth educators who were concerned that their birth clients were increasingly being denied access to a full range of birthing options.[33] Manhattan's only freestanding birth center, Elizabeth Seton Childbearing Center, had just been closed and midwifery services all across the city were being cut. As induction and cesarean section rates soared, it seemed that heavy medical management of birth was the only option. Women who wanted a natural birth, or who simply wanted to avoid unnecessary medical interventions, were finding it more and more difficult to identify providers and facilities that would honor their choices. In response, Choices in Childbirth has engaged in a number of education, outreach, and advocacy programs designed to inform the public (including families, the press, policy makers, students and medical professionals) about women's rights and options in maternity care.

Since 2006, Choices in Childbirth has annually published *The Guide to a Healthy Birth*, a free printed resource that began in New York City but that now has distribution in all fifty states. The guide is supplemented by an online database of mother-friendly providers and other local level resources accessible at http://www.choicesin childbirth.org. Choices in Childbirth provides three free monthly meetings for New York City families: Inspiring Birth Stories, Healthy Birth Choices, and the Sexy Moms Series.

In 2009, the National Quality Forum (NQF), perhaps the best-known and most respected national organization seeking to improve American healthcare, for the first time established quality measures for maternity care. These measures have been adopted by The Joint Commission, the organization that accredits and certifies U.S. hospitals. The effect of these new perinatal quality measures is that most hospitals will be looking for ways to decrease elective births before thirty-nine weeks, to decrease cesarean rates for low-risk women, and to increase the number of women exclusively breastfeeding their babies when they leave the hospital.

In 2006, Choices in Childbirth worked with the Public Advocate for the City of New York to ensure that all of the city's forty-four hospitals were providing obstetric intervention rates to the public in compliance with the Maternity Information Act. They also petitioned the New York State Department of Health to put the intervention data up on the state's website so that it'd be more readily accessible to a wider audience. In the same year, and continuing in the spirit of increased transparency in maternity care, Choices in Childbirth partnered with the Coalition for Improving Maternity Services (CIMS) to pilot *The Birth Survey*, a consumer feedback website where women provide information about the maternity care they received from specific practitioners and facilities.[34] The consumer feedback is then made available to other women in the community to aid them in choosing the birth practitioner and setting that's best for them. Since its pilot in New York City, *The Birth Survey* has continued to grow and is now available nationally at http//www.thebirthsurvey.com.

- **International Cesarean Awareness Network (ICAN)** is an advocacy group committed to improving maternal-child health by preventing unnecessary cesareans through education, providing support for cesarean recovery, and promoting vaginal birth after cesarean (VBAC).[35] ICAN's vision is that there will be a significant decrease in the cesarean rate, driven by women making evidence-based, risk-appropriate childbirth decisions. They believe, as we do, that the inappropriate overuse of cesarean surgery is jeopardizing the lives of mothers and babies. They also believe that the rate of maternal-request cesareans is exaggerated. For nearly three decades, ICAN has made significant contributions in raising awareness of the shocking rise in cesarean rates and helping put a face on the statistics by telling women's stories and highlighting the long-term, sometimes life-threatening consequences of cesarean surgery for women. Visit their website, http://www.ican-online.org, for more information.

Films You Should See

Two documentaries on birth have attracted a swirl of media attention as well as the attention of the American Congress of Obstetricians and Gynecologists (ACOG) and the American Medical Association (AMA). *The Business of Being Born* by Ricki Lake and Abby Epstein and *Pregnant in America: A Nation's Miscarriage* by Steve Buonaugurio challenge the current maternity care system by presenting historical and research evidence in graphic, personal ways. (See Recommended Resources.) Both documentaries make the case for a maternity care system that respects the natural process of birth and does not interfere in that process unless medically indicated. Debra Pascali-Bonaro's film *Orgasmic Birth* introduces a variety of women giving birth in hospitals and at home with deep pleasure and satisfaction. It too received wide media attention, including a segment on the acclaimed television news magazine program *20/20*.

> Professional, grassroots, and media advocacy efforts are making the safety issues related to standard U.S. maternity care more visible to the public.

CREATING HISTORY:
SHARING BIRTH STORIES

All birthing women are part of the same circle of mothers. When we share our stories, our wisdom, and our encouragement, we offer each other important tools for navigating our lives. In the realm of birth, we can learn from each other the purpose of labor pain, the rewards of those brief and intense hours that lead to cradling a baby.

We can help each other give birth with confidence, thereby gaining strength for future challenges along life's journey. New birth stories are created every hour around the world—stories about unique women in unique situations bringing unique human beings into the world. Every story is special; every one is important.

Children grow up treasuring the stories their parents have repeated to them. Knowledge of our past helps us understand who we are and where we've come from. In the same way, the sharing of birth stories reminds women of their shared strengths, hopes, and fears.

Even if you'll never hear a birth story from your mother or grandmother, there are numberless sources you can—and should—tap. You need birth information told from a variety of perspectives, and what you read in a memoir or hear from a trusted sister, aunt, or friend may be dramatically different from what you read in a birth manual, see in the media, or hear from a doctor.

In 1988, Kathryn Hall founded Birthing Project USA (BPUSA) in Sacramento, California,[36] to help at-risk African American pregnant women invest in their pregnancies and understand the importance of the hard work they're doing in pregnancy. Today, BPUSA pairs pregnant women across the U.S. with volunteer "sister friends" to improve the health and well-being of the young mother and her baby. BPUSA is a modern model of women helping women successfully enter the dance of motherhood.

Finding Out about Others' Birth Stories

Here are some questions you might want to ask other women who've given birth, as well as examples of answers you might receive:

* *How did you feel when you found out you were pregnant?*

   "I'd been using birth control pills for several years and began to wonder if my body would even know how to get pregnant. What a surprise to miss a period after just one month off the pill!"

- *Whom did you tell first?*

   "We'd been trying to get pregnant for a while, and when I found out we were, I couldn't bring myself to tell anyone. My husband broke the silence by sending three roses to the office where I worked. A few wise women got it right off."

- *What do you remember about your pregnancy?*

   "My mother never offered information to me about her pregnancies on her own. 'We were raised not to talk about it,' she told me, 'because it was related to sex!' As a result, I think she dismissed so much of her experiences that she lost a bit of herself."

- *Were you able to talk about your pregnancy with others?*

   "It can be a touchy thing, talking about your pregnancy. I worried about how one woman who couldn't get pregnant would feel hearing about my pregnancy. I'm so glad we're part of a church community where there are a lot of young parents. Once I began showing, a few women came alongside me and just sort of chatted their way into my life. They ended up lending me maternity clothes and books, and giving advice when I asked. It's not easy to find support sometimes. I was pretty grateful for those people."

- *Did you feel supported or alone during those months?*

   "I've had others tell me that when they became pregnant, all of the sudden they were seeing pregnant women everywhere! Of course, it's because we were suddenly so present and aware of babies growing inside us. It felt like a silent sisterhood. My husband was super supportive, even though I knew what he was experiencing was pretty different from what I was."

- *Who was your caregiver?*

   "I'd been seeing a midwife for my first pregnancy, but I labored too long according to the hospital protocol, and I can't tell you a thing about the intern who delivered my baby. It definitely shaped my decision to have my next baby at home, where I'd build a relationship with my caregivers that would last beyond the birth."

- *How did you choose your caregiver?*

   "It's so important to talk with other women with babies to find out about their birth experiences, who their docs were, how things went. There was one OB practice I 'un-chose' because of what two mothers shared about how they were treated."

- *How did you prepare for birth?*

  "A friend gave me a new little journal when she found out I was pregnant. I'm not much of a diary person, but I carried that book in my purse and got into the habit of jotting things down—everything from name ideas to fears that would creep into my head, to comments people would make to me, to what I wanted to collect and prepare in the baby's room. I've put the journal with my daughter's baby book for her to read someday."

- *Where did you have your baby?*

  "I'm one of few women, I think, who gave birth in the same hospital where she was born. But my experience was very different from my mother's. My baby never went into a windowed nursery—he was with me the entire time. No feeding schedule or formula given to him. And I actually requested that the baby not have a bath, and the nurse just washed his hair a bit while I held him. I didn't want to be separated from him, and it made me sad to think of someone else giving him his first bath. Besides, he smelled so good, I didn't want that washed away."

- *Who was in the room with you, and what did they do?*

  "I invited an older friend to be with us for our birth. I was afraid my mother would be freaked out. She was an old-school nurse with a lot of baggage from her training days about how women were being treated in maternity wards. My friend was such a quiet, steady presence to both of us. It turns out she'd had 'bad births' herself back in the day. I think she experienced a bit of healing by helping us."

- *How did your labor start?*

  "I hear so many women say they labored for thirty or more hours. That was me, with my first birth. It turns out I went to the hospital way too soon. I could have stayed home and walked and rested in the back yard that first day. That first labor is such an unknown, you think the baby will be born any minute, and really, your body is just getting warmed up for the work down the road."

- *How did you feel and what did you think about during labor?*

  "I remember thinking, 'This is not at ALL what I thought it would feel like!' No one can really put words to the essence of a contraction. No two women will describe it the same way. I don't think there is harder or richer work in the world that a woman will take on during those hours."

- *What was done to you during labor and birth?*

  "I loved how my midwife encouraged me to 'listen to the music in my body.' I would close my eyes and visualize that I was dancing with my baby in my arms. That helped get me on my feet and 'sway' my way through contractions, on the birth ball but also sometimes with my husband's arms around me from behind. He got into the dance with me."

- *What were your thoughts when you first saw your baby's face?*

  "Isn't it just so surreal to meet this person face to face, after feeling her move around inside me for so long? To finally put a name to that face and have her look at me with such deep interest. Wow!"

- *What was it like to breastfeed for the first time?*

  "My midwife was such a patient, quiet help to me as I got the hang of it. And I was blessed that my baby knew what she wanted. I can't imagine a more powerful moment of connection than that first feeding."

- *If you didn't breastfeed, why not?*

  "I tried, but I just don't think I was made for breastfeeding. My mom had told me beforehand how she had tried as well but it hadn't worked out. I planned on going back to work anyway, so it wasn't such a bad thing to have to switch from nursing to the bottle, which I've heard can be hard."

- *Was becoming a mother what you thought it would be?*

  "I had a rough few months with morning sickness that made me wonder if I was up to what I was getting into. And it's true, caring for a baby is not for the faint of heart. In a hundred ways, it's a richer experience that I could have predicted, but it's also more intense than I could have known. My life is not my own anymore. It's that 24/7 listening and being at the ready that changes everything."

Like most conversations, your sharing of thoughts and questions about birth will lead you down interesting pathways to new destinations. You may learn more than you were looking for. Perhaps you'll learn not only about pregnancy, labor, and birth, but also about caring for newborns, about mothers' feelings during those first days postpartum, about the presence or absence of fathers, or about how birth affects relationships. The possibilities are limitless.

"It was autumn 1912 when my mother was born to a German housewife, the ninth baby to enter the world in the cramped bedroom of her little Ohio farmhouse. There was no doctor present, no hospital in the sparsely settled area, no running water or electricity on the farm, no time for my grandmother to delight in her newborn. All too soon the care of her family, home, orchards, and garden pulled her back onto her feet.

In the same little town in 1949, my mother birthed me, her third and final child, in a scopolamine haze at the 'modern' hospital two blocks from her little house. A black-and-white hospital photo shows me swaddled in receiving blankets and sleeping in a little nursery box, a hand-printed sign reading 'Baby Jones' above my head. My mother could recall nothing about the night I was born. It was two weeks before she could leave her room to gather me in her arms and take me home.

In 1980, my mother stood in the living room of my little California house. It was the middle of the night, and she was cradling the baby boy I had just birthed with the quiet help of my midwife, my husband, and a trusted friend. Our son had already nursed, moments after he'd come into our world. The dimly lit room was shimmering with the holiness of his arrival.

Three generations of women—my grandmother, my mother, and me—did what women from the beginning of time have done. We stepped into the dance of motherhood in a changing world. We brought our histories, our gifts, and all our strength to those moments when new human beings emerged from our bodies and breathed air into their tiny lungs."

—Charlotte

Starting Your Own Story

The story of pregnancy and childbirth plays on in your body, as it does in all the women around the world who are pregnant alongside you now. Each story is worth telling, worth hearing, worth treasuring. Your story is no exception. It deserves a place of honor right next to all the stories of parents who, as children's advocate Fred Rogers said, "have loved us into being."[37]

No matter how well you understand the physical process of birth, it still holds a spiritual spark. How you decide to picture your pregnancy is an important choice. Is it a mechanical event that needs modern medicine to help it along? Or is it a natural unfolding of life and of your family history? Your answer to this question is sure to influence the course of your story.

Today, the stories of many births languish in medical files, written in scientific terms that too often increase fear rather than self-confidence. When birth stories are encoded in medical language, the truth about natural birth and the strength of women is usually lost.

You can prevent your story from being lost by sharing it with friends, family, and your child. You can ask those present at your baby's birth to write down what they've witnessed and give their tales to you for safekeeping. You can tell and read the stories on your child's birthday each year, affirming your child's worth and the importance of his or her entry into history. Such birth stories become treasures to children and parents alike. Remember that your birth story isn't just *your* story. It's also your *baby's* story. It's a story of new beginnings for you, for your family, and for the new person who's come into the world through you.

AND NOW THE CHOICES

This slow and powerful work of pregnancy, birth, and helping your child grow up is a beautiful and important bit of weaving in the fabric of humanity. It's a holy event that will be remembered, shared, and used in ways you can't predict, in a world you can't always understand. As former U.S. Supreme Court Justice Sandra Day O'Connor says, "We don't accomplish anything in this world alone...and whatever happens is the result of the whole tapestry of one's life and all the weavings of individual threads from one to another that creates something."

The threads of your own life began thousands of years ago when your ancestors brought their offspring safely into this world. Generation followed generation, and here you are today, ready to take your place in the tapestry of life and send another thread into the future through your child.

Because of the way maternity care has evolved in the U.S., you have two distinct options regarding how to view your pregnancy and birth. What you choose to believe about your ability to grow, birth, and nurture your baby will determine the color and pattern of your piece of the tapestry.

Chapter 3

YOU'RE PREGNANT!

Rely on your own inner resources,
trust your body's responses, and take joy
in preparing for the new life that is now
becoming a part of yours.
—Peggy O'Mara

The growth of your baby inside you is a natural and self-sufficient process. Perhaps the best thing you can do for both of you is pay attention. Listen to what your body tells you about how to care for yourself, how to prepare for your baby's arrival, and how to give

birth. You don't need to be a genius or highly educated to listen to what your body and heart are telling you. It's a simple matter of letting nature's perfect design unfold.

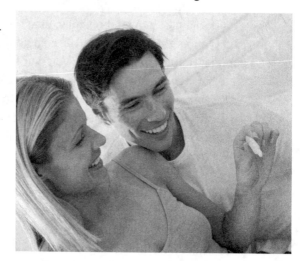

Message from Your Body: "You're Pregnant"

What was your first clue? Perhaps you missed a period, or you just had a hunch, or your belly felt sort of "busy." Maybe you sensed something different about your body, little changes you'd never noticed before. Or you found your emotions were strung a little tighter than usual. You wondered: "Could I be pregnant?"

Whether you confirmed your pregnancy with a home test or at a clinic, you likely knew beforehand that *something* was different by observing your body closely. That's just the first of many opportunities pregnancy offers you to be mindful—to pay close attention to your body, your environment, and your instincts. Being mindful during pregnancy is important because it helps you navigate the moments of your day.

During early pregnancy every moment is packed with drama. Beginning at conception (when egg and sperm join), your body undergoes an avalanche of change in a very short time. Even before the embryo (what your baby is called through eight weeks gestation) implants in your uterus, HCG (human chorionic gonadotropin, the hormone detected by pregnancy tests) levels rise. This is the beginning of hormonal changes that continue throughout pregnancy and breastfeeding. These hormonal shifts and your growing baby change your body in amazing ways.

If you take a quiet moment to stand before the mirror after a bath, you might note some changes in your breasts—darker, bigger, bumpier nipples; blood vessels you don't remember seeing before; a feeling of tenderness or heaviness. These early developments in your breasts are your body's first preparations for milk production.

You may be experiencing nausea in the mornings, at mealtimes, or more often. Pregnancy nausea (often called morning sickness) varies from woman to woman, and it can be unpleasant. Eat and drink whatever you think might help you deal with nausea—small, regular snacks that sound comforting and digestible. Take note of what goes down easily. For many women it's carbohydrates.

Research shows that about two-thirds of all pregnant women have some nausea, and that it may actually serve an important purpose: protecting mother and baby from harmful chemicals and food-borne illness.[1] Certain foods are common triggers for pregnancy nausea;

many expectant mothers feel sick when they consume or smell eggs, poultry, fish, meat, alcohol, or caffeinated beverages. A pregnant woman's body might perceive these items as threats to an embryo that hasn't finished making a good, strong attachment. (In the same way, her body might crave certain foods because it needs those nutrients.)

The first weeks of pregnancy are a time of deep tiredness for lots of women. Jennifer remembers wanting to crawl under her desk for a ten-o'clock nap at work: "Those mornings, I'd long to curl up and sleep—just out of the blue. It suddenly occurred to me that I'd *never* been like that! I'm a dancer, full of energy, ready to take on the day. That was my first real attention grabber." Since Jennifer's periods had never been regular, her tiredness was her first signal to begin looking for other changes in her body.

> If you're suffering from pregnancy nausea, one way to cope is to think of your baby getting strongly established in you, making his or her presence known, helping your body adjust to his or her needs. You might also keep this in mind: One researcher has said that the term *morning sickness* should really be changed to *wellness insurance*; pregnancy nausea may be linked to better birth weights for babies. If nothing else works, keep your eyes on the road ahead: Morning sickness *will* end eventually. For most women, it goes away somewhere between the third and fourth month.

Some women's emotions send them strong signals. You might find yourself snapping back in reply to a casual comment or ready to cry over some small matter. This sensitivity is a message from your baby: "Listen up! We've got work to do together, and I need your attention."

When you pay attention to your body's signals, you'll find them to be valuable information suppliers and bond builders. Midwife Pam England says that while a baby grows inside you without much effort from you, "the development of your parent-identity is not necessarily an automatic process of nature. If you want to help this happen, you'll have to play an active part."[2] As you listen and respond to your unborn baby's messages, you begin a lifetime of conversation with and learning from each other.

WHAT'S HAPPENING?

You and Baby Are in This Together

Pregnancy is not just the making of a baby. It's also the making of a mother. A mother's body and soul grow and adjust to parent each unique child she carries. During pregnancy mother's and child's bodies, rhythms, abilities, and cues develop together. For example:

- Your baby's heart, which begins beating three or four weeks after conception, is growing into the heart of the child you'll raise. Meanwhile, *your* heart is growing into the heart of the mother who'll love this unique human being.

- Your baby's eyes, which are protected by eyelids eight weeks after conception, are becoming eyes that'll behold the world as no other eyes have. Meanwhile, *your* eyes are becoming those of a mother who will see what no one else sees in this new person.

- Your baby's ears, which can hear your voice perhaps as early as nineteen weeks after conception will enter the world listening for familiar sounds. Meanwhile, *your* ears are developing into those of a mother attuned to the unique voice of this child.[3]

You may hear the word *trimester* (period of three months) a lot while you're pregnant. The division of pregnancy into three chunks of time provides a framework for thinking about your baby's growth and changes in your body.

During the first months of your pregnancy, what started out as a microscopic ball of cells is rapidly developing into a complete body with facial features and teeth and fingerprints, a full collection of systems from digestive to nervous, and the ability to move and feel. Your baby is nourished through his or her umbilical cord, which is attached to an organ called the placenta, which develops after the fertilized egg implants in the wall of your uterus.

In the first months of pregnancy your uterus grows to accommodate your growing baby. At about ten weeks you can feel the top of your uterus in your lower abdomen. (By the end of pregnancy, your uterus will be just under your ribs!) Your growing uterus and your high progesterone (pregnancy hormone) levels over the next months will cause a wide variety of physical changes. Even before you gain any weight, you'll notice your waist thickening as your ligaments loosen to help your belly expand. You may urinate more frequently. Your skin may look radiant, or you may develop acne. You may notice that your hair has never looked better. You may find that your breasts are larger, your nipples more erect, and your areolas darker. Your body is already preparing for breastfeeding.

About Due Dates

Calendars can be so comforting—helping us move through the paces of daily life and plan ahead for important events. Circling your baby's due date on your calendar can help you organize your preparations, can make your future more real and exciting, and can help your caregiver manage his or her schedule. But predicting *exactly* when your baby will arrive is not possible.

Though you and your caregiver might calculate a due date forty weeks from the first day of your last period, bear in mind that only about 5 percent of babies arrive on their due dates. Many factors make due dates difficult to pin down. For example, the formula described above assumes a woman has a twenty-eight–day cycle and ovulates on day fourteen, which isn't true for many women. And some babies just take more or less than forty weeks to be ready for the outside world.

Imagine making of a batch of popcorn. Most of the kernels pop during a few noisy moments. But there are lots of early and late poppers, too. All the popped kernels are perfect—but each needs a slightly different amount of time to be fully cooked. The same is true for babies.

Some caregivers are in a hurry to begin labor when they think a baby is fully developed. But only your baby knows when he or she is ready to be born. Your baby's chemistry communicates with yours to declare that all systems are go and that labor should begin. By adopting a relaxed attitude about your due date in early pregnancy (you might even think of it as your guess date), you're practicing patience and trust that'll serve you well as your pregnancy progresses.

WHAT CAN YOU DO?

The beauty of pregnancy is that for most women it just happens. As you go about your everyday life, a miracle occurs within you. Even if you know little about pregnancy and haven't seen a doctor or midwife, your body changes and your baby develops. You're creating a baby all by yourself.

Though pregnancy may not affect your daily routine much, you may view everyday events through a different lens. You may find your good and bad moods more pronounced. Your sleep patterns and dreams may change. Your appetite and your likes and dislikes may shift. Lovemaking may take on different meaning.

You may be wondering, "If pregnancy 'just happens,' is there anything I can *do* to support it?" Yes. You can use the brief days of your pregnancy to discover your strengths, to live well, and to change habits that might be damaging. The most important thing you can do to ensure a healthy you and a healthy baby is to stay healthy yourself. Eat well, rest, exercise, manage stress, and make time for fun.

Handle the Worry Habit

An old Swedish proverb says, "Worry gives a small thing a big shadow." Perhaps it's pregnancy's boost of emotional energy that feeds the specter of worry. No matter how fit you may feel, how much you may enjoy being pregnant, or how radiant you may look, worry can find a way to sneak into your psyche.

Worry is an equal-opportunity ghost, able to haunt any thought, any insecurity, any issue at all. You may worry about being up to the task of parenting. You may worry about how profoundly becoming a parent will change your life. You may worry about how you look and if you'll ever feel like you again. You may worry about how your child is developing, how you'll handle the pain and hard work of labor, how you'd cope with the hundreds of scary scenarios that come to your attention via conversation and the media.

> "I worried at every my comment my OB made, ever glance from the nurse. I was sick with worry at every appointment. And there was so little reassurance. If I could give myself a gift, it'd be to erase those worries from that time in my life."
>
> —Lori

You know that bristling feeling you get when someone says offhandedly, "Oh, c'mon, don't worry!" Not worrying is easier said than done, especially about matters of pregnancy and birth. After all, worry is a normal emotion and does serve a useful purpose. Naming your fears and examining them can help you understand them, put them in perspective, and develop coping strategies. If your nightmares come true, how might you respond? How might your partner or caregiver help you? How might you prevent or accept or improve the situation?

By all means, face your fears—but don't exaggerate them. Humans tend to grow their worries—to become preoccupied with possible pitfalls, rather than positive probabilities. We've all come through times of great worry in our lives, when fear overtook our thoughts and robbed us

> "I worried about everything. My mother was a great. She kept reminding me that there was no reason to expect trouble."
> —Anna

of peace and joy. Looking back on those times, we can see that our worries didn't change the eventual outcomes, and that we survived the challenges that felt insurmountable at the time.

Check In with Yourself Daily

Finding the time, energy, and peace to face your fears—or do anything that requires mental focus—is a challenge in our culture. One pregnant woman shared that after years of working at her office, she'd tuned out the sounds of phones ringing and computers clicking. She didn't even notice how noisy her office was until an older coworker looked at her across the bank of desks and said, "You're bringing this child into a world of sounds my babies never heard."

It's true: In just a decade or two, technology has changed the world dramatically. From cell phones to ATMs, from microwave ovens to Facebook friends, from high-definition DVDs to iPods, technology fills our days with vivid images and messages. It's a noisy, busy world that can crowd out the peace we need to connect with ourselves.

Connecting with yourself is an important task during your pregnancy. It's a big job to pay attention to all the physical, emotional, and spiritual changes you're experiencing. It takes concentration to envision a future that includes a new role and a new person. Finding a place of stillness for a few moments each day can help you do this crucial work.

Even if your space and your schedule are crowded, you can find a place and time to keep a daily appointment with yourself. Perhaps you can retreat to the corner

> "Crazy as it sounds, there was a storeroom in the office where I worked. I made a date with myself to slip away for five minutes in the afternoon to just be in the quiet darkness, to just breathe and relax."
> —Char

of your bedroom, the bathroom, a closet, or an empty room at your workplace. Perhaps you can sneak a moment before others wake up, after they've gone to bed, before you get in the shower, or during your lunch break. You might want to "check in" at the same time each day so you treat this appointment with yourself as the important time it is.

Your daily check-in may be a few moments of silence, meditation, or prayer. You can use this time to get in touch with not only your feelings, but also your body and the little one who is taking up more and more of it. Close your eyes for a moment and listen to your breathing, then take an inventory of yourself: Are there any tense areas in your body—neck, shoulders, throat, hands, back? Is anything nagging at your mind? Doing a full-body and -mind check will help you identify what needs to be released, relaxed, or dealt with.

Exercising is an excellent way to keep your mind and body healthy during pregnancy. It aids digestion, improves your mood, keeps you fit for the work ahead, and helps you sleep better. Must you exercise to have a healthy baby? No. Are you likely to feel better if you stay active? Yes. Find a regular time and a comfortable rhythm, and give it priority. You may find walking a simple and pleasant exercise during pregnancy. Or perhaps you enjoy swimming, dancing, or yoga. Let your body guide your choices. Do what feels right without pushing yourself to extremes.

> Yoga, an ancient form of exercise that includes breath control, meditation, and body postures, has become popular among pregnant women. It's easy to understand why: Many yoga exercises include movements that open the pelvis. Yoga also teaches rhythmic breathing, concentration, stamina building, and relaxation. Some women who do yoga report improved physical coordination and more balanced emotions.

Thomas Moore writes in *The Re-Enchantment of Everyday Life*, "It's difficult to imagine being busy and enchanted at the same time. Enchantment invites us to pause and be arrested by whatever is before us; instead of doing something, something is done to us."

We think pregnancy should be a time of enchantment. It's a time to pause, to step away from your crowded agenda, and to surrender to the delight and mystery of what is growing within you. This is a powerful and amazing thing that you and your baby are accomplishing, a dance unlike any other in the human experience.

Love Your Blooming Body

Midwife Ina May Gaskin encourages you to spend your pregnancy "loving your uterus and your body. I mean this literally. Positive energy makes a good birth outcome more likely, so go for it."[4] Early pregnancy is a great time to fall in love with your body and cheer its growth into a beautiful new shape.

Maternity clothing designers have finally figured out how to accentuate the pregnant women's body, allowing the world to acknowledge the beautiful woman standing at a crosswalk, her hands spread lovingly over her pregnant belly, wearing a clingy dress or playful pants and a shirt that accentuates, rather than hides, her shape. Thanks to today's maternity fashions and all the expectant mothers who've stepped out of their homes and into the public eye, the pregnant body has come to be seen as a thing of beauty.

Your pregnant body is carrying not only a growing baby, but a growing placenta, amniotic fluid, increased blood volume, and growing breasts and uterus. Your body is also storing the fat needed to make the perfect food for your baby—your breast milk. This is a time in your life when gaining weight is a good thing.

Remember this, too: A woman's good design includes a postpartum weight-loss mechanism. The months you devote to nourishing your baby with your own milk will burn off some of the fat your body stored protectively during your pregnancy. And as the active mother of a demanding newborn, you'll also sweat off some of the extra fluids your body needed in pregnancy. Pregnancy weight gain is nothing to fear. It's nature's way, and it results in a beautiful you and a healthy baby.

Make Changes for the Better

Consider whether any of the following changes might make sense in the early months of your pregnancy:

- **Changes in your schedule:** Are you striking a good balance between working and stopping work, between exercise and rest?
- **Changes in your diet:** Are you getting enough protein, fiber, iron, folic acid, and calcium? (For more on pregnancy nutrition, see page 74.) Proper nutrition is important not only for your baby, but also for you. It protects against a wide array of potential problems, from maternal nutrient depletion to low birth weight. Good food for your pregnant body needn't be expensive or out of

the ordinary—just wholesome and nutrient-rich. You choose what, when, and how much to eat, and try to make your choices as healthy and as balanced as possible. If you find it difficult to eat because of nausea, don't panic. Simply eat as well and as often as you can—your baby will make the most of whatever you're able to keep down. There is absolutely no evidence that either salt or calories should be restricted during pregnancy.

- **Changes in what you drink:** Are you drinking enough water? During pregnancy you need plenty of water to support your increased blood volume and your baby's amniotic fluid. Water can also help with problems like constipation, headache, nausea, muscle cramps, dry hair and skin, low energy, and much more. Drink when you're thirsty, and drink enough to satisfy your thirst. Although in the United States many doctors recommend that women drink no alcohol or caffeine at all while pregnant, there's no research supporting total abstinence. In fact, research shows that mild caffeine consumption (one to two cups of coffee per day) is safe.[5] *The Cochrane Library* believes there isn't suffi- cient evidence to recommend restricting caffeine.[6] And *A Guide to Effective Care in Pregnancy and Childbirth* says, "prohibition of all alcohol intake during pregnancy" is "not likely to be bene- ficial," but that "advice to avoid excessive alcohol consumption" is "likely to be beneficial."[7] What is "excessive"? *The Cochrane Library* suggests that consuming more than seven drinks a week on a regular basis is excessive.

- **Changes in your habits:** Do you smoke or use street drugs? Smoking during pregnancy may not only harm your health, it may also lead to serious health problems in your baby. The risk of prema- ture birth and low birth weight is nearly doubled for the baby of a smoking woman, and that baby inherits a higher risk of health problems. Smoking has also been linked with several birth defects. Here's the good news:

Many programs are available to help you stop smoking. The March of Dimes provides a prac- tical, helpful "Tips to Quit" checklist and links to other smoking cessation organizations at its website (http://www.marchofdimes.com). While you're trying to quit, stay away from places and activities that tempt you to smoke or that might expose you to secondhand smoke. And don't get discouraged if you can't quit cold turkey right away. Cut back as much as you can, and find someone who will support your efforts.

Stopping or substantially reducing your smoking and staying away from secondhand smoke can greatly improve your odds of having a healthy pregnancy and a healthy baby. Street drugs, too, can be harmful to your baby's health and growth. The placenta allows most drugs (street drugs and pharmaceuticals) to reach your baby's bloodstream. Drugs like cocaine and heroin can cause premature labor, as well as addiction, stunted growth, and behavioral and emotional problems in your baby. It's extremely important to get help if you can't stop yourself.

- **Changes in your planning:** Are you making informed choices about your care and your baby's birth, or are you simply "going with the program"? Remember: Choices that are made for you or happen by default really aren't choices. You're more likely to be satisfied with your journey to motherhood if you educate yourself and are actively involved in decision making about pregnancy and birth. Try to make changes during your pregnancy with confidence, not anxiety. Misinformation abounds in the media, old wives' tales, and on the internet, spawning a growing amount of unnecessary fear about foods, procedures, and activities that might threaten fetal health. How can you navigate this churning river of anxiety? Remember that much of the information is hearsay—it's incomplete, out-of-context, or not evidence-based. Get the full facts. (See Chapter 11 for tips and resources.) Make any changes in your lifestyle sensibly and positively, not anxiously and gullibly.

Find Good Prenatal Care

For most women, pregnancy and birth require no medical intervention of any kind, but it is important to have good prenatal care. Good prenatal care should help you move through pregnancy healthy and confident and help you prepare for the safe, healthy birth of your baby.

Your caregiver and birth site can dramatically influence how your pregnancy and birth go, so choose carefully. It isn't critical to see a caregiver the minute you suspect you're pregnant—unless you have a preexisting medical condition like diabetes or heart disease that adds risk to your pregnancy,

> "I called my gynecologist immediately after I realized I was pregnant. The first prenatal appointment I could get was at twelve weeks. Suddenly I realized I had time to think about my choices."
>
> —Angela

you suspect you have a sexually transmitted disease or other infection, or you have bleeding, pain, or severe vomiting, or plan to do early prenatal testing (see Chapter 5 information about early prenatal testing). Otherwise you have time, and you should take that time to think about the kind of prenatal care and birth you'd like and to find a caregiver and birth site that suit you.

Chapter 4

Choosing a Caregiver and Birth Site

*It is your choice. You can do what you think is best.
You don't have to agree. There is no right answer.
You can take more time to decide. It's okay to follow
your instincts. You can say no and still be respected.*
—Alessandra Godinho

Informed Choice

Is "What Is" What's Best for You?

There's probably a human tendency to assume that "what is" is "what is best." There must be a good reason why so many doctors require routine ultrasounds during pregnancy. Or why so many labors are induced. Or why so many women have epidurals.

It's easy to forget that just a few decades ago, hospitals routinely used practices that we now know are useless or even harmful. They banned partners from delivery rooms. Women received enemas at the onset of labor. Newborns were suspended upside down by their feet and smacked on their little bottoms. Women got injections after birth to prevent their breasts from making milk. These practices ended because women asked questions and challenged assumptions. Women's informed choices changed the status quo.

You have a wonderful opportunity before you to make informed choices about your body and your baby's birth. Remember that these are *your* choices, not your caregiver's, not your relatives' or friends', not the hospital's or clinic's or medical textbook's. Look beyond what is—what modern obstetrics and culture dictate—and you may discover better options for you and yours. You can make your pregnancy an empowering time of learning, discerning, and choosing as you plan for your baby's arrival.

Gathering and Analyzing Information

We live in a time when lots of information (both accurate and inaccurate) on just about any subject is readily available. Technology has increased our access not only to information, but also to goods and services—simultaneously widening and narrowing our everyday choices. For example, you can have a home entertainment system that offers hundreds of viewing options, but find that none of them is worth watching. You may be able to find exotic fruits from all over the globe in your neighborhood supermarket, but not a locally grown apple.

The same paradox exists in the realm of childbirth. In the United States pregnant women have the right to make informed choices about their maternity care. (For more on the rights of childbearing women, see Appendix C.) They're legally entitled to full and clear information from their caregivers about the benefits and risks of maternity care practices. But many don't get that crucial information.[1] And those who search for it on their own face the daunting task of distinguishing obstetric myth from fact.

To make matters worse, our medicalized culture bombards us with both subtle and direct messages that make it very hard to think independently about pregnancy and birth. Watch TV programs about birth, and you're bound to see a lot of dramatic hospital scenes. Open any mainstream pregnancy or parenting magazine, and you'll see page after page of formula ads. And then there are all the individual voices joining the din. As your pregnancy progresses, more and more people will talk to you about their pregnancies and births. As you listen to all these messages and stories and recommendations—which may contradict each other or what you're reading in this book—you may wonder what really is best for you and your baby.

Here are a couple of ideas to help you analyze all the information you're gathering:

- *In the media, hospitals and doctors generally take center stage in stories about birth, while mothers play supporting roles. Does this type of role suit you?* It happens in real life, too. If you've ever had a routine medical exam, you've probably found yourself perched on an examination table, shivering in a flimsy backless gown as staff swept in and out of the room wearing lab coats or scrubs and official ID tags. It's common to feel vulnerable, awkward, and out of place in moments like these, and such feelings can diminish your power to question a professional's opinion or to consider all the factors that contribute to making the best possible healthcare decision for you. Many a pregnant woman's labor and birth decisions are made by others, long before she writes a birth plan or arrives at the hospital—as though it's all from a generic script. Considering that you are *you*, not a generic patient, would you prefer to write your own script?

- *How did the stories you're hearing come about? How did the tellers of these stories arrive at—or forfeit—their choices?* Did they make informed choices or "go with the program"? Does their information agree or conflict with the information you've gathered? Were they pleased with their outcomes? Would those outcomes please you? If you respectfully ask for more details and compare what you hear with your own values and knowledge, you're likely to get a fuller picture and wind up better equipped to make your own choices.

> For more information about specific caregivers and birth sites, we highly recommend visiting the websites http://www.choicesinchildbirth.org and http//www.thebirthsurvey.com.

MYTHS ABOUT CAREGIVERS AND BIRTH SITES

Your choice of a caregiver and birth site (the two are usually linked) is one of the most important decisions you'll make during your pregnancy. The most important way to ensure a healthy, safe birth is to choose a caregiver and birth site that provide evidence-based maternity care and do not interfere in the natural, physiologic process of birth unless there's a compelling medical indication to do so. Your choices will profoundly influence the path of your pregnancy, birth, and early mothering. Because women typically make this decision very early in pregnancy, they rarely take enough time to make a truly informed decision. They often choose their caregivers and birth sites based on convenience or on misinformation they've picked up before becoming pregnant. We urge you to take your time, to deliberately gather and scrutinize information. To help you get started, let's first dispel some widespread myths about maternity care.

Myth 1: Pregnancy and childbirth are terribly risky.

Fact: Having a baby is a natural, healthy life event.
The World Health Organization (WHO) believes that 85 to 95 percent of pregnancies can be expected to go perfectly.[2] Most women enter pregnancy in good health, and this is a strong foundation for a healthy pregnancy.

Could you encounter trouble in pregnancy and labor? Yes. Should you expect it? No. Pregnancy and birth are perfectly designed by nature and are safer now than ever before—*not* because they're managed by doctors and hospitals but because women are healthier going into pregnancy and birth, because hygiene is better, and because antibiotics are widely available. If a healthy pregnant woman lets nature take its course, her baby and her body are well protected.

Of course, some pregnancies and births are riskier. Smoking, substance abuse, and physical and psychological stress can harm both women and their babies. But these are lifestyle issues, not problems that can be prevented or fixed by medicine. Only a small percentage of women enter pregnancy with preexisting health problems (such as diabetes) or develop complications during pregnancy or birth (such as pregnancy-induced hypertension). It is for these women that medical intervention makes pregnancy and birth safer.[3]

Myth 2: Birth is safest in a hospital with a doctor.

Fact: For most women, birth at home or at a birth center is as safe as—or safer than—at a hospital.
You may also hear that in order to ensure your safety, you should see a doctor for prenatal care and give birth in a hospital—preferably one with a neonatal intensive care unit (NICU). This better-safe-than-sorry myth has been evolving for about one hundred years.

In the early 1900s there was deep concern about the maternal mortality rate; many women were dying after birth of puerperal fever. Doctors argued that poorly trained midwives contributed to this problem and insisted that doctors provided safer care. Many years later research showed that women who had been attended by doctors were *more* likely to die from puerperal fever because doctors weren't washing their hands well enough at births. Midwifery care had actually been *safer* for women.[4]

This is an example of an iatrogenic problem (a problem caused by caregivers). Iatrogenic obstetric problems have played out over and over in the years since then. Here's one modern example: Many doctors believe that continuous electronic fetal monitoring (EFM) makes labor safer for babies, so they do it routinely. However, research shows that routine continuous EFM results in no fewer babies who have problems or die but more mothers who end up with cesareans.[5] So EFM makes birth riskier for mothers with no benefit for babies.

Continuous EFM is just one of many routine interventions that disrupt and create problems in otherwise normal labors and births. The medical attitude of expecting trouble, and the hospital policies that support this attitude, prevent women from giving birth easily and safely in the typical hospital and contribute to the alarming U.S. cesarean rates. Cesarean surgery increases risks for both mother and baby.[6]

No research confirms that the hospital is the safest place to give birth. The Cochrane Collaboration has this to say on the subject: "The change to planned hospital birth for low-risk pregnant women in many countries during this century was not supported by good evidence. Planned hospital birth may even increase unnecessary interventions and complications without any benefit for low-risk women."[7] In the last decade there have been several large studies of home birth in the Netherlands,[8] North America,[9] and Canada[10,11] that report similar findings. Compared to hospital births, home births are associated with fewer obstetric interventions and the same or better outcomes for mothers and for babies.

The most recent study by Janssen et al. is especially compelling because the same midwives provided care for both women planning home births and women planning hospital births.[12] There were fewer interventions and better outcomes when the midwives attended home births than when they attended hospital births, suggesting that the hospital restrictions and routine interventions influence outcomes even when the caregiver is the same.

In a very small percentage of pregnancies and births, complications like preexisting diabetes or heart disease, prematurity, or fetal distress during labor *should* be managed in a hospital by a doctor. But for most women, birth outside the hospital is as safe as—or safer than—hospital birth.

Myth 3: Giving birth outside a hospital or with a midwife means suffering needlessly

Fact: There are many ways to find comfort in labor without drugs, and this search for comfort helps move labor along. Pain serves an important purpose in labor, but that purpose isn't maternal suffering. On the contrary: One purpose is to compel mothers to actively seek comfort and, in doing so, to facilitate the progress of labor. See Chapter 9 for more information on finding comfort in labor.

When allowed and encouraged to, a woman will naturally move, moan, sway, change her breathing pattern, and rock to cope with contractions, eventually finding the right rhythm for her unique needs. Such active comfort-seeking helps her baby rotate and descend and helps prevent her labor from stalling. As her contractions get stronger, her body releases endorphins—nature's narcotic—to ease her pain.

Comfort methods like activity and rest, eating and drinking, showering and bathing, receiving continuous emotional and physical support, massage, relaxation, and applying heat and cold are more available to women who give birth outside the hospital and/or are attended by midwives. In hospital births, often the only pain relief available is a drug—typically an epidural. Simple comfort measures are frequently prohibited by staff who don't understand the purpose or the value of natural comfort-seeking. Women are expected to lie quietly in bed, attached to monitors and intravenous (IV) lines,

But what if you really *need* medication? Most midwives can prescribe medications, but they are more likely to encourage and provide for non-drug pain strategies than physicians are. Hospital midwives encourage you not to depend entirely on the epidural for pain relief, because epidurals change the normal process of labor and lead to a cascade of interventions (required to ensure that you and your baby are safe).[13] Outside the hospital there are many more options for finding comfort in labor. But, because of the medical risks of epidural and other pain medications, you will need to be in a hospital if you require or desire them.

with strict limits on the number of people who can stay with and support them. Without the freedom to use a wide variety of comfort measures in labor, it's no surprise that more than 90 percent of women in some hospitals choose an epidural!

Myth 4: Choosing midwife or out-of-hospital birth is an all-or-nothing decision.

Fact: A good midwife is a skilled member of a caregiving team.
Many women worry that if they choose midwifery care or out-of-hospital birth, they'll be in big trouble—with no options—if problems arise. They assume that midwives can't handle crises and reason that if there's any chance of labor complications, they'd better be in a hospital.

This line of thinking springs from inadequate understanding of the training and role of midwives. Most midwives in the U.S. today are certified nurse-midwives (CNMs). A CNM has advanced training (often a master's degree) beyond her nursing degree and has passed a rigorous certification exam. Two other types of nationally recognized midwife credentials are CM (certified midwife) and CPM (certified professional midwife). Neither is a nurse, but both are well-trained, knowledgeable, certified professionals.

All three types of certified midwives are carefully trained to provide primary care for healthy women as part of a team. Their expertise is in normal pregnancy and birth. Because they're trained to recognize what's normal and what's not and because they base their care on the evidence that birth usually goes best without interference, midwifery care is as safe or safer for healthy women than obstetric care.[14]

Midwives collaborate with obstetricians, who are specialists in managing pregnancy and childbirth complications. If a woman develops a health problem or requires surgery, her midwife will refer her to a doctor. All certified and licensed midwives have physician backup (doctors on call who have agreed to treat or consult with their patients who develop unexpected medical needs) and can admit women to hospitals if necessary.

Furthermore, midwives are qualified to manage many problems and emergencies in hospitals and outside the hospital. They administer oxygen, prescribe medication including antibiotics (although this varies from state to state), start IV fluids, repair tears, and perform both adult and infant cardiopulmonary resuscitation (CPR).

Choosing a midwife and/or an out-of-hospital birth is a choice that changes if circumstances change. Midwives provide primary care, collaborating with doctors if needed, using guidelines approved by both midwives and obstetricians. In the countries where this model is the norm, there are fewer medical interventions and fewer deaths of mothers and babies than there are in the U.S.[15]

For more information about midwifery care, visit http://cfmidwifery.org.

CHOOSING A CAREGIVER

What's It Like to Use a Midwife?

The hallmark of midwifery is strong confidence in the natural process of childbearing. A good midwife patiently observes, teaches, and supports you throughout your pregnancy and birth. By doing so, she helps prevent problems. However, she can quickly and accurately identify complications and call in her physician backup if necessary. She is vigilant but doesn't expect trouble. This above all defines the difference between midwifery and obstetric care.

A midwife typically has more time than a doctor has to offer patient, supportive care—not only because she cares for low-risk pregnancies, but also because her goals are different. She emphasizes staying healthy, reducing stress, building confidence, and enjoying your pregnancy. She presents prenatal testing as an option, not an unquestioned routine, and encourages you to think about what you'd do with the information.

A midwife will provide continuous hands-on help during your labor and birth and will intervene only when necessary, not routinely. She'll let your labor start, progress, and end on its own. She'll encourage you to eat, drink, and move about freely. All these practices help reduce your risk of birth injury, trauma, and cesarean surgery.[16]

"My prenatal visits with my midwife were long, leisurely, and conversational. I weighed myself, tested my own urine, listened to the baby's heart beat, and chatted with my midwife. Not at all your typical prenatal visit in an OB office. I have often heard women comment that it was the quality of the prenatal visits that convinced them to switch to a midwifery practice, or that it came as an extremely pleasant surprise once they had made the switch." —Sarah

Women cared for by midwives have fewer babies born prematurely or born with low birth weight or birth related injuries.[17] Industrialized countries where midwives are the primary maternity caregivers for healthy women have lower perinatal mortality rates and lower cesarean rates than the U.S.[18]

Only 10 percent of U.S. births are attended by midwives, but according to *Listening to Mothers II* (a 2006 survey report on American women's childbearing experiences), women with midwives are the most satisfied with their births.[19] Approximately one in ten midwife-attended births (one percent of births in the U.S.) is a home birth. (Almost all U.S. home births are attended by midwives—usually CPMs or CMs.) The other nine percent happen in hospitals or birth centers (most often with CNMs).

Today there's a growing concern that some midwives are practicing like obstetricians—that they're expecting trouble in pregnancy and birth and are acting accordingly. If you want to keep your birth as natural as possible, be wary of a midwife who's controlling and prescriptive, who frightens you, who's content to go along with restrictive hospital policies, who pressures you into prenatal testing, or who won't stay with you throughout your labor. You probably won't be happy with her.

"When people ask me why I have a midwife, I can only respond that not every situation needs to be medicalized. Here's what I mean: I arrived at Brigham and Women's Hospital fully dilated. While the admissions staff tried to get me to do paperwork, I lay stretched out on the floor trying to get into my hypno-birthing relaxation mode. The staff hit a code blue because they had no idea what I was doing; they thought something was wrong. As everyone scrambled around me, I heard a voice down the hall. It was Biddy, our midwife. I felt calm and relaxed the moment I heard her voice and felt her touch. She pressed my head into her chest and hugged me. There was no reason to think anything was wrong. I was in labor, the most natural process in the world! I just needed people to let me do the work that my body and my baby knew how to do. That's exactly what Biddy did. During Ryan's birth Biddy and Dennis supported me, but they let me do what I knew how to do. Ryan was born forty-five minutes later— a healthy little boy with gorgeous eyes and beautiful red hair. As I await the birth of our second child, I'm free of worry and fear. Biddy has taught me to trust myself and my baby."

—Michelle

What's It Like to Have an Obstetrician as a Primary Caregiver?

Obstetric training focuses on caring for women with complications or those who are at high risk for complications, so it's no surprise that most obstetricians view pregnancy as an illness and birth as fraught with danger. Obstetric prenatal care tends to focus on screening for abnormalities, and childbirth under obstetric care is usually closely monitored and controlled.[20] Obstetricians diagnose problems based on narrow definitions of normalcy. As a result, pregnancy and childbirth transform from a normal, natural process to an intervention-intensive medical event.

If you have complications, you truly do need an obstetrician's expertise for at least part of your maternity care. But if you're healthy and your pregnancy is low-risk (as is the case 85 to 95 percent of the time), you may not receive the most appropriate care in a typical obstetric practice.[21] After a long career of research, practice, and teaching in public health, epidemiologist and midwife Judith Rooks has concluded that in too many obstetric practices, "the level of surveillance and intervention well exceeds the elements of necessary care."[22] This may seem harmless, but an attitude of expecting trouble may actually increase your risk and probably will increase your fear.

Most obstetricians routinely order prenatal tests like ultrasound, multiple marker screening, and gestational diabetes screening. But many women don't receive full information about the accuracy of tests or the information that tests can and can't provide. And women are often pressured if they express misgivings or refuse prenatal testing. During labor, an obstetrician is likely to use routine interventions (like continuous EFM and IV lines), and you can expect your labor to be moved along quickly. And ironically, though obstetricians tend to expect trouble, an obstetrician probably won't stay with you throughout labor.

Research suggests that for all these reasons, there are few, if any, benefits of obstetric care for healthy, low-risk pregnancies. *A Guide to Effective Care in Pregnancy and Childbirth* summarizes the evidence: "It is inherently unwise, and perhaps unsafe, for women with normal pregnancies to be cared for by obstetric specialists."[23]

Even if you've been pleased with an ob-gyn's (obstetrician-gynecologist's) wellness care, you may not be equally pleased with his or her maternity care. Your needs change when you become pregnant, so it's important that you ask questions. For example:

- What prenatal testing is done routinely?
- What labor practices are used routinely?
- What are your doctor's rates of inductions, episiotomies (see page 155), instrument deliveries, and cesareans?
- What does he or she think about doulas?
- Does he or she seem to have more confidence in interventions than your ability to give birth?

Veteran midwife Ina May Gaskin advises, "If any of your questions provokes resentment, sarcasm, hostility, scare tactics, or vague or patronizing answers, keep shopping."[24] We add: Beware of doctors who simply tell you what you want to hear, who kindly brush aside your questions to get past them and move on to a more comfortable discussion.

What about a female obstetrician? Many women believe that female doctors are likely to practice more compassionately. This isn't a safe assumption. Though a woman may have firsthand experience of birth or may have a more sensitive manner, all obstetricians—regardless of gender—are trained to view birth as a medical event.

How Does a Doctor-Midwife Practice Work?

In a doctor-midwife partnership, an obstetrician employs a midwife to care for healthy, low-risk women, and the doctor cares for those who have complications or are at high risk for problems. The midwife and doctor work as a team to attend births—usually in hospitals, but sometimes in birth centers or homes.

A doctor-midwife practice isn't always the best of both worlds. If the midwife covers only office visits while the doctor manages births, or if the practice routinely uses labor interventions like continuous EFM or restrictions on eating and drinking, this might indicate a belief that birth is a medical event, not a natural process.

A practice like this can work very well, though. Biddy Fein directs a large midwifery service attending births at Boston's Brigham and Women's Hospital, one of the biggest and most respected maternity hospitals in the U.S. She says, "At Brigham and Women's we have a wonderful collaboration with the physicians. They take care of the women with medical problems, but we continue to see these women. We provide the care that ensures they will be confident, be able to work with their labors, be supported—none of these things goes out the window just because they have medical problems. These women need midwives even more."[25] We agree.

What's It Like to Have Maternity Care with a Family Doctor?

Family doctors provide comprehensive medical care with emphasis on the family unit. They used to provide a great deal of obstetric care in the U.S., especially in rural areas. (They still do in some areas.) Though all family doctors have some obstetric training, only about 30 percent include obstetrics in their practice. The cost of malpractice insurance, the fear of lawsuits, and the demands of attending births around the clock have all contributed to this decline.[26]

Many family doctors are concerned about the current level of routine obstetric intervention. The American Academy of Family Physicians (AAFP) encourages its members "to develop a style of obstetrical practice that recognizes that most pregnancies require no specific 'medical' intervention," and to forge "closer ties with the growing number of well-trained midwives."[27]

Some family doctors provide care that's very similar to typical obstetric care, while others provide care that's more like midwifery. Find out the style of a particular family doctor by asking questions. (See previous questions on page 57.)

"With my first baby, I'm sure I would have chosen the path that most women choose today—an obstetrician and a medically managed labor—if not for my friend Maureen. When her first baby was born a few years before mine, she used a CNM and had an unmedicated, low-tech birth. Maureen had fifty-six hours of back labor with this wonderful nine-pound girl, and she came away from it seeming so powerful and proud, not victimized and complaining like most other women I knew. She spoke about everything she did as if it were the normal way that women gave birth. She said labor was hard, but she was so high and felt so fine after her baby was born that I knew when I had my baby I would try to do it the same way. As I think about it now, I realize this is just what women did before the last few generations became so terrified of birth. I learned from a woman who had walked the path before me, and I felt confident."

—Allison

Making Your Choice

The best caregiver for you is the one who helps you feel the most confident and supported as you journey through pregnancy, labor, and birth. Whether you choose an obstetrician, a family doctor, or a midwife, it's important that he or she listen to you, respect your ideas and questions, and encourage you to make truly informed decisions.

Pay attention to your gut feelings. Be cautious about recommendations from friends and family. What's important to others may not be what's important to you. You may also be finding that your own priorities in pregnancy and birth are changing.

CHOOSING WHERE TO HAVE YOUR BABY

You may choose to have your baby at home, at a birth center (free-standing or within a hospital), or at a hospital. These environments are very different and will powerfully influence how your labor and birth progress. Your choice also shapes the preparation you must do to ensure that you'll feel confident and supported during labor. This choice will also influence how the hours and days unfold for you and your baby after the birth.

Questions to Ask

The Coalition for Improving Maternity Services (CIMS) suggests that when you're investigating birth sites, you should ask the following questions to learn more about your options at each site and to help you choose a birth site that is "mother friendly."[28]

- **Who can be with me during labor and birth?** Some support people you may want are your baby's father, your partner (if he or she isn't your baby's father), your children, other family members, friends, a doula, and/or a midwife. Can you have all, some, or none of these people with you?
- **What happens during labor?** You should be able to get statistics on every part of the birth process at the site. For example, how often is labor induced? What, if anything, is done to speed up labor and birth? How many cesareans are performed per year?
- **How does this site accommodate differences in culture and belief?** Families have widely varying values and customs regarding issues like who may witness a birth, ceremonies or rituals during

labor or after birth, symbolic or spiritual objects present in the room, and so on.

- **Can I walk and change positions during labor and pushing?** Being allowed to move about as you wish and to choose your position for pushing is important for your comfort and confidence.
- **What birth practices are used routinely?** Keep an eye out for common interventions, like those listed below, that have been proven ineffective or harmful for mothers or babies. (For more information, see Chapter 8, pages 122–27, and Appendix A, pages 241–42.)
  - * Continuous EFM that restricts a mother's mobility: Intermittent EFM or auscultation (listening to the baby's heart rate) provides equally useful information with less chance of misreading a printout and better mobility for the mother.
  - * Prohibiting or restricting food and drink during labor: This is an old practice that many hospitals have abandoned because research shows women need energy and hydration to do the hard work of labor.
  - * Shaving a mother's pubic hair or giving her an enema: These, too, are archaic practices shown to provide absolutely no benefits to a laboring woman.
  - * Insertion of an IV needle: Women are told that this provides quicker access to their bloodstream in case of emergency. But needles and IV lines can restrict mobility, and the sight and feel of them can increase stress.
- **Besides drugs, how will you help me deal with labor pain?** In most cases, non-drug coping methods give mothers more confidence and control and are safer for mothers and babies. Does the site offer a variety of methods to help you stay as comfortable as possible in labor? (Some non-drug comfort measures are helping you change positions, a warm bath or shower, massage, and providing a birth ball for rest and movement.) Or is the site inflexible, giving mothers no choice but to depend on medication for pain relief?
- **How will you help me with breastfeeding?** The WHO has made breastfeeding a priority in its policies for improving the health of babies around the world. In accordance with the WHO, a birth site should be telling all its maternity patients about the importance of breastfeeding, and it should have policies in place to ensure that babies nurse during the first hour of life and receive only breast milk, unless there's a valid medical reason a baby

can't. Mothers should be encouraged to feed their babies on demand. There should always be staff available who know how to help mothers with breastfeeding, and mothers should be given the name of a person or group to contact for support and information. A birth site should not give away free samples of baby formula.

More about Hospital Birth

Hospitals are designed to deal with illness. If you're among the 85 to 95 percent of pregnant women who are healthy and low-risk, you don't need to give birth in a hospital. But if you have preexisting health problems or develop serious complications during your pregnancy, labor, or birth, the hospital is exactly where you should be.

Some hospitals have worked hard to provide more homelike birthing rooms and to reduce the number of rules and restrictions, but you can still expect to have less freedom at a hospital than you would at home or at a birth center. A homelike birth unit doesn't translate into a homelike birth. Common hospital interventions like IV use, eating and drinking restrictions, and continuous EFM can make it harder to work actively with your labor. If you do choose to give birth in a hospital, you'll need a birth plan that helps you avoid or limit the negative effects of hospital policies. (See Chapter 10.)

Most women look forward to having help from a labor and delivery nurse in the hospital and expect her to be a calm, supportive presence throughout labor.[29] Research suggests that this is an unrealistic expectation. In today's high-tech birth culture, a labor and delivery nurse spends most of her time monitoring IV fluid intake, EFM, and induction; assisting at cesareans; and taking care of women with serious problems.[30] Although most labor nurses would like to stay at your side, they simply don't have the time.

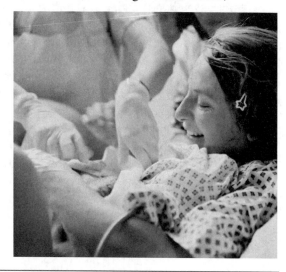

Because of this, if you choose a hospital birth, you'll need to supply your own continuous labor support. Consider hiring a doula in addition to having support from your partner,

"My spirits were high as the nurse announced that I was three centimeters dilated and 100 percent effaced. My doctor told me that if my labor didn't progress throughout the night, I would be induced in the morning. I wasn't worried; I had a strong feeling I'd give birth by then. I trusted my body and ignored all the horrendous stories of pain and cesareans, reminding myself of all the women who have gone through this life-changing, thrilling event.

The nurses didn't interfere much. Justin and I knew it was important for me to change positions and use the bathroom every hour, and that helped my contractions grow stronger. Lying on my back was uncomfortable, so I mostly labored on my sides, leaning against Justin, or sitting in the shower. We all dozed on and off.

As my contractions grew stronger, Justin and Chris, my doula, massaged me. I visualized being at the ocean, with waves of contractions washing over me, and the pain was manageable. I moved into the shower, and Justin stayed with me, telling me I was doing a wonderful job. I was relieved at how smoothly my labor had progressed and never considered pain meds, even when a nurse asked if I wanted any.

As my contractions began to double-peak, I vomited. I recognized this sign of transition and was excited to be closer to meeting my baby. I knew my body was working to get my baby safely out, and I remembered that this stage wouldn't last long. I kept thinking, 'After this contraction, there'll be one less I have to conquer.'

Then came the urge to push. I let my body tell me what to do. I decided the toilet would be most comfortable to push on, and Justin and Chris joined me there, massaging, comforting, and encouraging me. When the doctor came in to check me and said I could start pushing, he didn't realize I'd already been pushing for a half-hour.

I got on my hands and knees, and with lots more encouragement, pushing, and rocking, my son Dylan Alan was born on Sunday morning. He was so beautiful, with amazing cries, a full head of hair, and such a tiny face. He had a wonderful Apgar score, but because he was premature, I could hold him for only a moment before he was taken to the NICU. Justin followed him, and a kind nurse kept me informed about his condition.

After I was discharged, Dylan stayed in the hospital for a week and I became a boarder. He needed some time and help learning to breastfeed. But now he's happy and thriving on my milk. Although my birth didn't go exactly according to plan, I have good memories of it. I remember the visualizing I did during labor. Dylan's name means 'of the sea.' He is calm and flexible—an amazing, bright, and beautiful little boy. He is a gift, and it was a good birth."

—Claire

family, and/or friends. The presence of an experienced, knowledge-able, reassuring woman can help you remain confident during labor and work effectively with your contractions. A doula can also help your other support people help you. A doula may even help you feel more comfortable about staying at home for most of your labor. Research suggests that the longer you're in the hospital and the more interventions you have, the less satisfied with your birth you're likely to be.[31]

It is more challenging to labor and give birth in a hospital, but it's definitely possible with good planning and a confident attitude. Claire's story (see page 62) is a wonderful example of a hospital birth. She had personal and professional support, her obstetrician didn't interfere in the natural process, and in spite of her baby's prematurity, Claire was encouraged to breastfeed him.

More about Birth outside a Hospital

Most women who choose hospital birth do so because they believe that's the safest place to have a baby, "in case something goes wrong." Most health professionals believe this, too. This opinion is based on observing the poor outcomes of unplanned out-of-hospital births.[32] A closer look at the research tells a different story.

A number of studies compare hospital births and planned out-of-hospital births. *Planned* out-of-hospital births are safe (see Myth 2 on page 50). *A Guide to Effective Care in Pregnancy and Childbirth* concludes that "women who have no factors that con-traindicate a home birth, and who prefer a planned, attended home birth with facilities for prompt transfer to hospital if necessary, should not be advised against it."[33]

Birth at a Birth Center

A birth center may be either freestanding or located within a hospital. Birth centers provide many of the comforts of home plus a number of comforts that may not be available at home, like whirlpool tubs. At some birth centers, a variety of pain medications are available. Emergency equipment for mother and baby are always available. Every birth center has physician backup and a system for hospital trans-fer if complications arise.

> To find a birth center near you, call the National Association of Childbearing Centers (NACC) at 215-234-8068 or visit NACC's website at http://www.birthcenters.org.

The philosophy of a good birth center is that birth is a natural, healthy process and that women are capable of giving birth. A good birth center has no routine interventions and gives women freedom to respond to their contractions in any way that seems right. Be wary of a facility that calls itself a birth center but its rules and restrictions don't differ much (if at all) from the hospital.

Birth centers are usually staffed by midwives, but some doctors attend births in this setting. Although many women who choose birth centers hire doulas, they also receive continuous labor support from the nurses on staff. This is possible because with fewer restrictive rules, the nurses' time isn't consumed with managing medical interventions and complications. Typically women return home several hours after giving birth at a birth center.

"My daughter Mary had her first child at a hospital birth center. Mary labored for twelve hours, walking the quiet, carpeted halls, moving from birth ball to tub. Her midwife rocked in the corner, knitting patiently but watchfully. Her nurse waited quietly and patiently, too. Mary worked very hard, occasionally teetering on the edge of despair, but always supported and encouraged by her husband and me. After a few frantic contractions in the whirlpool, finally baby Nora rotated, descending at great speed. After her birth, Nora snuggled in the big bed with her mommy and daddy. Within thirty minutes the birthing room transformed into a party room. Trays of lasagna and salad arrived. Champagne corks popped. Two ecstatic families toasted Nora's birth and Mary's hard work. All the while, Nora nursed and slept in Mary's arms.

Mary had her second child at the same birth center two years later. This time, she arrived shortly after dawn, labored briefly in the tub, and gave birth quickly. Big sister Nora arrived soon after the birth, and several hours later everyone went home. The whole process—from labor starting to homecoming—took six hours. The party happened at home, with Mary and baby Molly tucked into their own bed."

—Judith

Birth at Home

The 1900s saw a dramatic shift from home birth to hospital birth, but there's growing interest in bringing birth back home. Why is this shift happening? Simply put: Research is showing that hospitals may not be the best places to have babies unless there are specific medical needs that can't be met at home.[34]

Birth is a natural process, and in the vast majority of pregnancies, there's no reason to expect problems. Any problem that might arise can be identified and handled promptly at home. A skilled caregiver sees warning signs well before there's serious danger. Most problems can be managed at home—by starting an IV, administering oxygen, and so on—or a doctor is consulted and the woman may be moved to a hospital.

The great advantage of giving birth at home is that home is where most women feel safest and most comfortable. It's where they can truly relax and be themselves. At home, it's so much easier to be undisturbed than it is at a facility full of unfamiliar people, sights, sounds, and smells. And at home, there are no hospital-borne supergerms to fear.

When you give birth at home, you don't have to worry about when to go to the hospital. You don't need to follow (or avoid) regulations that make sense in a large institution but make labor and birth more difficult. You have complete freedom to do whatever brings you comfort: curling up on your sofa, making a cup of tea, watching your favorite video, snuggling under your grandma's quilt, resting in your own bed. Your baby stays warm in your arms from the moment of birth—no whisking away for a bath, eye drops, or testing—and can nurse immediately. You choose the caregivers, family, and friends you want helping you, wear your own clothes, sleep in your own bed, eat your own food.

Not only is the birth different if you choose a home birth, but you can also expect your prenatal care to be strikingly different than if you receive prenatal care from an obstetrician and plan for a hospital birth. Most home birth midwives provide prenatal care in your home. Prenatal visits aren't just an opportunity for your midwife to check on you and your baby; they also provide the opportunity for getting to know each other well. There's time for long discussions, not just about your pregnancy and the upcoming birth but also about your worries, concerns, and whatever else is important to you. By the time your baby is born, you'll probably feel that you and your midwife know each other well.

> "Visits from my midwife were almost like what I think therapy must be. It was all about me. I loved it, and I missed her visits so much after my baby was born."
> —Melissa

"I no longer remember when I decided I wanted to give birth at home—it was certainly long before I ever became pregnant. It was almost a non-issue for me; just something I simply *knew* in the core of my being that I wanted to do, rather than something I decided to do. I am pretty certain this stems from my core feminist convictions. I knew giving birth was something I could do. I never doubted my body's ability or my inner strength.

After I became pregnant, I read a lot about home birth—Sheila Kitzinger's *Birth Your Way* was especially important to me. I was fortunate to find a wonderful home birth midwife. I knew that planning a home birth put me on the fringes of American society—not just hospital-centric, but really hospital-philic American society.

Frankly, the desire the give birth in a hospital is something I have never understood. It seems so unsafe, so *unnecessarily risky* to me. When I occasionally revealed my plans to give birth at home, I was typically met with horrified exclamations of "How could you?! Isn't that unsafe?!" I always felt that for me, these questions actually applied to the decision to give birth in a hospital.

As for pain, I just somehow knew I could give birth without drugs. After all, haven't women been doing so for millennia? If that long chain of women before me had done it, I could too. I was astonished during my first pregnancy when, unbidden, women would tell me, 'Go for the epidural,' as if they were handing me the keys to the kingdom of heaven. I was hungry for the whole experience of birth; I didn't want to drug my body, my mind, or my baby."

—Betsy

Is Home Birth Right for You?

The American College of Nurse-Midwives (ACNM) sees the choice of home birth as one that a woman and her midwife make together. If you'd like to have a home birth, you and your midwife should evaluate your overall health, obstetric history, nutritional status, home environment, and social support to make sure that you are low-risk (in other words, that you're very likely to have a healthy pregnancy and give birth with no serious problems).[35] Here are some questions to consider:

- Are you in good general health?
- Are you committed to maintaining a healthy pregnancy?
- Are you committed to birth without medication?
- Do you have an adequate social support network?

- Do you have privacy and physical and emotional safety at home?
- Are you willing to share responsibility for your maternity care?
- Do you have a midwife or doctor experienced in attending home births?
- Can your caregiver provide vigilant but low-intervention care?
- Does your caregiver have physician backup and hospital admitting privileges?
- Can you arrange for safe, quick transport to a hospital if necessary?
- Do you accept that if your circumstances change, a home birth might not be possible?

Complications that require hospital resources include substance abuse, multiple babies (usually), prematurity, fetal distress, and maternal insulin-dependent diabetes. Other conditions, like a pregnancy that goes well past its due date, can be handled in collaboration with a doctor. Clear and honest communication between a woman and her midwife are essential to determining whether home birth remains a safe choice. For more detailed information about planning a home birth, we recommend reading Sheila Kitzinger's *Birth Your Way*.[36]

A Few Tips As You Make Your Choice

The birth site you choose should be the one that makes you feel the most secure. But no matter where you give birth, a big chunk of your labor should take place at home. You'll need a plan to help labor along and to find comfort as you move through labor.

Know that the work of childbirth is usually more challenging in a hospital. Also keep in mind that an obstetrician is available whether he or she is your primary caregiver or your midwife's physician backup. Choosing out-of-hospital birth doesn't mean you won't need a hospital or that you can't go to a hospital. Every safe birth plan includes physician and hospital backup.

The most important way to ensure a safe, healthy birth is to choose a caregiver and birth site that does not interfere in the natural, physiologic process of birth unless there's a compelling medical indication to do so.

"The long summer days leading up to Mary's third birth were relaxed and easy. She ordered a birth kit from the internet. Miriam, her midwife, visited weekly. Big sisters Nora and Molly waited happily for the new baby. I asked Mary, 'Do you have everything ready?' She answered, 'What's to get ready?' This baby would slide easily into the rhythm of her family's life.

Miriam visited one morning, and Mary complained of some pressure. She felt big and tired. Miriam offered to stay. No, Mary wanted to take a shower and get on with her day. Her husband, Rob, had already planned to be home, and they called me to say something might be up. It was eleven o'clock.

When I arrived, Mary, freshly showered and dressed, was pacing and shaking her arms wildly—her usual ritual for coping with hard labor. Her girls were playing happily with their aunts upstairs. At 11:35 Mary said, 'I have to push.' Miriam was still in transit. Mary rocked and swayed and changed position. I was amazed at how serene we all were. I thought, 'I wonder what the neighbors will think when they realize a baby is being born here.' Miriam swept in the door at 11:40, filled a bowl with water, opened her birth kit, and turned down the air conditioner.

Mary said, 'This really hurts. I'm not doing so good.' We quietly, firmly encouraged her. Baby Maggie (all nine and a half pounds of her) was born at 11:50 as her sisters, aunts, and grandfather raced down the stairs and into the room. Everyone piled on the bed, exclaiming over the sweet baby already nursing happily. Molly, we learned later from the photos we'd taken, birthed and nursed her doll over and over during the next hours.

This birth happened so simply. There were no interventions, no vaginal exams, no episiotomy, no suctioning, no eye drops, no vitamin K, no sepa-ration, no speeding up delivery of the placenta—nothing to distract Mary from the work of labor or the joy of holding her baby.

An hour later, Miriam weighed Maggie and helped Mary to the shower. We put fresh sheets on the bed, then we all ate lunch. As Maggie nursed, Miriam fed Mary grapes and gave her sips of Gatorade. Maggie was alert and nursed off and on for almost three hours. It was very peaceful.

Later in the afternoon, the traditional party started. Mary and Maggie were tucked into bed, alternately dozing and joining the festivities. Family and close friends ate and toasted the miracle of this baby. Life moved effortlessly on. Mary and Rob gave us a gift that day: not just their beauti-ful baby girl, but also the chance to see just how simple birth really is."

—Judith

How Will You View Your Pregnancy?

Marilyn Curl, a midwife and childbirth educator, suggests that every pregnant woman visit both a midwife and a doctor before choosing a caregiver: "Midwives care for healthy women, and physicians care for the sick. Hopefully, a comparison visit would help women decide how to view pregnancy. I think most young women today consider themselves healthy and capable, and midwives are best suited to reinforce that view."

How will you view your pregnancy? We encourage you to choose a confident outlook. Instead of anxiously attending prenatal checkups to hear from others how you're doing, why not enjoy your growing baby, discover the changing you, and let your caregiver know how you're doing? Instead of worrying about your baby's due date, why not rest in the knowledge that your body and your baby will start labor at just the right time?

No matter who your caregiver is, he or she should acknowledge that you are the expert in your pregnancy and that you already know how to do the work you need to do. Whether you choose a hospital, birth center, or home, your labor and birth should be interfered with only if it's clear that the benefits of intervention outweigh the risks.

As your pregnancy progresses and birth approaches, you may find that the choices you've made don't feel as right as they once did. Trust your instincts, and don't be afraid to change your mind. Many women—even very late in pregnancy—change doctors or change to a midwife, change hospitals or decide to have a birth center birth. None of your decisions needs to be etched in stone.

> "I did the typical thing and went to my gynecologist as soon as I knew I was pregnant. I really liked her. But I slowly began to realize that I was on an assembly line. She laughed when I said I wanted a natural birth. She asked if I would have a root canal without Novocain. I thought, 'She doesn't get it.' So twenty-six weeks into my pregnancy, I switched to a midwife and home birth."
>
> —Lauren

Chapter 5

Moving through Pregnancy

The first home you have is your body.
—Ursula Knoki-Wilson

The Shape of Things in the Middle Months

In the early months of pregnancy, you learn to adjust as your body becomes home to a new little body inside you. The middle months also bring an avalanche of change for your body, but by now you're probably better at adjusting to the changes—you're more energized, sleeping better, and over your nausea. During these middle months, you could probably tackle most normal activities, just like before you were pregnant. It's almost as though your body has gotten the hang of what it's being asked to do. You and your baby have set up a nice, calm rhythm, both growing and getting ready for labor and birth in these golden, waiting months.

Physical Growth

Some of the changes you experience are physical. You may notice changes in the color of skin across your abdomen, where your flesh begins to show the effects of stretching to accommodate the growth underneath. Your breasts may be less sensitive than in prior months, and they're beginning to produce colostrum, their first milk. Stretch marks may show up there as well. Your complexion may either display its most radiant state or produce bothersome pimples. Increased blood volume and changes in hormone levels may lead to varicose veins in your legs, hemorrhoids, bleeding gums, or even nosebleeds—all normal responses from your body. Making smart, healthy choices will help, such as putting up your feet as much as possible, eating fiber-rich foods that will help with constipation, and gently brushing and flossing your teeth on a regular basis. Also, drinking plenty of liquids—especially water—will help prevent urinary tract infections and keep dry skin at bay. Wearing cotton underclothes and loose clothing will prevent increased fluid secretions from getting trapped and leading to vaginal infections.

Although you might not yet have that cumbersome feeling that comes with late pregnancy, backaches may become a growing complaint because of the shift in posture, belly size, and body proportions. Baths, warm compresses, massages, gentle exercise, and heating

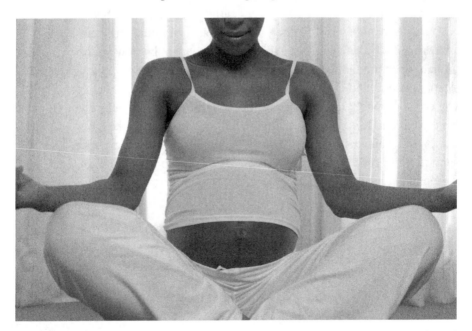

pads may help with the strain. Placing pillows between your knees or propping pillows behind your back or under your belly will provide relief when you lie down. Some women find relief for their backs by getting down on all fours and slowly arching their backs up, like a stretching cat, and doing pelvic tilts. This helps shift the weight down into the muscles a bit—a pleasant change from how things rest in the upright stance.

A daily walk builds stamina and tones pelvic muscles. It also oxygenates your body, aids in digestion and efficient calorie use, and may help you sleep better. And the gentleness of walking makes it the perfect preparation exercise for labor and birth. Taking a walk might be that daily appointment with yourself that we discussed in Chapter 3, a time for self-affirmation, relaxed breathing, and confidence building. You might also appreciate yoga as a stress release, a time for centering your busy mind, and a gentle opportunity to build stamina and confidence. Need some help learning how to do yoga? Pregnancy yoga videos are available in most public libraries, and you can enroll for classes in many communities. Many women testify to the benefits of yoga in pregnancy, especially because it can later become a technique for relaxation and centering attention in labor.

In these middle months you'll welcome the sensation of your baby's movements. You may describe the first flutterings (or quickening) you feel from your baby as bubbles popping or little fish darting about. Your baby has actually been moving about well before you were able to feel the sensation. But in these months, the baby has grown big enough to explore the little world inside you and make noticeable contact with the sides of your uterus. The baby's body grows to be up to ten inches long during this time, and the head, arms, and legs are more proportioned like a newborn's. He or she now has hair and blinking eyes. Along with all that growth comes a burst of activity. As the weeks go by, your baby will be up to all sorts of antics: kicking, sleeping, hiccupping, turning over, sucking that newly defined little thumb.

A Time for Emotional Growth, Too

These middle months bring heightened awareness of not only the physical and hormonal changes in pregnancy, but also the psychological impact of growing a baby. You may become intensely aware of all sorts of feelings, from sadness to elation, confidence to fear. Dreams may become more vivid, symbolic, or nonsensical than in prepregnancy.

These dreams are opportunities for growth, for self-discovery, for facing fears, and for learning new strengths and insights.

If painful memories or unresolved issues emerge, it's best to deal with them rather than ignore or dismiss them. Seek out support from a trusted friend or family member or a support group recommended by your caregiver, childbirth educator, library, or health club. It's a time to pay close attention to your emotions, but you don't have to navigate the sometimes choppy emotional waters of pregnancy alone.

Above all, you need to keep the lines of communication open and keep relationships healthy as your body, mind, and baby change and grow. Expressing hopes, fears, and concerns; facing tough questions; and figuring out strategies for coping are abilities that will accompany you into the challenging and exciting years of parenting ahead.

NOURISHING YOUR BODY

In the middle months, your appetite increases, often with cravings for certain foods, such as things that are sour or salty. You may not necessarily crave the foods that were your favorites before pregnancy. This is a pleasurable time of answering unique food cravings and following your body's lead, but it's also an important time to make simple choices for good nutrition. Pregnant or not, you benefit from healthy eating with better overall wellness, healthier skin and hair, and more energy.

Healthy Eating

That said, eating healthy isn't always easy, and the pleasure of eating well during pregnancy can get drowned out if you try to strictly follow a detailed diet. That's because many health practitioners don't agree on just what "good nutrition" is—how much of a particular food is right or how many calories and fat grams you should consume. In a world of different cultural foods and customs, it's clear that there's no single right diet for a pregnant woman to follow.

The best thing to do is remember that good eating need not be a complex ordeal. What's most important is that you enjoy what you eat, eat when you're hungry, and stop when you're full. Beyond that, nutritionist Jill Stansbury's simple suggestion for good nutrition is "eating a rainbow of natural food colors." Healthy amounts of vitamins C and B_6, iron, calcium, folic acid, protein, fiber, and unsaturated fats naturally show up in fresh fruits and vegetables, dairy foods, fresh nuts and grains, lean meats, poultry, and fish. Here are some basic suggestions for eating well, whether or not pregnancy is in the picture:

- Choose foods high in vitamin C, which strengthens blood vessels, aids in healing, and helps the body resist infection and absorb iron. Look for brightly colored vegetables (green and red peppers, broccoli, Brussels sprouts, squash, and sweet potatoes) and fresh fruits (oranges and kiwi fruit) and juices.

- Choose foods high in B_6, which aids body growth, brain and immune systems, hormone regulation, and blood cell production. Look for bananas, fresh vegetables, dried beans (limas, pintos, and chickpeas), and fresh nuts and cereals.

- Choose foods high in iron, the nutrient known as the red-blood-cell builder. Iron can be absorbed more easily by your body with the help of vitamin C. Some good sources are dark molasses (stirred into a glass of milk), brewer's yeast (stirred into juice or baked into muffins), dark green leafy vegetables, prunes, raisins, and nuts.

- Choose foods high in calcium, important not only for healthy bones and teeth (yours and baby's), but also for blood clotting and muscle function. Enough calcium now will help protect your bone health during your breastfeeding months and beyond. Pay attention to dairy foods, leafy vegetables, whole grains, carrot juice, tofu, and nuts. Yogurt is a great pregnancy food, especially if it contains live acidophilus, a good bacteria found naturally in your body. More than just a calcium provider, yogurt has been found to aid digestion, promote healthy skin and bones, help balance intestinal bacteria, and keep vaginal yeast in check.

- Choose foods high in folic acid (another B vitamin), which is essential to the formation of the baby's spinal cord and brain systems, tissue growth, and cell division. Eat plenty of broccoli, spinach, and other dark green leafy vegetables, as well as dried beans and peas, asparagus, sunflower seeds, oranges, berries, whole grains (especially in breads and pastas), and fortified cereals. The U.S. Public Health Service suggests that women need to be getting more folic acid even before they get pregnant. And *A Guide to Effective Care in Pregnancy and Childbirth* recommends paying close attention to folic acid in your diet (or taking a folic acid supplement) for two months before conceiving, especially if you have a family history of neural tube defects.[1]

- Choose foods high in protein, which, second only to water, makes up most of your body's essential weight. Protein accomplishes your body's general repairs and maintenance as well as builds muscles and skin. Lean meats, poultry, fish, eggs, soy and milk products, and nuts are good sources. Vegetarians know that eating whole grains and dried beans throughout the day, not necessarily together at the same meal, will satisfy protein needs.

- Choose "good" fats (essential fatty acids, found in fresh nuts, seeds, certain oils, and avocados) and avoid "bad" fats (animal fats and the saturated fats in processed and prepared foods). *Fat is often the bad word of diet-speak, but healthy fats help control blood pressure and aid hormone and cell production. Unhealthy fats, on the other hands, are present in so much of what we eat, despite our body's minimum need for them. For some women, those fatty foods may cause indigestion, skin problems, and unnecessary weight gain. Read food labels and look out for hydrogenated fats or "trans fats." These are empty calorie foods that are not worth your time.

- Choose foods high in fiber, which, along with drinking plenty of water, reduces constipation brought on by increased hormones that slow down digestion. Fiber is found only in plants—fruits, vegetables, and whole grains.

- And don't forget these miscellaneous gems: Ginger is a useful herb to help with nausea and settle the stomach after birth. Peppermint might work the same way. Teas are the best vehicles for ginger and peppermint. Garlic is also your friend, boosting your body's ability to stave off infection, aiding in healing and digestion, helping rid the body of toxins, and improving the health of your intestines, heart, and skin. Garlic has been defined as a food, an herb, a medicinal plant, and more. Fresh bulbs are inexpensive, and they'll improve the taste of soup, stew, vegetables, meat, poultry, or fish.

What about Supplemental Vitamins?

Should you take supplemental prenatal vitamins? The use of vitamins dates back to 1500 B.C. Since then, science has researched the needs for and uses of vitamins and other supplements, but our understanding is far from complete. Today there's little agreement about their necessity or about what vitamins to take and in what proportion. It seems for every news bulletin announcing a breakthrough discovery about how a certain vitamin improves health, there's another one down the road announcing that we shouldn't be taking so much of that vitamin after all.

Before commercial vitamin supplements came on the market, women were able, even in less-than-ideal dietary circumstances, to birth healthy babies. While a prenatal vitamin seems good "insurance" if you're not getting enough of the right stuff naturally from your diet, no research confirms the need for routine use of them.[2] Trying to get the "right" dosage of prenatal vitamins isn't an exact science. The best thing you can do is eat a well-balanced and varied diet of fresh, unprocessed foods.

What about Fad Diets?

While pregnancy can be a time of new cravings, it shouldn't be a time for new fad diets. Specialty diets that exclude certain food categories, such as carbohydrates, do not fulfill a pregnant women's nutritional needs. For example, carbohydrates have been called "universal building blocks." They have the important job of providing energy to cells in the body, and they make up many of the essential staple foods humans rely on around the world, such as rice, potatoes, corn, and wheat. Rather than eliminate carbs altogether, choose those that convert more slowly into glucose. Choose brown rice rather than white, whole wheat rather than white bread, whole juices rather than processed fruit drinks. In other words, choosing unprocessed foods rather than refined foods will ensure a healthy, balanced diet. Diet fads come and go. Now's not the time to dally in them.

What about Lattes and Chocolate Bars?

Visit one chat room, and you'll probably see an ever-growing list of pregnancy no-nos when it comes to foods. So what are the facts about two of our favorite vices—caffeine and chocolate?

There's no agreement about how much is too much caffeine during pregnancy. While some folks preach abstinence from all caffeine, there's no evidence that moderate amounts (one to two cups of coffee per day) have any effect on your baby[3] or that restricting caffeine affects outcomes.[4] If you get a great deal of pleasure from of a good cup of coffee, enjoy your latte.

Now, about chocolate—there's good news from Finland. Researchers there have found that six-month-old babies born to mothers who ate chocolate during pregnancy smiled and laughed more and showed milder reactions to stress than babies of mothers who abstained from chocolate. The researchers' conclusion: The chemicals in chocolate associated with positive moods might indeed pass from mother to baby during pregnancy.[5]

But What about Weight Gain?

With so much emphasis on eating, it's hard for some women not to worry about weight gain during pregnancy. But take a glance around,

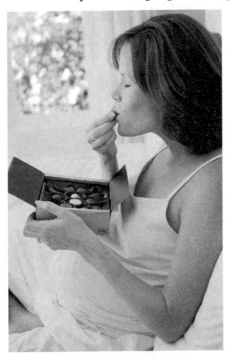

and you'll see that we all come in different sizes, especially during pregnancy. Even with similar diets and activity levels, women vary greatly in how much weight they gain (including how much is baby and how much is placenta and body fluids) and how their bodies carry that weight (all in front, on the sides, up high, or down low). There is no normal range of weight gain, although the American Congress of Obstetricians and Gynecologists (ACOG) recommends at least twenty-five to thirty-five pounds. Placing too much emphasis on pounds and a potential postpartum weight-loss struggle can lead to negative self-images.

Again, the best thing you can do is eat a healthy, balanced diet. Knowing you're eating well to nourish both you and your baby may help you feel better about your changing body. And don't forget that nature has a perfect plan for that extra fat you store during pregnancy: Nine hundred calories a day are used producing breast milk! But if negative feelings about how your body looks still overtake positive feelings about what your body is busy doing, talk with a trusted family member or friend, someone who can listen to your worries and encourage positive thoughts about how your growing body benefits both you and baby.

What about Food for Baby?

As you choose healthy food to nourish your body, your body is busy preparing the perfect food to nourish your baby after birth. Nature's plan for the nourishment and nurturing of your baby is breastfeeding. Only in the last century have babies who were not breastfed had any chance of living. And only in the last fifty years has research examined breastfeeding and breast milk in comparison to artificial infant formula. The differences are astounding. The value and importance of breastfeeding for babies and for mothers is so well documented that we no longer talk of the *benefits of breastfeeding* but rather the *risks of not breastfeeding*.[6] (To read more, see Appendix D.)

Breast milk is the perfect food for babies. No artificial infant formula comes close. Breast milk contains every nutrient your baby needs, in just the right amount. For example, breast milk contains many essential fatty acids not present in any formula. Since fat is essential for brain development, it's no surprise that a number of well-designed research studies have documented higher IQs in breastfed babies. Breast milk is also rich with antibodies and macrophages that destroy bacteria and protect the baby. So it's no surprise either that formula-fed babies are at greater risk for respiratory infections, diarrhea, ear infections, and sudden infant death syndrome (SIDS). Formula-fed babies also have a greater risk of developing allergies, juvenile diabetes, and childhood cancers later in life.

And breast milk changes to match your baby's needs. Colostrum is extremely rich in antibodies and nutrients—perfect food for a newborn's tiny stomach, which is only the size of a walnut. Mothers of premature babies produce milk that's higher in fat than mothers of full-term babies. As breastfeeding is established, milk is higher in fat at the end of a feed and during the night. As baby gets older, the composition of milk is different than it was when baby was a newborn.

Breastfeeding makes a difference for mothers, too. Breastfeeding helps contract the uterus and reduce postpartum bleeding. Women who breastfeed their babies are at less risk of developing breast cancer and osteoporosis later in life (and the longer you breastfeed and the more babies you breastfeed, the better). Not only does breastfeeding provide health benefits, but most breastfeeding mothers describe how enjoyable it is as well. Every time you sit down to nurse your baby, oxytocin and prolactin are released. You feel relaxed, even a bit sleepy, ready to settle down and enjoy being with your baby.

If baby is breastfed exclusively—no formula or water between breastfeeding—and around the clock, levels of prolactin stay high enough to decrease the mother's fertility. Once baby starts on other food and starts sleeping through the night, fertility gradually returns. As a result, in parts of the world where women breastfeed exclusively and have no other form of birth control, babies usually come every two to three years.

Breastfeeding is simply and beautifully designed. You don't need to do anything to prepare your body for breastfeeding. There is no need to toughen nipples. Breasts and nipples come in all sizes and many shapes, and they all work beautifully. Nipples that don't stick out usually do so once baby latches on and begins to suck. Your baby comes fully equipped to nurse. Your baby will nuzzle and snuggle, find your nipple, open wide, and self-attach. Your baby knows just what to do.

That said, if women in your family or your friends haven't breastfed, you may want to take this time now to seek out and spend some time with women who are breastfeeding. (You might also purchase a book about breastfeeding. See Recommended Resources.) Seeing breastfeeding in action and hearing how breastfeeding fits into women's busy lives is invaluable. You'll probably hear that many women let most of the "dos and don'ts" of breastfeeding go in one ear and out the other. There are no rules. Eat and drink what you like. Breastfeeding has been part of women's everyday lives since the beginning of time, so you'll see that it surely isn't meant to turn your life upside down. It's nature's perfect plan for the nourishment and nurturing of your baby.

PRENATAL CARE

By the time you've reached these middle months of pregnancy, you've chosen a caregiver, and a birth site. The issue of prenatal appointments and tests comes into play in the middle months. The number of prenatal appointments and the range of tests you will face vary greatly with your choice of caregiver and birth site. If you chose an obstetrician and a hospital birth, you may find yourself making many more appointments for exams and tests than if you chose a midwife and a home birth or birth center birth.

But prenatal care is more than exams and tests. Appointments should provide an opportunity for you to share how you're feeling and doing, and allow you to raise any concerns and questions that you have. Visits should provide an opportunity for you get to know your caregiver and should not increase your fears, but instead help you let go of worry and become confident in your ability to grow and birth your baby.

Obstetricians and midwives all do a number of tests that are considered basic and important. The following are facts about three tests you will encounter.

Blood Tests

Blood tests check for a number of things, such as blood type (including whether you are Rh negative or positive) and iron levels that might need boosting. Some tests will determine the presence of sexually transmitted diseases or an infection. These tests are considered standard and helpful.

Blood Pressure Checks

Blood pressure checks are considered essential components of prenatal care. High blood pressure may be related to stress or any number of other things, but in pregnancy, especially in the last trimester, it can mean preeclampsia. Controlling high blood pressure with bed rest and medication is sometimes necessary to keep it from developing into full-blown eclampsia, a very serious complication for mother and baby.

Baby Checks

At each prenatal visit, your baby's heartbeat will be monitored and your growing uterus measured as a way to evaluate your baby's growth. Another measure of your baby's growth is your weight gain. Your caregiver may also ask about fetal movement.

Facts about Other Prenatal Tests

The important thing about prenatal tests is to know what's being done and why—and that you have the right to refuse any test. Many tests were originally created for diagnosing problems in high-risk pregnancies. But with the increased medicalization of pregnancy, these tests have become routine for all pregnancies—high-risk or otherwise. This does not mean that the tests are risk-free. On the contrary: Some of them have not been thoroughly tested for safety, and some of them actually present risks to mother and baby. The American Academy of Pediatrics (AAP) is an organization of pediatricians and researchers who help improve health and safety for infants as well as children, adolescents, and young adults. When it comes to routine diagnostic prenatal testing, the AAP admits that "no test is perfect. There may be a problem even if the test does not show it. Also, a problem may not exist even if the test does show it."[7] This often presents an emotional risk. Because some tests can be unreliable, their unclear or misleading results can either decrease your confidence or give you a false assurance.

Cervical Checks

Cervical checks are seldom questioned by the women who go into a clinic or doctor's office, slip off their clothes, and don an exam gown every few weeks and then every week as they get closer to the birth. But these routine examinations are invasive and provide little useful information on their own in early or middle pregnancy. Pregnancy is a time to protect your body from intrusion. Once in labor, your caregiver may check your cervix for dilation, although it isn't necessary. Measuring dilation doesn't determine how labor will progress or how long it will last.

Ultrasound Examinations (Sonograms)

Ultrasounds use sound waves produced by a moving a transducer across the mother's abdomen to create a picture of the baby inside the womb. These are often routine and popular tests, but it's important to weigh the pros and cons before you choose to have one done.

Both the World Health Organization and the National Institutes of Health agree that routine ultrasound testing has not been sufficiently evaluated to let the practice go unquestioned. For one, caregivers strongly disagree about the effect of ultrasound waves on fetal brains. A recent statement from the Federal Drug Administration (FDA) says, "Ultrasound is a form of energy, and even at low levels, laboratory studies have shown it can produce physical effects in the tissue, such as jarring vibrations and a rise in temperature." Because of this, the FDA declares that "prenatal ultrasounds can't be considered completely innocuous."[8] Although, some small studies in Europe and the United States have found an association between ultrasound in pregnancy and developmental delays, including speech delays, a large systematic review did not confirm this finding.[9] *The Cochrane Library* does not recommend routine use of ultrasound in pregnancy, noting that while there are clear benefits to the judicious use of ultrasound, and there is no sound evidence that ultrasound is harmful in pregnancy, theoretical concern about potential hazards remains.[10]

Perhaps more importantly, ultrasounds give imperfect information. An "abnormal" finding on an ultrasound is very likely to turn out to be a false alarm. But the suggestion that the baby is anything other than perfectly healthy can cause a great deal of anxiety for you and for your family. It can also lead to follow-up testing, and some of those tests, such as amniocentesis, carry risks to the mother, the growing baby, or both. On the flip side of the coin, a "normal" ultrasound can't guarantee a healthy baby. While ultrasound is a good tool for finding problems, sometimes even the best ultrasound technician can miss something of concern.

On a more personal note, expectant mothers approach ultrasound with different expectations and different emotions. It's wise to examine for your own feelings and motives before you make your decision. Some mothers choose to have ultrasounds because they're eager to "see" their babies and hear their heartbeats. It can be a tangible yet magical step toward building confidence and attachment, and they look forward to having photos of their babies in utero. Other mothers are much more hesitant, viewing ultrasound as an invasion of their babies' privacy and a "sciencing" of the intimate knowledge and ownership of pregnancy. They feel it's one more aspect of medicalization that lowers confidence in the natural ability of women's bodies to do the work of pregnancy and birth.

If you do wish to obtain an ultrasound photo of the baby, talk to your caregiver. Be leery of the new crop of unregulated, commercial sonogram shops. These "fun ultrasound" shops lure parents with the opportunity to "meet their baby" and the promise of "baby's first picture" as "a nice addition to any family album." Birth activist Marsden Wagner sounds the safety alarm: "At present, there is no known training or certification for users of ultrasound apparatus in any country. In other words, the birth machine has no license test for its drivers."[11]

Another aspect of ultrasound testing that meets mixed reactions is the opportunity to learn the baby's sex. Some mothers look forward to this important discovery, seeing it as a chance to know more about the babies growing inside them. They appreciate learning the sex early in the process, rather than in the emotional moments after the hard work of labor and birth. Some mothers value having the extra time to digest the information before their babies arrive. In contrast, other mothers want to preserve this surprise at all costs. They consider learning their babies' sex a beautiful reward after labor and birth.

To them, finding out the sex is, again, an invasion of the special privacy of pregnancy. However you feel about this issue, know that using ultrasound to learn your baby's sex is an imperfect science, just like using ultrasound to calculate due dates and diagnose problems. For example, many parents have been told during ultrasounds that their babies are girls, only to be surprised to be holding boys in the moments after birth. As with all aspects of prenatal testing, think about what you'll do with the information if you choose to learn your baby's sex. And if you choose to have an ultrasound but not learn your baby's sex, make your wishes known to your caregiver so no one will unwittingly spoil the surprise during the procedure.

As you consider ultrasound testing and all its aspects, do it with the knowledge that it's an option—not a *requirement*—and that you have the right to refuse it. Since much of the information provided by ultrasounds does not ensure a baby's health and safety and is often subjectively evaluated, why routinely subject baby and mother to a procedure that has not been proven to be risk-free? Many women have stated that when they questioned or refused ultrasound testing, their caregivers made them feel guilty. These women were led to believe that choosing *not* to have the procedure done might endanger their babies. Heather shared her reaction after having an ultrasound: "I was surprised to find myself crying, and these were not tears of happiness," she recalled. "I felt like I'd given in on having the procedure done, not really believing it was necessary or right." If you feel undue pressure from a caregiver to have an ultrasound, consider seeking care elsewhere.

First Trimester Serum Screening (Nuchal Translucency Sonogram or Combined Test)

This test estimates the chance that the fetus has Down syndrome. It's done between the tenth and fourteenth weeks of pregnancy, although the most reliable results are at eleven to thirteen weeks. The combined test includes a blood test to provide a more accurate assessment. As in any screening test, there are false positives (results indicating there's something wrong when there isn't), and there are also false negatives. If the test is positive, a diagnostic test like amniocentesis is offered. Before doing this test, you should think about what you will do with the information.

Multiple Marker Screening

Multiple marker tests (also known as maternal serum screening, triple test, triple screen, quad screen) look for the presence of proteins or hormones in the mother's blood that may signal a developmental problem (neural tube defects, Down syndrome, and a few other chromosomal conditions). These tests are done between fifteen and twenty weeks. They have a high rate of false positives, which are discovered when further testing yields different results or when babies are born healthy despite the emotional toll the incorrect results placed on the mother. Before allowing this blood test to be done, you should think about what you would do with the information. You have a right to refuse this test. And if you have a positive result, you have the right to refuse further diagnostic testing (for example, an amniocentesis).

Amniocentesis

Amniocentesis is a procedure in which a small amount of fluid and cells are collected from the amniotic sac surrounding the fetus. Some caregivers warn women, especially those over the arbitrary age of thirty-five, that by not having an amniocentesis done, they are "at risk" of not finding out whether their babies have Down syndrome or other birth defects. What they may not emphasize is that this invasive test puts a woman's body and baby at risk of infection, bleeding, amniotic fluid leakage, fetal distress, and miscarriage. Because of these risks, it is *most* important to think about what you will do with the information before you agree to the procedure.

Glucose Tolerance Test

The glucose tolerance test screens for gestational diabetes. The mother drinks a special sugar mixture, and the level of glucose in her blood is measured. Many Canadian doctors have stopped using this test because research has not shown it to be necessary. Because women are overdiagnosed with gestational diabetes (at least 25 percent of pregnant women are treated for it in the U.S.) and because there's no evidence that taking preventive measures against gestational diabetes is beneficial ("untreated" women with high blood sugar have somewhat larger babies but no increased risk of cesarean or difficult labor), "it's probably not a good idea to be doing it routinely," says University of Washington family doctor Alfred Berg, who headed a government task force questioning the benefits of some prenatal testing.[12] *A Guide to Effective Care in Pregnancy and Childbirth* has this to say: "The available data provide no evidence to support the wide recommendation that all pregnant women should be screened for 'gestational diabetes' let alone that they be treated with insulin."[13]

Group B Streptococcus (GBS) Test

GBS is a harmless bacteria that's present in the vagina and rectum of 10 to 30 percent of all pregnant women. During labor, especially if the membranes have ruptured, the baby is exposed to the bacteria. Although harmless in women, GBS can cause serious, but very rare, infections in the newborn. Because of this risk, the United States Centers for Disease Control (CDC) recommends that all women be tested for GBS between the thirty-fifth and thirty-seventh weeks of pregnancy, and that women who test positive for the bacteria receive one (or two) doses of antibiotics in labor.[14]

For most GBS positive women (90 percent of all pregnant women who are GBS positive), one dose of antibiotics is effective in reducing the exposure of the baby to the bacteria during labor. If labor is preterm, if your membranes have been ruptured for more than eighteen hours, or if you have a fever in labor, the risks are a bit higher, but at least one to two hours of antibiotics during labor significantly reduces the risk of GBS newborn infection.[15]

The Danger of "Spoiling" Your Pregnancy

Sociologist Barbara Katz Rothman, who has studied the enviable Dutch system of birth, states that some Dutch midwives use the phrase "spoiling the pregnancy" when grappling with the issue of routine prenatal testing. They feel testing—especially misleading tests with false positives—robs the mother of joy, peace, and a relaxed relationship with the baby she's carrying inside.[16] One midwife Rothman interviewed said that after a baby is born, there will always be concerns throughout life—threats of accidents or illness and so on. The midwife mused, "It is a process, all life long, isn't it? Somehow or somewhere you have to let it go, you cannot control everything, and maybe you have to start to let it go at the beginning." Rothman writes, "Americans cannot see the costs of ruining a pregnancy, of taking out a piece of the joy."[17]

But many women *are* making the choice to trust in their pregnancies and decline some of the prenatal tests recommended to them. It's important to know that the tests presented to you as being "absolutely necessary" in one country may not be so in another country where

"During both of my pregnancies, I was offered the option of having a level three ultrasound at twenty weeks because I had a sister who died at ten days. She was born two-and-a-half years before me, and she was missing a valve in her heart. The ultrasound was supposed to give the docs a really good look at the heart—but of course, they checked many other things as well. I wasn't worried about the heart business, because no one else in my family has anything like what my sister had.

When we went in for the ultrasound for my second pregnancy, the perinatologist came in to have a look. She told us that the heart looked fine and many other things looked fine, but that there were two physical markers she noticed that have shown a correlation with Down syndrome: Tate's little finger seemed a bit crooked and there were some cysts in the cerebral/spinal fluid, which occur at a very specific time during some pregnancies and then disappear without explanation. By themselves, these markers weren't dangerous. I think the doctor said that my chances of having a baby with Down syndrome were now 1 in 100.

I remember the doctor talking to us about our options, and my shock that abortion was an option at this point. She also gave us some sobering statistics about people with Down syndrome, about how many of them are institutionalized. It was a lot to absorb in a half-hour appointment!

I chose to have an amniocentesis, which caused quite a bit of stress on our marriage because Pete didn't feel that it was necessary and thought it was risky (which it is—1 in 100 cause a miscarriage). At that point, I felt like I *had* to know and prepare myself for whatever came next. I mostly remember the emotions involved: fear, worry, pain, suffocation, loss of control. I remember telling my mom as she laid next to me, trying to help me go to sleep, that I felt like there was a monster inside me. I even forced myself to go online and read chat rooms for parents of Down syndrome children so that I would be a little bit prepared.

My parents and friends were great. I prayed a lot, mostly bargaining. When I got the results of the test ten days later, it was like a weight had been lifted. I hadn't planned to find out the sex of the baby, then in a moment of weakness the woman giving me the results of the test asked me if I wanted to know and I said yes. I think I still had a little nagging worry until he was actually out of my body and I could *look* at him."

—Lauri

the benefits and disadvantages have been better weighed. Also know that if an obstetrician believes a test is absolutely necessary, it may not be what a midwife believes. And it may not be what *you* believe.

Ripening and Readying: The Final Months

For some, the final months are the longest days of pregnancy. As your body grows into a ripened fruit, with your abdomen stretching to accommodate a growing baby inside you, you may feel beautiful but uncomfortable. Along with your hearty appetite, you may have indigestion from the pressure against your stomach. Pressure against your bladder and increased beverage consumption, which ensures healthy fluid exchange for the baby, bring frequent urination. Increased pressure in your abdomen and decreased blood return from your extremities may produce swelling in your ankles and feet. Backaches may be more frequent in response to the heaviness and positioning of the baby. Some women complain of leg cramps during times of rest, which may be caused by challenged calcium levels in their bodies.

For many mothers, the tiredness they felt during early pregnancy returns. The baby requires more and more of your assistance to run his or her body systems, and your energy wanes from carting around a little human being at every moment. The need for short periods of rest to let your body catch up with itself is just as important as the need for gentle exercise. Elevating your feet and propping up with pillows while lying on your left side will provide good support and blood flow for you and baby. (Lying on your left side takes the uterus's pressure off the main vein that passes through your body.)

Once the baby settles head-down in your uterus in the weeks before birth, you will notice less pressure on your lungs and stomach. You'll no longer feel a shortness of breath, but you'll feel a need to urinate more often. Your hormones are busy at work, helping your breasts produce colostrum in preparation for breastfeeding. The tissues in your pelvis are ripening and softening to prepare the birth canal for the baby's passage. The amniotic sac (also called the membrane or bag of waters) that surrounds the baby with protective fluid is busy exchanging its contents every six hours.

To help baby settle into the best position for labor, in the last weeks of pregnancy. it may help if you avoid semi-reclining, such as when you're lying on the sofa watching TV, slouched in the bucket seat of your car, or propped up in bed reading. A semi-reclined position may make it easier for baby to slide around into a posterior position, which in turn makes labor more difficult. So it may help, and it won't hurt, to try to sit upright, supported by pillows when watching TV or traveling by car, and sleep on your side rather than propped on your back.

In the last weeks, you may begin to notice your uterus tightening. These are called Braxton-Hicks contractions. Your uterus has been tightening and releasing throughout pregnancy, but now it's noticeable. You are most likely to notice the tightening when you sit and relax or when you're moving quickly during the day. You also may notice an increase in vaginal discharge as your due date approaches. These signs all are part of nature's plan for the last weeks of pregnancy. (Note: Lots of contractions, a low backache, and an increase in vaginal discharge well before the last weeks of your pregnancy could mean preterm labor, and you should see your caregiver.)

The baby, who enjoyed a dance inside you in the earlier months, will continue some of those entertaining and athletic movements, but he or she may have quieter times as the birth draws closer and there's less and less space to explore. The baby will continue to grow toward the birth weight (a half-pound a week), and the heart, lung, and digestive systems will grow more and more able to independently function. The senses can already respond to light and sound and touch, and the sucking reflex matures as baby rehearses for the first meal at mama's breasts, which are busy readying milk that's full of nutrients and antibodies.

Recent research suggests that the baby's brain is only two-thirds developed at thirty-five weeks.[18] Those last few weeks are very important not just for lung development but also for brain development. Babies that are born even a day too soon (usually because mother was induced or had a planned cesarean) are at greater risk for health problems.[19]

These final months are a time to pay loving attention to the work at hand of birthing your baby. Pregnancy should not be on the "back burner" of your life. If your maternity leave is limited and you're feeling well, you may choose to work until labor starts. Or you might choose to step back from work to center your mind and body, to rest and gather the energy for the birth ahead, and to "nest"—quietly attend to the final details of preparing your heart and home for this new family member. Throughout pregnancy, you've had to accommodate the changing shape of your body; now it's time to accommodate the changing shape of your life in general: How might the hours of your days (and nights) change in the months and years ahead? What are reasonable expectations about your home and appearance? What might lie ahead in relationships with your partner, your friends, and your extended family as you learn to accept and seek help in settling into your new role? What can you learn from this baby about yourself, your values, and your lifestyle? Now's the time to refigure what's most important.

What about Lovemaking These Days?

There was a time when pregnant women were told that intercourse in the last months might cause membrane rupture (breaking the bag of waters) and preterm labor. But there's no evidence that lovemaking in the last three months of pregnancy causes a difference in the length of pregnancy or the baby's birth weight or health.

This is good news for couples during this intense time in a relationship. Many couples feel the need to share physical affection in the final months of pregnancy, and having sex may lead to new ways of pleasuring each other and discovering each other's sexuality. It's an important time to affirm your love for each other, especially in a modern culture where thinness can be a commodity. The shape of a your fully pregnant body might make you feel unattractive, and your partner may fear that lovemaking will be awkward or that it might harm the baby, but there is nothing like sensitive and caring lovemaking to keep intimate lines of communication open. Use good sense in intimacy to find what works and feels best.

LAYING OUT CLOTHES FOR THE BIG DANCE

Some women buy, borrow, and collect everything they think they'll

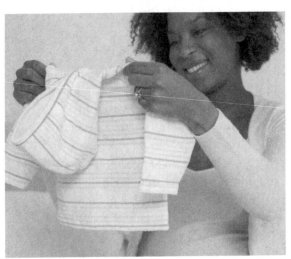

need for the baby's room and wardrobe long before the third trimester. Other women prefer to wait until they are closer to the baby's arrival, be it a matter of energy levels, cultural preferences, or superstition. Likewise, some women will gather a roomful of brand-new items for their brand-new baby—T-shirts, onesies, sleepers, sweaters, hats, blankets, outfits, cloth or disposable diapers. Others will gladly receive used items from friends, family, yard sales, and secondhand stores. A lot depends on habit, value systems, and income levels. But no matter when and how you assemble your baby's layette, laundering, folding, and arranging a newborn's clothes is good therapy for the last weeks.

Don't forget to collect a few items for yourself. These are the last days of maternity clothes—for better or worse. Your new body and new role after birth will no doubt require special clothes. One young mother shared her delight when her older sister bought her a stack of roomy, white cotton T-shirts, something she appreciated herself when nursing her own newborn. A clean T-shirt is relaxing, soft, and breathable; it goes with just about anything; and it makes things easily accessible during those first weeks of breastfeeding. "My sister looked back fondly on those first summer days with her little baby, when she'd shower and slip on one of those shirts and plop down to nurse, relaxed and refreshed," she shared.

AN ALTERNATIVE TO BABY SHOWERS

Our modern world can be so fast-paced that we forget to take thoughtful time to celebrate and honor important life transitions, such as the one you face during these last days of pregnancy. The modern baby shower came into vogue after World War II, possibly in response to the baby boom of that era, but there's evidence that ancient Egyptians and Romans practiced gift-giving to newborns.

Although baby showers allow friends and family to share in the joy of welcoming a new life, they—like so many of our modern celebrations—often fail to really address the importance of the event they celebrate. These gatherings should be times of inspiration, encouragement, and strengthening for a mother-to-be, but they seem to have become marketable events that the baby-goods industry has capitalized on.

We need to take the time to do a more ritual honoring of a pregnant woman and the work she's doing and is about to do. Kathryn Hall of the Birthing Project (see page 28) tells of a naming ceremony celebrated with parents of newborns, but it's an event you could modify and incorporate into a baby shower during the last months of pregnancy. "I learned of the naming ceremony from a woman from Ghana, but it's used all over the world in different ways. It calls people together to educate, to inspire, and to support them when they're getting ready to do something different, something new. And having a baby is something new!" says Hall.[20] Rather than just eating, unwrapping gifts, and playing games like usual, adding elements of the naming ceremony lends some symbolic importance to your gathering.

A naming ceremony gathers (or creates) a mother's support group—people who will support you and your child during the life journey that lies ahead. Hall suggests the group form a circle and help pass around items that have special meaning about the future with your baby:

- A little bowl of cinnamon for you to taste from, symbolizing the bitter things you won't like, the difficulties you'll encounter;
- A little bowl of sugar, symbolizing the things you'll love about being a mother;
- A little bowl of salt, symbolizing individuality—the way you'll use your unique judgment;
- A little bowl of honey, symbolizing the richness and the hard but rewarding work that lies ahead; and
- A bowl of water to drink from, symbolizing the things over which you'll have no control in the years ahead.

After the tasting comes an important part of the ceremony—the empty crystal bowl. Hall explains that the empty bowl symbolizes that when we come into the world, we are empty. "And as you go through life, things will eventually come into your bowl and *that* will be who you are." The bowl is passed around, and each person places a symbolic stone into it, perhaps sharing a word of encouragement or support to the mother. When the Birthing Project's "Sister Friends" step into a relationship with a pregnant woman, they place into the bowl small stones that symbolize prayer—the prayers they commit to offer for this new life. This becomes a powerful statement affirming that this baby truly belongs to a community, that this mother does not have to care for the baby all by herself, and that others stand beside her with their love and prayers.

Candles are also symbolic items in the Birthing Project community, and you can adapt their special candle ritual for your own event as well. "Prior to the birth of the baby, special candles are given to a group of people who are going to pray for the baby while it's being born," says Hall. "So a mother would identify five to ten people who will have this special role in her life. She gives them the birth candle, and at the point when she goes into active labor, someone will be instructed to call the rest of the folks who have a candle. They'll light it and keep it going until they hear that the baby has arrived here safely." These people then save their candleholders and give them to the child when he or she is older, perhaps at a birthday celebration or a difficult time. This symbol lets the child know that he or she was valued and thought of right from the beginning. So, you may wish to be a gift-giver at your own shower, placing candles into your shower attendees' hands with a request that they light them when your labor begins.

CAN YOU HEAR THE MUSIC?

These final weeks before birth are like a preparation for a big dance. The dance floor is ready—the past nine months of eating well, exercising, and resting have been a time for preparation. The musicians are practiced and gathered—mother and baby have been warming up for months, learning how to make the best music together. And at just the right time, when things are completely ready, the dance of labor and birth will begin, and the players who have been rehearsing for all these weeks will delight in seeing each other's faces. For now, enjoy the last days before the dance, and take heart in the confidence that you are ready and able to do this very good work of giving birth.

Chapter 6

PREPARING FOR LABOR AND BIRTH

That is what learning is.
You suddenly understand something
you've understood all your life,
but in a new way.
–Doris Lessing

You may not realize it yet, but you have been preparing for the work of labor and birth throughout your pregnancy—in fact, throughout your life. The power and wisdom you need to give birth is already in you. But like most women, you may need to do some thinking, talking, reading, and more thinking to find and use these resources.

Everyday life is excellent training for childbirth. Chances are you've done plenty of simple (and not-so-simple) hard work over the years. Every challenge you face and every demand you meet prepares you for the work of birth and mothering. You'll draw on all that you are as you help your baby out of your belly and into your arms. And you may well find that this work transforms you into a stronger, more capable, more confident woman.

Listen to Your Body

Throughout your pregnancy you react to what you feel physically and emotionally. You move differently in response to your changing size and shape. You eat differently in response to nausea, sensitivity to smells, and changing tastes. You sleep differently in response to

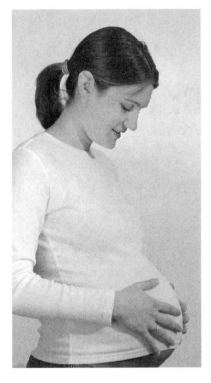

increasing fatigue or discomfort. You pat, stroke, and talk to your belly when you feel your baby squirm and kick. Your body tells you what to do and when to do it, and you are free to listen and follow your body's lead.

In the same way, your body will lead you into and guide you through labor and birth. During the last months of your pregnancy, a precisely choreographed dance takes place inside you. Your hormones shift, your uterus begins to contract, and your cervix softens. Your baby stores fat and his or her lungs mature. As your baby begins to outgrow your womb, he or she turns head-down and drops lower in your pelvis. Your baby's getting ready to leave the warm protection of your womb, and you're getting ready to care for your baby in a new way.

Listen to Other Women

While on a basic level, all you really need to do is listen to your body and follow its lead, giving birth isn't meant to be taken for granted. You'll naturally have questions as you approach birth. You may wonder, "How will I know I'm in labor? What will it feel like? What should I do?"

Getting answers to these questions can help you learn what to expect, tune in to your body, and build confidence in your ability to do the work your body's designed for. In the past women learned the details of labor and birth from their own mothers and from women who had become wise about birth from years of childbearing and attending to birthing women.

Judith's Story of Learning about Birth

In 1917 my grandmother Nora, who was expecting her first child, asked her mother, Nellie, about birth. And my great-grandmother Nellie shared her five birth stories with Nora. Over time, surrounded by the quiet comfort and encouragement of her mother and sisters, Nora birthed six children in the bed where they were conceived.

By the time Nora's daughter Ruth, my mother, grew into a woman, babies were brought into the world differently. My mother gave birth to her own six children in a hospital, alone except for the medical staff who told her what to do and who were, in reality, strangers. Nora, having had her babies naturally and at home, had little advice to offer my mother. She knew nothing about "modern" hospital birth. Although my mother, like Nora, labored without medication, she was anesthetized for all six births because that was standard hospital procedure.

The birth culture of my mother's childbearing years disconnected her from the birth wisdom of her own family. The lost stories included not just Nora's and Nellie's, but also my mother's own story. My mother never shared her birth stories with me or my sisters. Robbed of consciousness, joy, and the ability to remember her births, she felt she had nothing to share.

I grew up to be a nurse. Despite my nursing training, I learned my most important lesson about birth when I attended one—just one—woman who gave birth without medication and with her husband at her side. It was 1966, and I was a nursing student. From that day on I carried with me the life-changing image of a strong woman laboring and birthing naturally.

When I became pregnant and wanted more information about the experience of pregnancy and childbirth, I signed up for a Lamaze class. My nursing classes had taught me the facts of anatomy and physiology. And my Lamaze classes went on to teach me about the stages of labor and how to deal with the pain of contractions. But that one woman birthing naturally in 1966 taught me my most valuable lesson: the lesson of confidence in my body and in my innate ability to give birth.

After considering all that I'd learned, I chose to give birth naturally. And like my great-grandmother Nellie, I shared my birth stories with my daughters. I believe that sharing my confidence and my knowledge of women's ability to give birth naturally is among the most important things I have given them. My daughters have learned about birth in simple faith, by listening to birth stories and being surrounded their whole lives by women and men who trust birth.

When my eldest daughter, Mary, became pregnant, she asked me the same questions my grandmother Nora had asked my great-grandmother Nellie in 1917. Like Nora, Mary got her questions answered. And I, like many generations of mothers before me, stood beside my daughter during her pregnancy, labor, and birth to offer encouragement, comfort, and support. Though we couldn't restore our family's lost stories, we did restore our family's tradition of women helping women on the road to motherhood. Our broken link in the circle of birthing women was repaired.

With confidence in her abilities and help from her family, Mary gave birth to a daughter and blessed her with the ancestral name of Nora. In time she had four more daughters: Molly, Maggie, Cate, and Claire. (For Mary's first three birth stories, see pages 64 and 68.)

Mary now shares her story again and again with her sisters, her friends, and you. And Mary has already shared her birth wisdom with her little daughters. When Cate was born, six-year-old Nora sat at her mother's side and welcomed her sister into the world. Molly and Maggie, wide-eyed and joyful, helped dry Cate and place her in their mother's arms. And when Claire was born two-year-old Cate insisted on wearing her party shoes for the birth and was just as wide-eyed and joyful as her sisters had been at her birth.

Learning from Women You Know

If you want to give birth naturally, and you know women who've experienced normal birth, they will be your most important teachers. Talk with them. Ask the women in your family about their births. If your family has lived in the United States for a while, you may have to go back a few generations to written birth records or handed-down family stories. If your parents or grandparents grew up in other countries, you may be fortunate enough to hear family stories of natural birth firsthand. In such stories, there's a wealth of knowledge to be uncovered and reclaimed. (Take the time to read the birth stories in Chapter 11.)

And what about stories from women who've experienced medical birth? Listen to these, too; you'll learn a lot from them. But don't let them frighten you; remember that the women telling these stories probably see birth through a different lens than you do.

Note how these stories differ from the stories of women who have given birth normally.

As you listen to and learn from women who've gone before you, think about whether their strengths and hopes resemble yours. You may be surprised at what emerges—ways you'd like to emulate, ways you'd like to do things differently, ways you can make positive progress in your journey toward birth.

CONSIDER CHILDBIRTH EDUCATION

Chances are you're wondering how childbirth education fits into the scheme of preparing for normal birth. Formal childbirth education sprang up to fill the void created when several decades of birth stories were lost. During the first half of the twentieth century, most women were heavily medicated for labor and anesthetized for birth, and they simply had little—if any—memory or practical information about childbirth to share.

When Lamaze and other childbirth classes were first offered in the early 1960s, they gave women basic information about birth physiology and coping strategies, like breathing and relaxing, to enable them to labor and give birth without medication. Husbands attended classes, too, and learned to "coach" their wives through contractions and provide emotional support throughout labor. The information was basic, and the skills were simple. In the 1960s and 1970s, that was all women needed to give birth confidently.

But times have changed. Though some harmful and/or useless medical birth practices have fallen by the wayside since 1960, new ones have appeared to take their place. The technology that has grown up around U.S. birth during the past fifty years has made it progressively harder to give birth without intervention. Though a growing body of research supports the value of natural birth and a growing number of women are learning about, experiencing, and sharing stories about natural birth, many more women continue to hand over their births to obstetricians and hospitals.

The other change is the internet, which has opened up the world of medicine to the world at large and has given women the ability to easily access medical information about pregnancy and birth. Unlike any time in history, women today are able to access information that was accessible only from doctors, if at all.

Today, childbirth education needs to provide more than basic knowledge and skills. The most valuable childbirth classes will also help women understand the possible negative influence of technology on their ability to give birth safely and equip them with strategies to minimize unnecessary interventions. Most importantly, childbirth classes can help you make sense of the vast amount of information about pregnancy and birth that you have probably accessed on the internet, read in the countless books on birth, and heard from women of all ages. Childbirth education can help simplify birth and help you make sense of information, let go of your fears, make informed maternity care decisions, and get the safe, healthy birth you want in the current maternity care environment.

Should You Attend Childbirth Classes?

Ideally, women shouldn't have to take formal classes to give birth confidently. But we aren't living in an ideal world. In a culture that relies on technology in both health and illness, formal childbirth classes and online groups can do much to help you recognize your own abilities and help you have a safe, healthy birth.

Our great-grandmothers, surrounded by the birth wisdom of women who'd gone before them, didn't need childbirth classes. But they also didn't face the cultural challenges birthing women face today. Should you attend childbirth classes? We recommend that you ask yourself the following questions to help you decide.

- Did you grow up believing that your body works beautifully? That its functions are normal, natural, and healthy in general—and in particular regarding childbirth?
- Do you know and trust women who have given birth naturally and confidently?
- Have you talked with a woman who had a baby with a midwife's help?
- Do you know other people who believe women's ability to birth naturally?
- Have you chosen a caregiver who provides evidence-based care and does not interfere in the natural process of birth unless there's a clear medical indication?
- Will your birth site allow you freedom to respond to your body's signals however you need to as you move through labor?
- Will you be supported during birth by family and/or friends who are confident and knowledgeable, like you?

If you've answered yes to all these questions, then you might not need formal childbirth education. If not, classes may help you.

What to Look for in an Educator

If you want to give birth naturally, you should look for a childbirth educator who's both knowledgeable about and committed to safe, healthy, natural birth. She should believe, with you, that you can do the work of labor and birth without medical intervention. She should respect your ability to make decisions that are right for you. She should be an advocate who shares *all* the information you need to make truly informed decisions.

How do you know if your teacher has the necessary knowledge and skill? Many childbirth educators are nurses, but not all good teachers are nurses—and not all nurses are good teachers. There are many organizations that train childbirth educators, including independent Lamaze-accredited childbirth educator programs, but Lamaze International offers the only certification examination for childbirth educators that's accredited by the National Commission for Certifying Agencies (NCCA). Accreditation by NCCA is assurance that the Lamaze childbirth educator certification examination meets the highest possible standards for assessing professional competence. If your teacher is a Lamaze Certified Childbirth Educator (LCCE), she has demonstrated her competence by passing this rigorous examination. She has proven her ability to:

- promote childbearing as a natural, healthy process that profoundly affects women and their families;
- help women and families discover and use strategies that facilitate natural, healthy pregnancy, birth, breastfeeding, and early parenting;
- help women and families understand how interventions and complications influence the normal course of pregnancy, birth, breastfeeding, and early parenting;
- give information and support that encourage attachment between babies and their families;
- help women and their families make informed birth decisions;
- advocate for women and families who want natural, safe, healthy childbirth;
- design, teach, and evaluate a course in Lamaze preparation that increases women's confidence and ability to give birth.

There are, of course, other excellent teachers who are not Lamaze certified. What's most important is that your educator trusts birth, is a good teacher, and has confidence in you. With those qualities will come the inspiration and motivation you need to help you prepare for the birth of your baby.

What to Look for in a Class

Like a favorite class you had growing up, on a subject you loved with a teacher you admired, the right childbirth class should make you smile, relax, and embrace what you're learning. It's not a place for lectures or tests. Rather, it's a place for discovery, questions, discussion, and confident anticipation. The best classes needn't provide vast amounts of technical information, but they should help you untangle the web of modern obstetrics and figure out what's best for you. You should leave your class assured rather than fearful.

What should you learn in a childbirth class? We believe that overall, childbirth classes should provide knowledge and skills that build your confidence in your ability to give birth. The most important thing you should learn is the simple story of birth (see Chapter 7). You should discuss how to keep birth as safe and healthy as possible (see Chapter 8). You should learn and practice ways to find comfort during labor (see Chapter 9). Classes should also include basic breastfeeding information and tips on communicating with caregivers. A good childbirth class gives you not just all the information you need to make truly informed decisions, but also the opportunity to develop specific strategies you might need to advocate for yourself with your caregiver and place of birth (see Chapter 11). Finally, good classes are small (preferably no more than ten couples) and interactive.

We recommend that you avoid taking a class that undermines your confidence in any way. Be wary of classes that focus on hospital protocols, possible complications, and medical interventions; learning about labor and childbirth shouldn't focus on what might go wrong. Be wary of a teacher who's quick to remind the class that the doctor and hospital always know what's best for you; only you know what's best for you, and medical practices aren't always based on best evidence. Be wary of large class sizes, which are likely to prevent your questions and concerns from being addressed adequately. Be wary of classes that suggest that birth is safe only in a hospital, that routine interventions are necessary for a safe birth, that epidurals do not affect babies, or that pain plays no role in labor; these claims simply aren't true.

If you're considering attending a "Lamaze" class in your area, make sure it's genuine Lamaze. A real Lamaze course is taught by a Lamaze Certified Childbirth Educator and is based on the Lamaze commitment to present evidence-based information. The hallmark of today's Lamaze classes are the six Healthy Birth Practices. (See Chapter 8 and Appendix A.) Lamaze classes prepare women for a safe, healthy birth by providing the most current, evidence-based information about birth, simplifying birth, and helping women navigate the maze of modern obstetrics. Be wary of "Lamaze" classes that spend a lot of time practicing relaxation and breathing and little or no time building your confidence or discussing how to keep things simple and how to have the safe, healthy birth you want in the birth setting you have chosen.

When to Start Childbirth Education

As soon as they learn they're pregnant, women are on the internet and reading books about labor and birth. So, right from the beginning of pregnancy, childbirth education has begun! Lamaze childbirth education starts at the beginning of pregnancy, too. Here are just a few of the online resources you'll find at http://www.lamaze.org: Sign up for the weekly pregnancy e-newsletter, *Lamaze...Building Confidence Week by Week*. Become part of "Ask Henci," Lamaze's ask-the-expert forum. Read Lamaze's Healthy Birth Practice papers. View the videos *Everyday Miracles* and *Healthy Birth Practices*. Follow the blogs *Giving Birth with Confidence* (http://givingbirth withconfidence.org/) and *Science & Sensibility* (http://www.science andsensibility.org/).

Several other organizations' websites are excellent sources of information, including Citizens for Midwifery, Childbirth Connection, Coalition for Improving Maternity Services (CIMS), DONA International, and the International Cesarean Awareness Network (ICAN). It's also important to visit http://cfmidwifery.org and http//www.thebirthsurvey.com to learn more about maternity services in your area. (See Recommended Resources for details).

What about formal classes? Lamaze's vision for the future is that formal childbirth education, in person and online, should start early in pregnancy. If you can attend a class early in your pregnancy, it will make choosing a caregiver and place of birth easier for you and will help you understand all the choices you have. Most importantly, if you are fearful, classes will help you let go of fear and increase your confidence in your ability to grow, birth, and nurture your baby.

Classes in the middle of your pregnancy can help you move through pregnancy more easily. The comfort-, relaxation-, and confidence-building strategies you learn will be useful in pregnancy as well as in labor. Classes all through pregnancy will provide information that's credible, reliable, and useful; most importantly, they can help you make sense of information so you can make informed decisions. By the time you reach the end of your pregnancy (when formal childbirth education traditionally begins), you'll already be confident and able to make specific plans for labor, birth, and getting to know your baby.

Making Your Choice

As you choose a birth class, talk to a few women who've taken classes in different settings. Talk to a midwife or other caregiver. Talk with the childbirth educators themselves. Ask yourself how the class you're considering fits your values. And remember that if the class you choose turns out to be a poor fit, you can change classes.

The following chapters provide a quick snapshot of the information that's important to know as you prepare for labor and birth. Your classes will provide a forum for discussion, for questioning, for strengthening your communication skills, for practicing comfort measures, and for building your confidence.

Be especially cautious if you are considering attending classes at a hospital. Many hospital classes are simply too large, and hospital administrators often pressure teachers to prepare women for the birth experience in that particular hospital. As a result, teachers must often withhold evidence and options. For instance, if a hospital's policy is continuous electronic fetal monitoring (EFM) for all women, its teachers are expected to discuss the importance of EFM for safety. And naturally, they're expected *not* to discuss the important evidence that continuous EFM doesn't benefit babies and increases maternal risks. The women who attend these classes never learn the full story.

THE SIMPLE STORY OF BIRTH

When I crossed the finish line of my first marathon,
I felt exactly the same exhilaration I felt when Ben was born.
I did it! The feeling of accomplishment I experienced after natural
childbirth gave me strength and confidence for years afterward,
whenever I wasn't sure I was up to a new challenge. The positive
struggle of working with your body in labor and birth can be a
reward in itself. And then add the joy of having a healthy baby!
—Debby Amis

HERE'S WHAT HAPPENS

During the last weeks of pregnancy a series of physical changes sets the stage for your baby's birth. The changes happen slowly but predictably, and each change is a vitally important event in the drama of labor and birth. Your baby is ready to be born. And your body knows this. Together, your body and your baby dance into motion.

Dramatic hormonal shifts orchestrate this entire process. In the final weeks of pregnancy, your body begins to release more prostaglandins to soften your cervix. Your baby settles lower in your pelvis. This is very early labor, and nature has designed it to happen gradually and deliberately. You may notice strong (but typically not painful) uterine contractions. Sometimes they become rhythmic, then go away. This is exactly what your body needs to do.

You may not realize you're in labor at first. Women who do recognize early labor contractions often describe them as mild, cramplike pains that start deep in the abdomen and move downward toward the groin. If the back of your baby's head is facing your back (occiput posterior position), you may feel early contractions as back pain.

Labor—especially early labor—is a process that's easily affected by your surroundings. Most mammals seek quiet and privacy when they're in labor, and if they sense danger of any kind, labor stops. This frees them to move to safety, or lets them wait until danger passes to deliver their babies. Human labor fits this pattern: Early on, it can be shut down by anxiety, fear, or anything that makes you feel unsafe. That's why it's important to choose a birth site and caregiver that help you feel confident and secure.

As labor progresses, your body releases increasing amounts of oxytocin to make your uterus contract (tighten and relax) in a steady rhythm. As your body releases more and more oxytocin, your contractions grow stronger and stronger. These contractions slowly efface (thin) and dilate (open) your softened cervix and encourage your baby to inch downward in your pelvis.

Contractions are like waves at the beach. Early contractions are like gentle waves. Gradually, the contractions grow stronger and closer together—the waves grow higher and deeper and more difficult to ride. When your contractions are lasting a minute long and are less than five minutes apart (from the beginning of one contraction to the beginning of the next), and are gaining strength, you're in active labor. It can take anywhere from a few hours to a few days to reach this point in labor.

As oxytocin surges and your contractions grow more painful, the high oxytocin and pain levels signal your brain to release hormones called endorphins. Endorphins decrease pain perception, moderate oxytocin release (giving you and your uterus little rest breaks), and help you enter a dreamlike state. Endorphins help you turn inward, act more intuitively, and find a rhythm as you cope with contractions.

At exactly the right time, as your baby rotates and descends through your pelvis, you begin to feel an urge to push. Pushing is a reflex, and like other reflexive behaviors (such as sneezing), it doesn't need to be taught. It happens naturally and is, in fact, difficult to stop. Responding to this urge, you move and change position frequently to find the best position for pushing. If you follow your instincts, you're likely to give birth upright to take advantage of gravity, and you may squat or get into other positions that enlarge your pelvis.

It's common to feel anxious during the pushing stage. This sudden anxiety stimulates the release of catecholamines (stress hormones) in you and your baby. At this stage, unlike in early labor, stress hormones actually help the process. French obstetrician Michel Odent theorizes that a mammal far along in labor is very vulnerable to predators, so it's essential for mammals to deliver their young quickly.[1] A catecholamine surge helps hasten birth.

Catecholamines make you more alert, more focused, and extremely strong to help you push your baby out. Your baby emerges face-down, then rotates ninety degrees so his or her shoulders can deliver one at a time. The rest of your baby's body slides out quickly. This trip through the birth canal squeezes amniotic fluid out of your baby's lungs to make room for air. The cooler temperature outside your body, a slight decrease in oxygen from you, and high catecholamines cause your baby to take an instinctive first breath. Catecholamines also make your newborn baby very alert.

When your baby is placed on your abdomen, his or her weight helps your uterus contract to deliver your placenta. Your body heat keeps your baby warm. Skin-to-skin with you, your baby's breathing and heart rate stay more stable than they would if he or she were separated from you and placed in a warming bed. Your baby's head and hand movements stimulate your body to produce prolactin, which helps your breasts make milk, and to continue producing oxytocin, which keeps your uterus tight to prevent bleeding and also helps your milk let down. If your baby is left undisturbed, skin-to-skin with you, he or she will slowly and methodically crawl to your breast and latch on.[2]

High levels of all these hormones—endorphins, catecholamines, oxytocin, and prolactin—contribute to the euphoria you feel holding your baby right after birth. And high levels of endorphins in your breast milk ease your baby's transition to life outside your womb.

In this story of birth, labor unfolds quite naturally. No machines time or rate your progress. No experts tell you what to do or what not to do. No one takes your baby from you. It's an ancient story of a strong, confident woman and a competent baby who both know just what to do. It's all good news.

PAIN WITH A PURPOSE

What may *not* seem like good news is the pain woven throughout this story. Most pregnant women worry about the pain of labor and birth. No one enjoys pain, and people go to great lengths to avoid it. But make no mistake: Pain is a normal, healthy, and necessary part of childbirth. In fact, pain is *central* to the elegant design of birth; it's not an unfortunate side effect.

At the beginning of labor, pain lets you know that it's not just another day. Knowing you're in labor gives you time to gather the help you need and to go to a safe, secure place. Without pain to signal the start of labor, many more babies would be born in cars, shopping malls, and on the street.

Like other pain in your life, childbirth pain protects you. If you accidentally touch a hot stove, the pain makes you instinctively pull your hand away to prevent a burn. If you develop a blister on your foot, the pain makes you change the way you walk to protect your foot from further injury. If you're in labor, the pain of a contraction makes you move, rub, or moan in an effort to get comfortable. Your actions ease the pain a bit and help you get from one contraction to the next—even stronger—contraction.

Coping with pain gives your body the green light to increase oxytocin release, which causes stronger, more effective, and more painful contractions—and ultimately the release of endorphins, "nature's narcotic." At the same time, your movement helps your baby rotate and descend gradually and gently. Every time you move, the diameter of your pelvis changes, giving your baby a little room to wiggle through your birth canal.

Medicating the pain away disrupts labor. If you can't feel the pain of contractions or the pressure of your baby's descent, you can't respond to it. Your body doesn't know to release more oxytocin, and your birth canal is more vulnerable to damage. Removing labor pain also prevents endorphin release, depriving you of the natural high of childbirth. Remove the pain at any point in the journey, and you remove the signals your body needs to keep labor progressing and to protect itself and your baby.

Why should you face and feel labor pain? The answer is simple: Pain is a key element of nature's perfect plan for birth. Pain promotes the progress of labor, protects the birth canal and the baby from trauma, and ensures high levels of oxytocin and endorphins. Coping with labor pain naturally improves your odds for a faster and easier birth, an alert baby, a healthy you, and a successful start to breastfeeding.

TRUST: A TRUSTY TOOL

"Self-trust is the first secret of success...," writes Ralph Waldo Emerson. We agree. Trust in the natural process of birth and in your ability to give birth is the best tool you have in your quest for a healthy, satisfying birth. In other words: Time is your friend in labor. Fear is not.

How long does labor last? Exactly as long as it needs to. There's wide variation in the length of labor. How your labor goes depends on many factors. The strength of your contractions and the size and position of your baby are two obvious ones. But other factors are equally important: security, confidence, freedom to move and find comfort however you like, emotional and physical support. All these things help labor progress.

British anthropologist Sheila Kitzinger believes that the most destructive technology used in birth is the clock.[3] Only in the Western world (particularly in the United States) is labor described in terms of time. For most of the world's women, clocks aren't central to birth. It takes time—sometimes lots of it—for your cervix to soften, for your hormones to rise, for your baby to maneuver, and for you to get into a laboring mind.[4] You can expect early labor to take longer and active labor to move more quickly. But outside these expectations, it makes sense to forget the clock and appreciate the time labor takes.

Remember that women have been doing this work forever. You have every reason to feel safe and confident. You are made for giving birth. Like countless generations of women before you, you will know what to do as your labor progresses. We encourage you to let go of worry and trust your body and soul. We bet you'll be glad you did.

Chapter 8

KEEPING YOUR BIRTH
SAFE AND HEALTHY

One cannot actively help a woman give birth.
The goal is to avoid disturbing her unnecessarily.
—Michel Odent

Today's typical American maternity care aims to help birthing women—but much of it actually disturbs them and makes labor more difficult and complicated. Research has clearly identified many birth practices that are ineffective or harmful, as well as many that promote, protect, and support the natural process of birth. We explain both in this chapter, with tips on how to avoid the former and achieve the latter.

The helpful care practices described on the following pages are simple and backed by strong evidence, but unfortunately, they're relatively uncommon in American obstetrics. We realize that these care practices may be unfamiliar to you and/or your caregiver, so we cite a great deal of research to support the claims we make.

Lamaze's six Healthy Birth Practices are a guide for creating a birth environment that lets you tap into all you need to work with your body in labor. (See Appendix A. The practice papers are also available on http://www.lamaze.org, as are the *Healthy Birth Practices* videos). Regardless of your baby's size, your labor's length and complexity, or your confidence level, these birth practices will help you keep your labor and birth as safe and healthy as possible.

LAMAZE'S SIX HEALTHY BIRTH PRACTICES

1. Let Labor Begin on Its Own

Letting your body go into labor spontaneously is almost always the best way to know that your baby is ready to be born and that your body is ready for labor. In the vast majority of pregnancies, labor will start only when all the players—your baby, your uterus, your hormones, and your placenta—are ready. Naturally, labor usually goes better and mother and baby usually end up healthier when all systems are go for birth.

Every Day Is Important

Every day of the last weeks of pregnancy is vital to your baby's and body's preparation for birth. During this time you pass antibodies to your baby to help him or her fight infections. Your baby gains weight and strength, stores iron, and his or her suck-and-swallow coordination matures. Your baby's lungs mature, too, and begin to produce a substance called surfactant, which helps the tiny alveoli (air sacs) stay inflated after birth.

Your maturing baby and aging placenta trigger a prostaglandin increase, which softens your cervix, and an estrogen increase and progesterone decrease, which make your uterus more sensitive to oxytocin. Your uterus contracts in response to the oxytocin, which makes your cervix efface (thin) and dilate (open). Your baby moves down into your pelvis.

New physical sensations at the end of pregnancy may make you feel antsy for birth. You may notice more vaginal secretions, colostrum leaking from your breasts, and interrupted sleep. After your baby drops, your clothes may fit differently, you may feel less short of breath, and you may have to urinate more often because your baby is crowding your bladder. You may also notice a burst of energy. This "nesting" urge is nature's way of helping you finish up baby preparations.

As labor approaches, you may notice some bloody show (blood-tinged vaginal discharge) or you may lose the mucous plug that sealed off the small opening of your cervix throughout pregnancy. Passing your mucous plug doesn't cause pain or discomfort, and it doesn't necessarily mean labor is about to start. You may also have diarrhea or very soft bowel movements; this is nature's way of making room in your pelvis.

Early Labor: Do Not Disturb

Many people believe that labor always begins with a woman's water breaking. Actually, only about one in six labors starts this way. (For most women the bag of water breaks sometime in active labor, and for some women it doesn't happen until the baby's head emerges.) If your water does break before contractions start, contractions will most likely start within twenty-four hours. When water breaks on its own, it's usually a small tear that only leaks during a contraction. So even if your water breaks early in labor, your amniotic sac continues to cushion your baby and your birth canal.

In early labor you're likely to feel contractions that are gentle and irregular, although they may become strong enough to stop you in your tracks and then fade. Such contractions may make you think you're in active labor, but chances are you're not. Active labor is marked by strong, regular contractions that do not fade, but rather grow stronger and closer together.

Early labor contractions can come and go for days or even weeks. Off-and-on contractions are sometimes called false labor, but really, there's nothing false about early labor. A long, sporadic early labor is normal, and it helps your body accomplish important preliminary work.

You may be quite unaware of your early labor, and it may go fairly quickly. Or you may find it long and tiring. Fatigue and frustration can make a long early labor difficult. It helps to alternate rest and activity to conserve your strength. It also helps to remember that this early stage is both important and normal.

It's very important not only to let your labor start on its own, but also to be undisturbed early in your labor. If you feel safe and secure and have some measure of privacy, your stress hormones stay low and your labor can progress unhindered.

When you're at home supported by family, friends, or a professional doula—people who understand and trust birth—you're more likely to feel safe and relaxed. Stay at home as long as you continue to feel safe and secure there. Here are some easy things you can do to help you through early labor:

- Eat and drink to keep up your energy.
- Alternate rest and activity.
- Remind yourself that your body knows what to do.

Anthropologist Sheila Kitzinger recalls a midwife's story of early labor from a birth she attended: "We spent much of the first stage in the garden, putting in bedding plants together. Then we came in and made some cookies and cleaned up the kitchen. By that time, I could tell from her breathing that she was nearly fully dilated."[1]

If you're not planning a home birth, remember that going to the hospital too soon starts a medical clock ticking and increases your risk of medical intervention.

It's time to travel to your birth center or hospital when your contractions are close together, are growing and staying stronger, and are increasingly difficult to handle.

When Labor Is Induced

If your labor is induced (started artificially), it becomes a medical event and proceeds quite differently from spontaneous labor. There are valid health reasons for induction (see page 115), but most inductions today are elective (chosen for non-medical reasons).

Most inductions today are done for social reasons: Women are tired of being pregnant and eager to meet their babies, caregivers prefer to schedule births during the week and during the day, or women want to schedule births for convenient dates. Many women are told elective induction has no downside. This is not true. Perhaps most disturbing is that more and more women are pressured into agreeing to induction as a result of warnings from their caregivers that the baby is getting too large; however, this is not an indication for induction.

Elective induction carries many risks and disadvantages. The important events of late pregnancy and early labor do not have a chance to unfold. Your cervix may not be sufficiently soft. Your uterus may not be highly sensitive to oxytocin. Your baby may not be mature enough. A baby who's even slightly early is more likely than a full-term baby to have problems adjusting to life outside the womb. Your baby may have trouble breastfeeding and is three times more likely to die in the first year of life than a full-term baby.[2] Elective inductions increase the use of medication, including epidurals, and also the incidence of non-reassuring fetal heart rate patterns, shoulder dystocia, instrument delivery, and cesareans.[3]

Labor is usually induced with intravenous (IV) Pitocin, a synthetic oxytocin. Pitocin contractions feel stronger and peak more quickly than natural contractions. Also, your uterus never totally relaxes between contractions, which puts more stress on both your uterus and your baby. Pitocin doesn't cross the blood-brain barrier, so your brain doesn't get the message (as it would with natural oxytocin) to release endorphins. Without endorphins, you have no natural pain relief and thus have a greater need for pain medication. When your labor is induced, you also require IV fluids, continuous electronic fetal monitoring (EFM), and sometimes a bladder catheter. Finally, you'll likely be restricted to bed and prevented from actively working with your labor.

Labor induction alters not only the process of labor and birth, but also the days after your baby is born. Pitocin short-circuits your natural hormone release, so neither you nor your baby experience the catecholamine surge necessary for energy and alertness after birth. Your baby is less likely to crawl to your breast and latch on and is less likely to make the hand and head movements on your chest that stimulate continued oxytocin release, which controls bleeding and helps your milk let down. This can complicate the start of breastfeeding.

There are, of course, some good reasons for inducing labor. The American Congress of Obstetricians and Gynecologists (ACOG) believes labor should be induced only when it's riskier for baby to stay in the uterus than to be born. This is true when the water breaks and labor doesn't begin, when pregnancy has reached forty-two weeks, when mother's blood pressure is high and can't be controlled by medication and bed rest, when mother has health problems (like diabetes) that can't be controlled and could harm her baby, when mother has a uterine infection, or when baby has a growth problem.[4] Suspecting a very large baby (macrosomia) is *not* a good reason for induction.[5] Research shows that inducing for "overdue" babies (before a full forty-two weeks) increases labor complications and cesareans without improving neonatal outcomes.[6]

Unless you or your baby has a health problem that necessitates induction, it makes sense to wait patiently for your labor to start on its own. Even if your due date has passed and you're longing to hold your baby, remember that nature has good reasons for the wait. It is safer and healthier for mother and baby to let labor begin on its own.

2. Walk, Move Around, and Change Positions Throughout Labor

Why Movement Works

Moving in labor serves two very important purposes. First, it helps you cope with increasingly strong and painful contractions, which signals your body to keep labor going. Second, it helps gently wiggle your baby into your pelvis and through your birth canal.

When allowed to move freely, women instinctively respond to labor pains the same way we deal with pain in our daily lives: squirming to find a comfortable position in an uncomfortable chair, walking differently to protect a blistered toe, rocking to ease gas pains, rubbing to relieve a headache. Walking, changing position, squatting, rocking, rubbing, and swaying are effective ways to work with many kinds of pain, not just labor pain. Without freedom of movement, it's difficult to cope with ordinary pain—and nearly impossible to handle labor without medical interventions.

In labor, movement provides other benefits, too: Not only does it help you find comfort, it also hastens your baby's journey through your body in a way that protects both of you from injury. Regardless of your pelvis size or your baby's size, your baby must rotate to get through your pelvis. Your uterus contracts more efficiently[7] and your baby rotates and descends more effectively when you move than when you keep still during labor.

According to birth activist and midwife Mary Kroger, "Often instinctively a mother will assume a position that favors faster, more effective labor.[8] Without direction, a woman in labor will follow her body's lead to move among standing, sitting, crouching, squatting, and kneeling. And she'll move more as the birth of her baby approaches.[9]

Research supports that walking, movement,

"When my daughter Mary was in labor, she rapidly and rhythmically shook her arms and hands with each contraction—a movement she'd never done before. My great-aunt Esther chanted, 'Oh my God! Oh Mama!' as she walked around her dining room table. Rhythmic movement like rocking, swaying, or slow dancing is an excellent way to relax and distract yourself from labor pain. It stimulates mechanoreceptors in your brain, which decreases your pain perception. Incidentally, hugging, kissing, and hand-holding do the same thing. No wonder they feel so good!"   —Judith and changing positions may shorten labor, are effective forms of pain relief, and are associated with fewer non-reassuring fetal heart rate patterns; in addition, walking in the first stage of labor decreases the likelihood of having a cesarean.[10] *The Cochrane Library* says that there is evidence that walking and upright positions in the first stage of labor reduce the length of labor. Women should be encouraged to use whatever position they find most comfortable.[11] Unfortunately, the *Listening to Mothers II* survey found that only 25 percent of women had freedom of movement in labor. The reason women gave most often for not moving in labor was "being hooked up to machines."[12] Imagine trying to navigate a dance floor tethered to an IV pole!

Movement and Your Baby's Position

The best birth position for your baby is occiput anterior (head down, with the back of the head against your belly). However, some babies assume an occiput posterior position (head down, with the back of the head against your back), which often results in a longer, more painful labor.

In the last weeks of pregnancy, your posture may affect your baby's position in your uterus. (Research on this is just beginning.) Semi-reclining may encourage your baby into a posterior position, so it's a good idea to avoid semi-reclining: Skip lounging on the couch, sleeping propped up with pillows, and kicking back in your chair at the office. If your car has bucket seats, straighten up your driving posture with a small pillow behind your back. When you're sitting in a chair, lean forward. Better yet, sit on a stool or a birth ball instead. Rest and sleep on your side.

If your baby is in a posterior position when labor starts, you may feel your contractions as back pain. This happens because the back of your baby's head is pressing on your spine. You may not get the relief between contractions that's typical in labor. Also, your labor may last longer because your baby needs to rotate more to fit under your pubic bone and needs more wiggle room to descend through your pelvis.

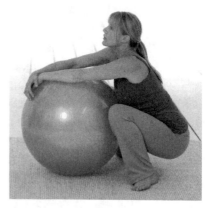

Movement and posture during labor are especially important with a posterior baby. You'll feel least comfortable on your back, because gravity will press your baby's head on your spine. (Actually, you'll feel least comfortable on your back regardless of your baby's position.[13]) Any position that widens your pelvis—such as climbing stairs two at a time, squatting, sitting on a birth ball, or kneeling on all fours with legs spread—will help your baby rotate and descend. If you have freedom of movement, you'll find yourself trying a variety of positions, searching for the one that feels best at the moment. Even if you don't find that perfect position, your movement will bring you some comfort and help keep labor moving.

Preventing Fatigue

Actively working with labor can be challenging and tiring. It's important to prevent fatigue so you can keep working with your labor for as long as it takes. Movement in labor doesn't mean endless hallway pacing, stair climbing, or floor washing. You could do all these things if you want to, but it's probably wiser to conserve your energy.

Here are a few ways you can stay active while your body is supported and relaxed:

- Rock in a comfortable rocking chair.
- Sit and sway on a birth ball.
- Bounce, rock, or sway while kneeling and leaning forward over a birth ball.
- Slow dance to music while your partner hugs and supports you.
- Lie on your side or sit in a tub of warm water. Because the water supports your entire body, you can easily roll from side to side, raise and lower your body, and move your limbs. The pressure and warmth decrease pain perception and increase circulation and oxygenation.

If you talk to friends who have given birth naturally, you'll hear stories of labors spent dancing, doing pelvic rocks, stomping, squatting, or sitting on the toilet. Though each story will be unique, they'll all share the element of freedom—freedom to respond to each contraction in whatever way felt right. Partners, doulas, and caregivers can suggest specific movements and positions, but only you will know what helps you—and what helps you may change from moment to moment. That's why unrestricted mobility is so valuable.

3. Bring a Loved One, Friend, or Doula for Continuous Support

Women, unlike other mammals, don't naturally labor alone. Why? Because our upright posture makes it more difficult for a baby to move through a woman's pelvis. The position changes that help our babies rotate and descend often require physical help. And in childbirth, as in many aspects of life, we humans do better when we're surrounded by those we trust, people who tell us we're doing well and encourage us forward.

Throughout time and across cultures, women have traditionally attended other women during labor and birth. Most births have happened at home, attended by community midwives. According to Sheila Kitzinger, "Woman to woman help in childbirth is the norm almost everywhere in the world."[14] The United States is one glaring exception. When U.S. birth moved from home to hospital, women lost the valuable support their ancestors had enjoyed—and their sisters in other countries continue to enjoy.

Two systematic reviews of research found that compared to women who receive typical hospital care, women who receive continuous, one-to-one support throughout labor are less likely to request pain medication or use Pitocin during labor, are less likely to have a cesarean and more likely to have a spontaneous vaginal birth, and are more satisfied with their births and less likely to have severe pain in the days after the birth.[15] Positive outcomes are more pronounced if support begins early in labor and is provided in settings where epidurals aren't routinely available. The results are better when support is provided by people present expressly to offer support, rather than hospital staff such as midwives or nurses.[16]

Modern hospitals make it difficult for staff to give birthing mothers continuous support. As birth has become more medicalized, the focus of nurses' work has shifted from providing comfort to supervising medical interventions such as routine EFM, IV lines, epidurals, inductions, and cesareans. Although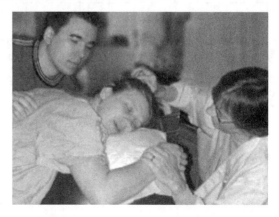

women expect their labor nurses to provide information, comfort, and support,[17] research shows that less than 5 percent of nurses' time is spent doing those activities.[18]

What Is Good Labor Support?

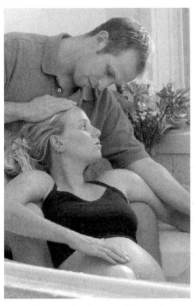

Good labor support is *not* watching the clock and checking IV lines and EFM printouts. It's making sure you're not disturbed, respecting the time that labor takes, and reminding you that you know how to birth your baby. Your helpers should spin a cocoon around you while you're in labor—create a space where you feel safe and secure and can do the hard work of labor without worry.

Good labor support can include reminding you to eat and drink, wiping your face, brushing your hair. It can mean helping you change position, putting a blanket around your shoulders when you're cold, taking it away when you're hot, whispering words of encouragement.

Good labor support can be your mother sitting in the corner, silently praying. It can be your partner holding your hand and reminding you what a great job you're doing. It can be your caregiver focusing complete attention on you as you cope with each contraction. Good labor support tries to respond to all your physical and emotional needs throughout labor.

"My grandmother Nora always lit a candle in front of a statue of the Sacred Heart of Jesus when her daughters went into labor. Each candle stayed lit until the baby's birth. My mother and aunts knew that Nora was praying and caring for them, even if she was hundreds of miles away. My husband prayed the rosary over and over again as our daughter labored with her first baby. In New York City, Haitian grandmothers make a paste of papaya leaves and massage their daughters in labor. They also brew a special tea for strength and nourishment. Orthodox Jewish men recite ancient prayers as their wives labor. Family rituals like these support women in powerful ways."

—Judith

Doulas Make a Difference

Who's a good candidate to support you during labor? You may want the familiar touch of your partner, your mother, or a close friend. You'll need someone you trust wholeheartedly, someone whose mere presence helps you relax. You'll also need someone who trusts birth, who won't be intimidated, and who won't lose self-confidence or confidence in you. That's a tall order.

A doula may fill any gaps you may have in your labor support team. In ancient Greece, doulas were important servants who helped their mistresses with all aspects of household management. Today, a doula is a woman trained to provide continuous physical, emotional, and informational support to a mother before, during, and just after she gives birth.

Doulas are well educated about birth, believe that birth is a normal and natural process, and have confidence in women's ability to give birth. A doula makes a point of getting to know you before your birth so she can provide better emotional and physical help. If you give birth in a hospital, she joins you, along with the other members of your labor support team.

Doulas don't replace the loving encouragement of your partner or the caring of your mother, sister, or friend. The special value of a doula is that she knows birth well. With her understanding of and strategies for nearly every situation, she can make the difference between being able to work with your labor and not being able to. Even more important is the quiet confidence she brings to your birth environment, which can help you and the other members of your support team feel relaxed enough to give your very best. Research has shown doulas to be so effective that neonatologist and researcher John Kennell says, "If a doula were a drug, it would be unethical *not* to use it."[19]

If you're interested in hiring a doula, ask your midwife, doctor, hospital, birth center, or childbirth educator for a referral. DONA International (is an excellent resource for learning more about doulas and finding a doula in your community. (For more information on DONA International, see Appendix E or visit http://www.dona.org.)

It's important that you feel comfortable with your doula, and every good doula knows that. She'll expect you to want to get to know her before you decide whether to hire her.

4. Avoid Interventions That Aren't Medically Necessary

Although research shows that routine and unnecessary interference in the natural process of labor and birth is not likely to be beneficial—and may indeed be harmful[20]—most U.S. births today are intervention-intensive. A majority of women surveyed for *Listening to Mothers II* (all gave birth in 2005) experienced the following interventions during labor:

- Continuous EFM (93 percent)
- Restrictions on eating (85 percent)
- IV fluids (80 percent)
- Restrictions on drinking (60 percent)
- Epidural anesthesia (76 percent)
- Artificially ruptured membranes (59 percent)
- Artificial oxytocin augmentation (55 percent)
- Episiotomy (25 percent)[21]

Common Practices You May Need to Question

Each of the following interventions has unintended effects. When interventions are used routinely, they set the stage for a cascade of other interventions. As a result, the physiologic process of labor and birth is disrupted, and women and babies are exposed to unnecessary risks.

Eating and Drinking Restrictions

Restricting oral intake is a long-standing obstetric tradition. It began in the 1940s, when women often gave birth under general anesthesia without airway protection. The rationale was that fasting reduces the chance of stomach contents entering the lungs (aspiration) in case of vomiting. However, there's no evidence to support this belief.[22] Today epidural rather than general anesthesia is used when possible, which reduces the risk of vomiting and is safer for mother and baby. Also, airway protection is now standard medical practice for general anesthesia, so even if a patient does vomit under general anesthesia, the risk of aspiration is extremely small.[23] In other words: General anesthesia is rare in modern obstetrics, and aspiration is rare in modern general anesthesia. Furthermore, fasting doesn't guarantee an empty stomach, and clear liquids leave the stomach almost immediately. So really, there's no valid reason for tightly restricting eating and drinking in labor.

Various medical organizations have published sensible, evidence-based guidelines for oral intake during childbirth. The American Society of Anesthesiologists (ASA) and ACOG say women with no complications may be allowed to drink clear liquids during labor.[24] The American College of Nurse-Midwives (ACNM) recommends that healthy women experiencing normal labors determine appropriate intake for themselves.[25] The Cochrane Pregnancy and Childbirth Group recommends that women should be free to eat or drink in labor as they wish.[26]

Despite all the evidence and advice to the contrary, many doctors and hospitals *still* restrict oral intake in labor. If your caregiver or birth site is one of these, labor at home—where you can eat and drink as needed—as long as possible.

Overall, we encourage you to eat and drink in labor if your body tells you to. If your labor is short and intense, you may not be hungry or thirsty. You probably will be if your labor is long, and you should eat and drink whatever appeals to you.

IV Fluids

IV fluids are used to prevent dehydration in women restricted from eating and drinking and to provide quick access to a vein in case of emergency. IV therapy has been a routine labor procedure since the late 1970s, but its value and safety are questionable.[27]

While an IV may lower the risk of dehydration in a woman who's truly unable to eat or drink in labor, it has drawbacks, too. It prevents her from moving freely, it may raise her stress level, it may cause fluid overload, and it doesn't ensure adequate nutrient and fluid balance for the demands of labor.[28] Because life-threatening emergencies and the need to restrict oral intake in laboring women are rare, research suggests that routine IV use is not likely to be beneficial.[29] In fact, no studies have demonstrated the routinely placing an IV in healthy women averts poor outcomes.[30]

Continuous EFM

Your baby's heart rate can be monitored either continuously or intermittently, using any of the following devices:

- A **fetoscope** is a stethoscope with a large head designed for listening to fetal heartbeats.
- A **Doppler** is a hand-held ultrasound device that transmits fetal heartbeats to a speaker.

- **External EFM** is an ultrasound device held against a mother's abdomen with a belt. The belt is connected to a large machine that measures and records both contractions and fetal heartbeats.
- **Telemetry EFM** is a wireless version of external EFM.
- **Internal EFM** uses an electrode inserted in the baby's scalp to read his or her pulse and a catheter inserted in the uterus to detect pressure. These are connected by wires to a machine that measures and records contractions and fetal heartbeats.

Electronic fetal monitoring was introduced into obstetrics in the 1970s and quickly became standard practice for all hospital births, even though there was no research at the time to support its value for low-risk births. EFM does provide more information than a fetoscope or Doppler: It shows how contractions affect your baby's heart rate. But does this extra information lead to better outcomes?

A great deal of research done well after EFM was introduced compares fetoscope and Doppler use with continuous EFM. Evidence shows no difference in outcomes for babies and a higher rate of cesareans and operative vaginal deliveries for mothers with continuous EFM. Why? It's difficult to interpret EFM printouts. Misread printouts lead to mistaken conclusions, and caregivers often intervene unnecessarily when labor is actually progressing normally and baby is doing fine. In other words: For most labors, more intensive monitoring increases obstetric intervention (and risk) with no clear benefit for babies.[31] Compared with the intermittent use of Doppler, the routine use of continuous EFM increases the likelihood of needing an instrument delivery or a cesarean, but does not reduce the incidence of problems for your baby (like admission to the neonatal intensive care unit, low Apgar scores, cerebral palsy, and death).[32]

Unfortunately, this evidence is largely ignored in U.S. birth. Most women are willing and happy to be closely monitored because they believe it makes birth safer for their babies. But continuous EFM not only increases the risk of cesarean with no benefit to babies, in most cases it also severely restricts maternal mobility. Unless telemetry is used, continuous EFM requires you to stay in bed and restricts your ability to change positions. It also restricts your access to comfort measures like a shower, bath, or birth ball. And despite your support team's best efforts, they'll probably find themselves focusing more on the monitor than on you, the one who's actually doing the work shown on the printout.

If you have a health complication, if you're given Pitocin, if you have an epidural, or if your baby is developing a problem, you'll need continuous EFM. Otherwise, intermittent monitoring with a stethoscope, a Doppler, or EFM is better. The ACOG supports both intermittent auscultation and EFM for women without complications.[33] The Association of Women's Health, Obstetric and Neonatal Nurses (AWHONN) recommends intermittent listening with a Doppler or fetoscope, rather than continuous EFM, for women with no complications.[34]

Speeding Up Labor Artificially

Speeding up labor may sound appealing, but research shows that routinely interfering with the pace and length of labor is not likely to be beneficial.[35] Each labor is unique; it's hard to say when a labor has gone on too long or not long enough. The length of your labor is influenced by many factors, including your baby's size and position, your confidence, your ability to move freely, your access to a variety of comfort measures, and the quality of your labor support.

There's strong evidence that breaking your water (manually rupturing your amniotic sac) will shorten your labor if your labor is prolonged or contractions are very slow, but it carries risks, too. When your membranes are broken manually, both you and your baby are exposed to greater risk of pressure injury as well as greater risk of infection. Research also shows an increase in cesareans with early rupture of membranes.[36]

Because having ruptured membranes for a long period of time raises your risk of infection, the medical clock starts ticking once your water breaks. If your labor doesn't progress rapidly, your caregiver will probably suggest artificial oxytocin (Pitocin) to speed things up. And then the cascade of interventions begins.

Current data doesn't show that liberal Pitocin use to speed up labor clearly benefits the women and babies receiving it.[37] It makes contractions stronger and harder to handle. It doesn't trigger endorphin release, so there's no decrease in pain perception. It also necessitates continuous EFM, an IV, and sometimes a bladder catheter. The stronger contractions, the loss of endorphins, the additional interventions, and the restricted mobility brought on by Pitocin all increase the possibility that you'll need an epidural—which carries risks of its own (see page 126).

A systematic review of the research suggests that only women with truly abnormal labor progress should have their water broken, and that only women with truly prolonged labors and sluggish uterine activity should receive Pitocin.[38] Neither intervention should be used routinely. According to the Cochrane Collaboration, letting women move around and eat and drink as they please may be at least as effective—and certainly more pleasant—for many women who need augmentation.[39] In most cases, eating, drinking, urinating, and movement can get a sluggish labor going.

Epidural Anesthesia and Analgesia

Most women fear childbirth pain and are eager to use pain medication—especially epidurals, which are very effective at relieving pain. In some hospitals over 90 percent of laboring women have epidurals. Among the women surveyed for *Listening to Mothers II*, 76 percent reported having an epidural.[40]

If you have an epidural, your pelvic muscles relax and don't offer the resistance your baby needs to rotate and descend with each contraction. Since you have no need to cope with pain naturally, your body may not get the signal to keep labor going by releasing more oxytocin, and you may need Pitocin. If you have an epidural, you'll require continuous EFM, an IV, and possibly a bladder catheter.[41] The changes in the physical process of birth and the interventions required to ensure safety during an epidural introduce several risks.

Research clearly links epidurals with fewer normal vaginal deliveries, more instrument deliveries, and longer labors, particularly for first-time mothers. Women with epidurals are also more likely to have fever during labor, and as a result, their babies are more likely to be evaluated and treated for infection. This means mother and baby get separated.[42] There's some evidence that epidural use—especially by first-time mothers—increases the risk of cesarean.[43]

You may be told that epidural medication does not reach the baby. This isn't true: Baby gets it within seconds of administration. There's increasing evidence that all labor pain medications disturb newborn behaviors like hand-to-mouth movements and sucking, which can harm breastfeeding initiation.[44] Also, babies of medicated mothers tend to cry longer and have higher temperatures than babies of unmedicated mothers.[45]

We advise you to weigh the risks and benefits of epidurals carefully before deciding whether to have one. You'll want to consider your unique circumstances, too. For example, you or your baby may have a health problem that necessitates a cesarean, and an epidural is usually the best anesthesia for this surgery. Or your labor may be especially long and exhausting, in which case an epidural may give you a much-needed break.

If you can work actively with labor and if you have continuous emotional and physical support, you'll be less likely to need an epidural—or you'll need it later in your labor. Getting less epidural medication, getting it later in labor, and waiting patiently for your baby to move through the birth canal ("laboring down") before you push go a long way toward reducing the risks of epidurals.

5. Avoid Giving Birth on the Back and Follow the Body's Urges to Push

Many doctors and nurses discourage a woman from pushing until her cervix is completely dilated and/or encourage her to hold her breath and push as hard as she can without a natural urge once her cervix is fully dilated (called "directed pushing"). There's no research to support these practices. Breath holding without the natural urge to do so is exhausting and deprives a baby of much-needed oxygen. In fact, recent research suggests that directed pushing is more stressful for the baby and is associated with increased risk of pelvic floor problems for the mother in the months and years after the birth.[46]

It's almost too obvious, isn't it? The signal that it's time to push is feeling the urge to push. If your baby is low in your pelvis, you may feel the urge to push before or at the time of full dilation. But if your baby is high in your pelvis at full dilation, you probably won't feel the urge to push until your baby's head moves well down in your pelvis. As your baby moves lower in your pelvis—especially when your baby's head touches your pelvic floor muscles (the tissue that forms the floor of your pelvis)—you'll find yourself involuntarily holding your breath during contractions. You may also naturally grunt and groan during pushing contractions.

How long will the pushing take? As long as it takes. Pushing shouldn't be limited as long as you and your baby are doing well. Like Silly Putty, your perineum takes time and effort to soften and stretch. Once it's soft and stretchy, your baby is easily born. Some caregivers interrupt this process and do an episiotomy (cut the perineum to enlarge the vaginal opening). Research shows that routine episiotomy is harmful.[47]

Pushing Positions

Throughout history and around the world, women have used both upright and gravity-neutral positions to push their babies out. They've often used objects like posts, ropes, and trees to get better leverage. They've also used birth supports or stools made from bricks, wood, or stone to help them squat, crouch, or kneel. Before birth forceps were invented in the 1600s, women were never shown giving birth on their backs.

Today, 92 percent of American women give birth in supine positions (lying on their backs) or only slightly sitting up.[48] They're encouraged to give birth this way even though research shows it's harmful.[49] Lying on the back can lower a laboring woman's blood pressure, and the weight of her uterus on major blood vessels can reduce blood flow to her baby.

On the flip side, research supports traditional birth positions. Studies show that pushing in upright postures shortens the pushing stage and decreases the incidence of severe maternal pain when pushing and abnormal fetal heart rate.[50] There are also fewer forceps or vacuum deliveries and fewer episiotomies.[51] Squatting widens the pelvic diameter, creating more room for the baby to descend.[52]

The best position for your birth is the one that's most comfortable for you at any given moment. By responding to what you feel, you make birth easier for you and your baby. You may change positions often, moving from kneeling upright to kneeling on all fours, or from standing to squatting. Or you may find yourself tightening and relaxing vaginal and perineal muscles as you sway from side to side or rock back and forth.

Using a variety of positions lets you respond to your baby's changing position as he or she descends, rotates, and extends in an effort to be born. Standing, kneeling, and squatting help gravity pull your baby down and protect your birth canal and baby from excessive pressure. Gravity-neutral positions—kneeling on all fours, side-lying, and semi-sitting—are perfect for resting between contractions and may help you if you're exhausted.

If your baby enters your pelvis in the occiput posterior position (see page 117), kneeling on all fours takes the pressure of the back of your baby's head off your spine and may give your baby enough room to rotate to the occiput anterior position. Dangling in a supported squat, with a helper supporting you under your arms and with no weight on your legs or feet, lengthens your torso and allows your pelvis to move freely.

When it's time to push your baby out, remember that instinct, tradition, and science are all on your side. Current evidence shows that letting you assume whatever position you find most comfortable, encouraging you to push in response to what you feel, and letting you push as long as you and your baby are doing well are all beneficial practices.[53] The safest and healthiest way to push your baby into the world is in positions other than on your back and only when you feel the urge.

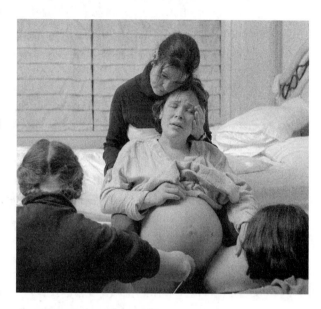

6. Keep Mother and Baby Together—It's Best for Mother, Baby, and Breastfeeding

Throughout most of human history, mothers and babies have stayed together from the moment of birth. Close to their mothers, babies stay warm and safe and can nurse frequently.

When U.S. births moved from home to hospital in the 1900s, for the first time in history mothers and newborns were routinely separated. Babies were kept in nurseries and brought to their mothers only for scheduled feedings. Mothers waited long hours to see and hold their babies, and often they didn't even see their newborns unclothed until they went home days or weeks after birth.

Recent research supports the traditional practice of keeping mothers and newborns together.[54] Evidence shows that this is a key element of nature's plan. Women experiencing natural birth have high levels of catecholamines, oxytocin, and endorphins. Catecholamines ensure that mother and baby are alert and ready to get to know each other. Oxytocin helps raise a mother's breast temperature and helps her feel calm and responsive.[55] As she holds her baby skin-to-skin, her baby's hand and head movements stimulate more oxytocin and endorphin release. The oxytocin helps her uterus stay contracted, which prevents excessive bleeding, and also increases milk production. The endorphins keep her calm and relaxed, and through her breast milk, they help her baby stay calm and relaxed, too. Physiologically, mothers and babies are meant to be together.

Experts now recommend that right after birth, a healthy newborn should be placed skin-to-skin on the mother's abdomen or chest and should be dried and covered with warm blankets.[56] The mother's temperature adjusts naturally to keep her baby warm.[57] Newborns (including premature babies) held skin-to-skin by their mothers cry less and stay warmer than newborns placed in warming cribs.[58] Skin-to-skin contact also exposes babies to their mothers' normal bacteria instead of hospital germs, which lowers their risk of getting sick.[59]

Other benefits of skin-to-skin contact for newborns are easier, more regular breathing; higher, more stable blood sugar levels; and a natural progression to breastfeeding.[60] Most babies kept skin-to-skin with their mothers after birth instinctively crawl to the breast, latch on, and start nursing all by themselves. Even brief separation can interfere with their ability to do this.[61]

Any care that needs to be done immediately after birth can be done with your baby skin-to-skin on your chest, with a light, warmed blanket over you both. Weighing and measuring can be delayed for several hours. As midwife Ina May Gaskin says, you're entitled to "keep your prize."[62]

Keeping your baby with you from the moment of birth is not just a nice option. Rather, keeping your baby close makes the early hours and days after birth safer and healthier for you both.

Chapter 9

FINDING COMFORT IN LABOR

We have a secret in our culture,
and it's not that birth is painful.
It's that women are strong.
—Laura Stavoe Harm

Having continuous emotional and physical support and being able to move in response to what you feel go a long way toward helping you find comfort during labor. But there's an array of additional simple comfort measures that can help you, too. This chapter explains what they are and how they work.

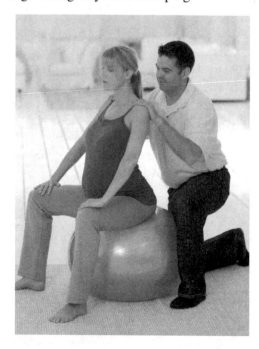

VIEW LABOR AS A TASK, NOT A TRIAL

One of the first—not to mention easiest—things you can do to bring comfort to your labor is to approach it with a positive attitude. View labor as an important job that only you can do, instead of an ordeal you must simply endure and would rather avoid.

Yes, labor is hard work, but hard work surely isn't new to you. It's a basic element of most women's lives; we put in long hours, hold demanding jobs, cram for exams, care for small children, and much more. And for many of us, leisure involves work, too: running, hiking, exercising at the gym, skiing, swimming.

The hard work of our daily lives is different from our great-grandmothers' work, but the work of labor and birth hasn't changed a bit over the years. Our great-grandmothers had to find ways to conserve strength and stay as comfortable as possible from one contraction to the next. So do we.

Here's some good news: This is work we innately know how to do, and we do it beautifully. Many of the comfort measures that helped our great-grandmothers and the generations of women before them still work well in labor and birth today. Women still reap the same great rewards for their efforts, too: satisfaction, confidence, empowerment, joy, and a new baby.

There's no way you can be *completely* comfortable in this work. But simply by searching for comfort—by accepting the job of working actively with your labor—you'll manage the pain of your contractions, keep labor going, and come out of labor richer in many ways.

"All the way through labor, Kate kept her positive attitude. Several times she said, 'This is very hard,' but she kept on going. After thirty minutes of squatting, she pushed her baby out into the world. He was put on Kate's belly, where he rested, quiet and wide-eyed. When she was ready, she confidently put her baby to breast and he latched like a pro. I marveled at the ease…it never occurred to this mother that it would be any other way. It was birth as it should be."

—Jennifer

CREATE A COMFORTABLE ENVIRONMENT

No matter what we're up to, we humans almost always feel better and do better in a safe environment—in a place safe from harm and threat, in a place safe from judgment and control, in a place where we're respected and cared for. For women in labor, this safe place is a private place

Even though we (unlike other mammals) don't naturally give birth alone, we don't naturally give birth onstage either. As in other intimate and important activities, in labor we relax and focus better if we don't feel observed, evaluated, or interrupted.

If you are disturbed or feel observed, if you have to worry or think too deeply about what's going on around you, or if you're surrounded by unfamiliar and discouraging sights, sounds, smells, and people, your body launches a stress response. It releases large amounts of adrenaline to help you face what your brain perceives as a threat. The body gears up to either stand and fight the threat or turn and run to escape it.

Adrenaline tells your muscles to tense up, your senses to pay close attention, and your heart to pump blood rapidly to all parts of your body. You're suddenly on guard and ready for anything. If you've ever swerved or slammed your brakes while driving to avoid an accident, or tripped and caught yourself before falling, you know what a stress response feels like. That sort of tense anxiety can shut down labor or make it a lot more difficult.

The quest for safety in birth can be a double-edged sword. Most women choose to give birth in hospitals because they believe hospitals are the safest place to give birth. But ironically, hospitals are *not* safer than birth centers and homes for the great majority of births. (See pages 50 and 63.) And hospitals make it more difficult for birthing women to feel safe in the way they truly need.

If you're giving birth in a hospital, you'll need to plan for privacy, support, and a comfortable environment. You should consider hiring a doula, and you should stay at home for most of your labor. When you leave for the hospital, bring with you some sights and smells of home: your pillow, your own nightgown and clothes, a stuffed animal from your childhood, a picture of your family. At the hospital, create as much privacy as possible by shutting doors and restricting the comings and goings of staff.

No matter where you give birth, make it a comfort zone. Do simple things that always help you feel better. Labor is hard work, but it shouldn't be torture. To make sure it's not, be good to yourself and let others take care of you. For example, in early labor take a shower or a long, leisurely bath, shave your legs, wash your hair, get into comfortable clothes. As labor progresses, brushing your teeth and having your face washed or your hair brushed are great pick-me-ups. Urinating often helps you stay comfortable and helps keep labor progressing. Eating and drinking give you the energy you need to finish the journey.

REDUCE YOUR PAIN PERCEPTION

You already know a lot about pain; everyone experiences some degree of pain in life. You already know what to do about it, too: You either eliminate its cause or somehow reduce your perception of it. If you've ever walked, rocked, or moaned with menstrual cramps, or hobbled slowly with blisters from a new pair of shoes, you've had practice reducing your pain perception.

What you may not know is why such tactics work. Research has revealed many specific mental and physical factors that reduce pain perception, such as:

- Relaxation
- Movement
- Smell
- Temperature change
- Distraction

Pain messages travel to the brain on thinner nerves, and sensory messages on thicker nerves. Thicker nerves transmit information faster, so if a pain message and a sensory message are sent at the same time, the brain gets the sensory message first. That's why rubbing an ache (which sends a sensory message) eases the pain.

There are many ways you can use this knowledge to reduce your pain perception in labor. On the following pages, we'll give you ideas to get you started. Use them to create your own dance of rhythm, ritual, and relaxation. These "three Rs of childbirth" are a time-tested recipe for coping effectively with contractions.

Your Usual Tension Tamers

Are there certain things you do in daily life to reduce stress or take a break? Spend some time thinking about what helps you truly relax. These same things are likely to help you in early labor.

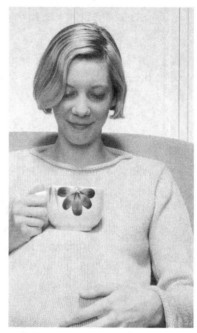

Maybe you're soothed by making a cup of tea—filling the kettle, waiting for the water to boil, adding the tea, letting it steep, pouring the tea into a favorite mug, adding sugar and milk, and finally taking that first wonderful sip. Or perhaps you have a bath ritual—turning the hot water on, carefully adding bubble bath, waiting for the tub to fill, and then soaking luxuriously. Maybe you have a calming daydream—imagining your next vacation, seeing yourself at the beach, hearing the waves, smelling the sea, feeling the warm breeze.

Reading a book, watching TV, and listening to music are other common ways to relax. More active methods like taking long walks, dancing, and singing are popular, too. Even cleaning the house works for some people! Whatever your usual tension tamers may be, they're bound to work well in early labor. We recommend that you stay home and use them as long as they're effective.

As your labor progresses, getting comfortable and staying relaxed will be more challenging, and you may want to try some of the following methods. In preparation for childbirth, practice them when you're stressed out trying to make an appointment on time, when you're frustrated and stuck in traffic, or when you have a headache or a charley horse.

> "When I felt a contraction come on, my silent mantra was, 'Open, open, open.' I didn't want to clench and contract in fear. I wanted the contractions to be fruitful, holy openings. I wanted my body to open, my mind to open, and my spirit to open to this experience."
>
> —Ashley

Conscious Breathing

Conscious breathing (especially slow breathing) reduces heart rate, anxiety, and pain perception. It works in part because when breathing becomes a focus, other sensations (such as labor pain) move to the edge of your awareness.

Conscious breathing is an especially useful labor tool because it not only keeps you and your baby well oxygenated, it's also easy to learn and use. It's naturally rhythmic and easy to incorporate into a ritual. And best of all, breathing is the one coping strategy that can't be taken away from you—even if you're stuck in bed attached to an electronic fetal monitor and intravenous fluids.

Conscious (or patterned) breathing used to be the hallmark of Lamaze childbirth education. For many women, it's still an important way to stay relaxed and stay on top of their contractions. It's true that conscious breathing can help you relax and feel less pain during contractions. There's no "right" way to breathe in labor, despite what others may tell you. Slow, deep breathing helps most women manage the pain of contractions. But the right way for *you* to breathe is whatever feels right to you. Issues like your number of breaths per minute, breathing through your nose or your mouth, or making sounds (like *hee-hee*) with your breaths are only important if they make a difference for you.

It may help you to have a visual focus to accompany your conscious breathing. You can recall an image with your eyes closed, focus on a picture or special object from home, keep your eyes on your partner, or simply stare at a spot on the wall. You may also find that as labor progresses, faster, shallower breathing—like a dog gently panting—feels better. You'll figure out what works best for you. And what works best will probably change as you move through labor.

Many women "practice" breathing during pregnancy by using conscious breathing when everyday life presents stressful situations, like being caught in traffic, running late for an important meeting, or worrying about any number of things.

Tension Release

Most people don't know how physically tense they are from moment to moment. It's likely that you're usually a lot more tense than you think you are. Spend some time becoming more aware of body tension, and then practice consciously letting it go. Systematically tensing and then releasing specific body parts can increase your awareness of tension.

Childbirth educator, doula, and birth counselor Penny Simkin calls this the "roving body check."[1] Here's how to do it: Find a comfortable position in which your entire body is supported. Starting with your head and moving down to your toes, slowly tense and then release one body part at a time. You can also do this exercise with your labor partner. Your partner touches a part of your body, and you tense it. Then you release the tension.

The roving body check not only helps you identify physical tension, but it also helps you learn to consciously release that tension. If you can consciously relax in labor, especially between contractions, childbirth will seem more doable.

Music and Other Sounds

The sounds that surround you in labor are important. Some women need quiet, while others prefer noise of some kind. Sounds that create natural images—like running water, waves, birds, wind, or rain—often comfort and empower laboring women. So does music.

Listening to music is a simple and pleasant way to change your mood, forget your troubles, lighten your heart, and focus your mind. Music can fire you up or settle you down, inspire you or sadden you. As you move from one contraction to another in labor, music can relax you, energize you, or help you find a rhythm.

As you get ready for labor and birth, don't forget to prepare some music and something to play it on. Collect music that gets you going (perhaps Latin or African music, percussive music, or upbeat symphonic music) as well as music that helps you focus and settle down (perhaps chamber music, folk songs, choral works, or lullabies). When you put it to use, it'll get you instinctively moving, swaying, rocking, and opening up.

> "My sister had compiled several hours of classical music for me, but it was the first piece that saved me. It was a soft, simple violin solo with piano accompaniment, and as the piece began, it was as if each note held my body in a tender embrace. My heart swelled and tears filled my eyes. My shoulders shook as I let myself break down and cry. Soon my sobs turned to calm silence, and I felt a new strength and serenity flow through me. I rested my head on my arms, closed my eyes, and breathed as I focused inward."
>
> —Elizabeth

Whatever your sound preferences and wherever you give birth, you'll need to find a way to keep unwanted noises from distracting and disturbing you. Keep your door shut, turn off the ringer on your phone, unplug the TV—do whatever it takes to help you focus.

Heat and Cold

You'll probably find your body temperature fluctuating during labor. One minute you're shivering; the next you're hot enough to fling all your clothes off.

If you're cold, have someone warm a blanket for you. (At home, just toss the blanket in your clothes dryer for a few minutes.) Ask for a shawl or light sweater over your shoulders. Snuggle up with a hot water bottle or a heating pad. Fill a cotton sock with uncooked rice and microwave it for three minutes; it'll provide moist heat for thirty minutes afterward.

If you're hot, shed some or all of your clothes. Have someone press a cold pack, a cold soda can, or a cool compress on your face, neck, and hands. If you're at a hospital, an ice-filled glove will bring quick relief.

Heat and cold are both pain relievers. If you have back pain, alternate heat and cold against your back. The temperature changes will reduce your pain perception by stimulating thermoreceptor sites in your brain.

Water

For most of us, a warm bath is more for relaxation than cleansing. The water massages our muscles to ease tension. It supports our bodies so we can change position easily. We feel weightless. It's easy to see why water is a friend to laboring women.

Some birthing women like the soothing sound and feel of water swishing in a bath. Others like the cleansing, rain-like sound and feel of a shower. In either form, water is a valuable way to reduce your pain perception, help you focus, and move your labor along. As you prepare for your baby's birth, make sure that a bathtub, shower, whirlpool, or birth pool will be available at your birth site.

Smell

Smell is a very powerful sense. When scents stimulate chemoreceptors in the brain, pain perception decreases. Scents can also trigger good or bad memories.

For most people, typical hospital smells are unfamiliar and associated with illness. Obviously, such smells aren't helpful for laboring women. In labor it helps to be surrounded with familiar and pleasant smells.

If you give birth in a hospital, wear your own clothes, bring your favorite pillow or blanket from home, and wear a fragrance you love. You may also want to have flowers, herbs, spices, essential oils, or other aromatic items that evoke good memories or bring pleasant images to mind. Some women find the scent of lavender or jasmine soothing.

Guided Imagery

We all daydream—we find ourselves unintentionally looking forward to vacations, reliving special family events, imagining our futures, and so on. Daydreaming frees you from an unpleasant reality, like a long commute, an all-night study session, or a sleepless night. When you mentally travel to another place or time, you recapture the joy or peace you found there once before.

You can take advantage of this in labor by using guided imagery to take you to a place where you feel peaceful, relaxed, and confident. The only difference between daydreams and guided imagery is planning where to go and how to get there. Will a picture, a smell, or a sound help you? Can you simply close your eyes and be there?

Guided imagery is also a good strategy to help labor progress. Imagining your cervix opening, your baby descending through your pelvis, and your baby nursing in your arms is an empowering way to cope with contractions. One woman recalls that during her first childbirth, her midwife suggested that she imagine her baby's first birthday.

Guided imagery is often more necessary at a hospital than at home. If you give birth in a hospital, you may find that home-based imagery works best to help you feel calm and confident.

"Each time a contraction started, my voice vocalized the sensation, and I remember making a conscious effort to keep my voice low in order to help my cervix open. Sitting on the birth ball felt really good because it provided me with great support and with enough give at the same time. At some point my midwives suggested I get up, and they helped me take off my nightdress. I remember picturing myself as a big tree: My legs were the roots, my body the trunk, and my head the branches. For some reason, this picture helped. It didn't matter whether I could see anything; the room was dimly lit, and I felt comfortable. All I needed to do was concentrate on feeling."

—Jessica

Touch

Touch is an ancient comfort strategy. It eases pain as it conveys sympathy and understanding.[2] Sympathy and understanding are, of course, crucial for women in labor.

Comforting touch in labor is as simple as having a hand to hold, a shoulder to lean on, or arms to support you as you stand, squat, or kneel. It can be firm pressure in the right place on your aching back. It can be stroking your brow or brushing your hair off your face. It can be wiping your neck with a cool cloth as you slow dance with your partner. It can be supporting your shoulders as you sit on a birth ball.

Comforting touch can be massage. Hand and foot massage feels good, is relaxing, and may stimulate acupressure points that bring you pain relief. Shoulders tend to hold a lot of tension, and a massage there can help you release some of it.

Counterpressure is especially helpful if you have back labor. Firm pressure against your back with a fist, a cold soda can, or a tennis ball wherever it hurts the most (the spot changes as your baby rotates and descends) can relieve some of your pain.

A rebozo (traditional Mexican shawl) can provide both pressure and support. A helper places the center of the rebozo against your back, forehead, belly, or whatever body part needs attention. Then he or she brings the ends around your body and pulls tightly. You can buy a rebozo from many online sources or simply use a large scarf or shawl. If you're in a hospital, you can use a sheet folded in half.

Touch doesn't have to be physical. It can be a blessing, like a mother lighting sacred candles while her daughter labors or an

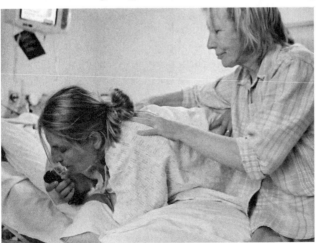

Orthodox Jewish man saying an ancient prayer as his wife gives birth. It can also be the vigilant watching, patient waiting, and complete attention of everyone who's with you.

What about Drugs?

Drugs have appropriate uses, and they can help you manage a difficult labor, especially if your labor is very long and you're exhausted. Women who labor in hospitals that restrict their ability to work actively with labor often find it very hard to manage without some medication.

However, it's important to know that *all* labor drugs—including the epidural—affect babies and alter the course of labor and birth. See Chapter 10 for ways to minimize the risks to you and your baby if you need drugs.

One "medication" that won't affect your baby or the course of your labor is a sterile water block.[3] A tiny amount of sterile water is injected just under the skin at four points on the lower back. The injection stings for a few minutes and then provides excellent relief of back pain for hours.

PACE YOURSELF

Although women worry most about the pain of labor, it's actually fatigue that often presents the greatest challenge. There's absolutely nothing you can do to change the pace or pattern of your contractions, and they do, of course, eventually need to become strong and powerful. But you can pace your activity to conserve strength and energy.

Assume you'll have a long labor. (If you don't, it'll be a pleasant surprise.) Alternate rest and activity throughout labor. In early labor, rest and conserve your energy as much as possible. In active labor, use supported positions and comfort strategies that don't use up all your strength. Remember to eat and drink; your body needs fuel for this journey.

FIND YOUR RHYTHM

At some point in labor, you'll "find your rhythm" or "get in a groove," much like a marathon runner does. You'll be living in the moment, doing without thinking.

To others you'll appear to be in another world. Your movements will be rhythmic; you'll relax between contractions; you'll respond to contractions in the same way over and over again, perhaps shaking your arms, rolling your head, breathing slowly, chanting, or praying.

You'll be totally focused, but you won't necessarily look comfortable. You'll look like you're working very, very hard—which you are.

When this happens, you'll know endorphins are working their magic—dulling your pain and helping you ride your contractions intuitively. You'll be doing exactly what you need to do. You won't need to be rescued; in fact, the worst thing that could happen to you at this point is to be disturbed or interrupted. A healthy dose of encouragement, support, and respect are all you'll need from your support team.

GET REAL ABOUT LABOR PAIN

No matter how your labor unfolds or what comfort measures you use, you definitely won't feel like you're drifting off to sleep in a comfortable bed after a relaxing bath. (That comes later, with your baby in your arms!) But labor isn't meant to be hopeless, endless, lonely agony either.

Nature rewards you for working actively with labor. Strong, powerful contractions bring endorphin release and, with that, a measure of physical and emotional relief. Through your own efforts, you figure out what you need to do from one contraction to the next and you learn how to make the most of the time—however brief—between contractions.

Your support team helps you stay warm, cool off, save energy, move, and rest. Their words of encouragement keep you going.

It's realistic to expect that labor will be hard work, and it's also realistic to expect that you can do this work. Expect to be amazed at your own power and strength!

Chapter 10

BIRTH PLANS
AND BABY PLANS

Nothing happens unless first a dream.
—Carl Sandburg

The first step in making decisions and planning for your baby's birth is learning about the natural process of birth and about the choices you'll face. If you've read this book, gathered birth stories, and consulted other resources for information about birth, you've already taken this first step. You know about safe, healthy birth, and you understand what helps facilitate the process of birth as well as what hinders it. This chapter is designed to help you take the next step.

Many of the birth plans you may see in books or birth classes are simply checklists of medical procedures you do or don't want. To be truly useful, a birth plan should include much more. If you want to have a safe and healthy birth, you'll need to develop strategies for making it happen. You'll also need to talk with your support team and your caregiver as your plans take shape. The more restrictive your birth site is, the more carefully you'll need to plan and the harder you'll have to work to protect you and your baby.

Remember, though, that your birth plan isn't an agenda. Creating a birth plan is like planning for a vacation. You read, talk to friends, and share ideas with your traveling companion. Together you sort through options and make some decisions. You settle on a beach vacation. You decide where and when to go. You make airline and hotel reservations. You know you want to rest, relax, and eat wonderful food, but you have no idea exactly how your vacation will unfold. You may eat every meal alfresco, take long walks on the beach, and watch breathtaking sunrises and sunsets. Or it might rain the whole time, so you might watch old movies, sleep late, read, and spend a lot of time in elegant restaurants. No matter how your vacation unfolds, you'll rest, relax, eat well, and have a wonderful time.

Your planning should focus on creating a space in which you feel safe enough to labor without worry and free enough to work with your unique labor. But as with a vacation, it's counterproductive to plan the details of birth too carefully. As poet Robert Burns says, "the best laid schemes o' mice and men often go awry." Your labor may unfold differently than you expect. And you will probably respond to your labor in ways that feel right but aren't planned.

Best Laid Schemes

Betsy had carefully planned and prepared for a home birth, but circumstances changed when she went into labor before thirty-seven weeks. With the support of her midwife and nurses, Betsy was able to have a safe, healthy birth, in spite of needing to be transferred to a hospital. (See her story below.) Her midwife was able to provide seamless care in a hospital that didn't restrict Betsy to bed, didn't force her to push on her back, and didn't separate her from her baby.

The following pages outline some key facts, options, and advice you might consider as you plan for your birth and the early days with your baby. In this chapter we summarize both the practices that are helpful during labor and birth and those that can make it much more difficult. (For more information on these healthy birth practices, see Chapter 8.) We also provide guidelines for appropriate use of interventions and suggestions for keeping birth as safe and healthy as possible if your labor and birth require medical intervention. Use our suggestions to create your own plans for birth and the early days with your baby.

Betsy's Story

I woke up just after midnight. I'd been asleep only thirty minutes or so, and I knew instantly that I was in labor. I wish I could say that my initial reaction to this realization was joy or relief or something positive, but instead I thought, "Oh no, this can't be happening." I knew I was in labor because my water had broken—I could feel fluid gushing out between my legs. This was just how my first labor had begun (and at just about the same hour, too). I didn't want to be in labor because (1) I was still more than three weeks away from my due date, (2) I wasn't ready to have the baby (I had just moved into a new house the week before), (3) my four-year-old daughter was away from me (she was looking forward to watching the baby be born), and (4) I knew that my home birth midwife's protocol for preterm labor would mean that I'd have to go to the hospital.

I was utterly alone in a house cluttered with boxes. So I took a deep breath, blinked back the tears that stung my eyes, and sat up on the edge of the bed. When I did, amniotic fluid came gushing out of me. This was no trickle. I reached for my phone and called my midwife, Louise. I was thirty-six weeks and four days. She confirmed what I already knew: I was in labor, and we would have to go to the hospital for the baby to be born. I choked back more tears and called my mother, who lived about three hours away. I told her the baby was coming, and through the fog of her sleepiness, she promised that she was on her way.

Somehow my body seems to hatch my babies early. My first child was born at home at thirty-seven weeks and four days. I remember crying when I realized I was in labor then, too—I didn't feel ready to give birth or have a baby. I was counting on those final weeks of pregnancy to get a lot done, to get my life in order, to finally be ready for the baby. But Lilly had other plans and arrived when she decided it was time to be born. Now this baby was following in her footsteps. And just as with Lilly, I went into hard and fast labor pretty quickly.

Now I needed to get ready to go to the hospital, not something I had planned. I took off my soaking nightgown and found a T-shirt and pair of shorts. I was in active labor, no gradual build up of contractions. I was alone, so I had to be my own labor support person. I was separated from my husband, who had left me just after I told him that I was pregnant with this baby. I lumbered around my room, trying to concentrate on what I needed to take to the hospital: clothes for me, clothes for the baby, my camera, my cell phone and its charger, a journal, a nursing bra, a container for the placenta. I walked from the basement to the second floor and back again, trying to find the boxes where various things were still packed away. When the contractions were strong and hard, I sang the ABCs to myself. I don't know why I did this. I was all alone and it was just what occurred to me.

I kept checking in by phone with Louise. At 3 A.M., the contractions were every two minutes, but lasting just twenty to thirty seconds each. Louise listened to me breathe through a couple of contractions on the phone and said she thought it was time to go to the hospital. She asked me if I thought I could drive myself, and I answered no. It took all my concentration to get through each contraction, by leaning against the wall and singing, "ABCDEFGHIJKLMNOPQRSTUVWXYZ." Louise said she was on her way and told me to find my box of home birth supplies and bring it in

Betsy's Story cont.

the car with us, just in case. I had received the box that week—it wasn't even opened yet.

Louise must have gotten to my house around 3:30 A.M. She didn't even come inside; she left her car running, came to the door, grabbed my bag and my box of birth supplies, and helped me out to the car. I was walking, but it took great effort to make it through each contraction.

We arrived at the hospital at 4 A.M. I was fully dilated and in a lot of pain and not coping very well. I remember that I kept crying that I had forgotten how much it hurts. The L&D nurses were great; one of them had even had a home birth, attended by Louise. The most high-tech thing anybody did to me was put an oxygen mask on me briefly. Before long, I felt the urge to push. My baby was born at 4:42 A.M. I gave birth kneeling upright on the hospital bed; I remember holding on tightly to the rail at the head of the bed as I pushed. I was barely aware of who was in the room, but I knew my mother had arrived, about twenty minutes before the baby was born.

As it turned out, my son was born on July 13, the eighth anniversary of my beloved grandfather's death. Because my own father had left when I was young, I grew up thinking of my grandfather as the father figure in my life. The last time I saw my grandfather alive was at my wedding, eight years earlier. He died suddenly six weeks later. He was buried wearing the tuxedo he wore at my wedding. Now, as my marriage was ending unexpectedly, my son was born. I think Henry arrived on July 13 to bestow a new meaning on that date.

PLANNING FOR BIRTH

What Helps Labor

A good birth plan addresses the ways you'll help your labor along. This is the most important part of your birth plan. Regardless of the path your labor takes, how will you develop and maintain confidence in your ability to give birth? How will you find comfort and cope with contractions? What support will you need, and who will provide it?

Confidence

You'll surely discover a lot of ways to be confident on your own, but here are some ideas from other women to get you started:
- Talk with women who've had satisfying births.
- Read Chapter 7 to learn about birth. Watch the documentary *The Business of Being Born.*

- Watch videos about natural birth, such as *Everyday Miracles* and *Orgasmic Birth*. (You can expect to see these and other videos in your childbirth class. For more information on these and other videos, see Recommended Resources.)
- Recite and think about the birth affirmations below.
- Stay away from anyone who makes you frightened about birth.
- Read the book *Ina May's Guide to Childbirth*, especially the birth stories. (For more information, see Recommended Resources.)
- Talk to women who've given birth at home or at birth centers.

> **Birth Affirmations**
> - My body knows how to give birth.
> - I'm strong and powerful.
> - I'm surrounded by people who care about me.
> - The work I'm doing is important.
> - Women have been doing this work forever.
> - The existence of birth technology doesn't mean I can't give birth safely without it.

Comfort

You aren't meant to suffer in labor. Nature intends that you respond to your contractions, not lie passively and feel tortured by them. As with other types of pain in your life, you should try to relieve labor pain in a variety of ways until you find something that works. Following are just some of the many comfort strategies you can try. (See Chapter 9 for more.)

- Move to ease your discomfort.
- Listen to music.
- Relax in a bath or shower.
- Get a hand or foot massage.
- Walk.
- Rock.
- Try some guided imagery.
- Sit and sway on a birth ball.
- Slow dance with or without a partner.
- Eat or drink when you're hungry or thirsty.
- Stay home as long as you feel comfortable there.
- Have your hair brushed.
- Sip tea.
- Keep your lips moist with lip balm.
- Brush your teeth every few hours.
- Have your face and neck wiped with cool water.

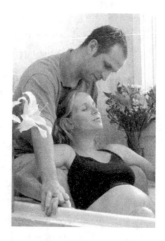

- Use a warm rice sock (see page 138) on your neck or lower back or under your belly.
- Stay active.
- Sit on the toilet.
- Change positions often.
- Breathe slowly.
- Moan with contractions.
- Pray.
- Push when your body tells you to.
- Use medication wisely.

Take some time to think about what might work well for you. But keep in mind that when labor is underway, you may find yourself responding to your contractions in ways you couldn't have imagined, tapping into a wisdom (really!) you didn't know you had.

Support

Research shows that labor is easier and birth outcomes are better if women receive continuous emotional and physical support.[1] Most women give birth in hospitals and expect doctors and nurses to provide this support. But in reality they see little of either, and when hospital staff are present, they're usually attending to or watching for complications, not comfort needs.

Regardless of where you give birth, you'll need minute-to-minute support. The following are just some of the ways you can plan for support:

- Have your partner attend childbirth classes with you.
- Tell your partner that his or her presence at birth is very important to you.
- Read *The Doula Book*. (For more information, see Recommended Resources.)
- Interview doulas and hire one who suits you.
- Ask your mother, your sister, or a close friend to be with you in labor.
- Tell your helpers that you want company at all times during labor and birth.
- Let your caregiver and support team know what kind of support you want, such as encouragement, comfort measures, help with changing positions, and advocating for you with hospital staff.
- Don't be afraid to ask nurses for help with non-medical needs.
- Stay at home, where support is easier to get, as long as you can.

What Hinders Labor

Many common medical interventions can hinder the process of birth by prolonging labor, discouraging you, and interfering with your ability to find comfort. These interventions can certainly be beneficial if they're used appropriately, when complications develop or the risk for complications is high. But they're often used inappropriately on healthy women whose labors are progressing normally. (See Chapter 8 for more details.)

To avoid interventions that hinder labor, you'll need some basic knowledge about their appropriate use and strategies for preventing inappropriate use. You'll also need to know how you can minimize the negative effects of truly necessary interventions and keep your labor as undisturbed and safe as possible. The following pages give you key information and suggestions to consider.

Continuous Electronic Fetal Monitoring (EFM)

What to Know

- Routine continuous EFM provides no benefit for babies and increases the risk of cesarean for mothers.[2]
- The American Congress of Obstetricians and Gynecologists (ACOG) says either intermittent listening with a stethoscope or EFM may be used for healthy, low-risk women (that is, almost all women). Intermittent listening with a stethoscope should be done every thirty minutes in active labor and every fifteen minutes during pushing.
- The World Heath Organization (WHO) encourages intermittent listening with a stethoscope or Doppler and warns that EFM is often used inappropriately.
- *You'll need continuous EFM if:*
    * Your labor is induced or speeded up with Pitocin.
    * You have an epidural.
    * Your baby's heart rate changes.
    * You or your baby has a health problem.

How to Avoid Unnecessary Use

- Remember that routine use of continuous EFM doesn't make labor safer for your baby.
- Find a caregiver who doesn't use continuous EFM routinely.
- Talk to your caregiver about intermittent fetal monitoring.
- Stay at home as long as possible in labor.

How to Keep Labor as Safe as Possible If You Need EFM

- Remember that your body knows how to protect your baby during labor.
- Continue to move as much as possible, both in and out of bed.
- Ask staff to turn off the monitor's sound.
- Ask staff to turn the monitor away from you and your helpers so it doesn't distract you.
- Ask for a telemetry monitor (that is, one that's not attached by wires to the machine).
- Ask to be disconnected from the monitor for regular trips to the toilet.
- Remind your helpers that *you* are the one in labor, not the machine.

Routine Intravenous (IV) Fluids and Oral Intake Restriction

What to Know

- Routine IV use restricts movement, decreases confidence, may over-hydrate mothers, and may contribute to low blood sugar in newborns.
- Restricting eating and drinking in labor depletes a woman's energy when she needs it most.[3]
- The WHO recommends offering women fluids by mouth and eliminating routine IV use during labor.
- The American Society of Anesthesiologists (ASA) and the ACOG recommend that low-risk laboring women be allowed to drink clear liquids (such as water, juice, carbonated drinks, clear tea, and black coffee).[4]
- *You'll need an IV if:*
  * You develop health problems or complications before or during labor.
  * You're at high risk for complications.
  * Your labor is induced or speeded up with Pitocin.
  * You have an epidural.
  * You're receiving medication such as antibiotics in labor.

How to Avoid Unnecessary Use

- Choose your caregiver and birth site carefully.
- Talk to your caregiver about your desire to eat, drink, and avoid unnecessary IV use.
- Confidently eat and drink while you labor at home.
- Labor at home as long as possible.

How to Keep Labor as Safe as Possible If You Need an IV

- Labor at home as long as possible.
- Eat and drink as your body commands while you're at home.
- Suck on ice chips, Popsicles, or lollipops during labor.
- Walk around with your IV pole.
- Stay as active as possible.
- If you need the IV at only certain times (such as for medications), have the IV tube disconnected between doses.
- Ask to have the IV placed in your forearm rather than your wrist or near your elbow so that you can still move around easily.

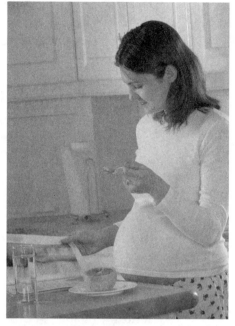

Movement Restrictions

What to Know

- Research shows that restricting movement reduces the effectiveness of contractions, prolongs labor, and increases Pitocin use.[5]
- The WHO encourages freedom of position and movement and discourages the supine (back-lying) position during labor.
- The ACOG encourages women to change position often.
- *You'll need to stay in bed or have help moving if:*
  - * You're having preterm labor.
  - * You have severe pregnancy-induced hypertension.
  - * You have epidural or spinal medication.
  - * You have narcotic medication through an IV.

How to Avoid Unnecessary Restrictions

- Discuss movement with your caregiver.
- Find out if your birth site restricts walking and movement during labor.
- Consider changing your birth site if it will restrict your movement.
- Choose a birth site that has showers and tubs available to all women
- Labor at home as long as possible, walking and moving freely.
- Have a doula or other support person.
- Remember that walking, moving, and changing positions help your labor progress.

How to Keep Labor as Safe as Possible If Your Movement Is Restricted

- Labor at home as long as possible, walking, moving, and changing positions freely.
- Change positions often in bed:
  * Move from side to side.
  * Sit on the side of the bed.
  * Kneel while leaning your head and shoulders against the raised head of the bed.
  * Lie in different directions; for example, move your head to the foot of the bed.
  * Squat while supported.
- Remember that the more you move, the more efficient your contractions will be.

Artificial Rupture of Membranes

What to Know

- An intact amniotic sac protects your baby's head and your vagina during labor.
- Artificially rupturing the sac increases your risk of infection and interventions (Pitocin, EFM, IV, restricted movement, and cesarean).
- Research shows that movement and hydration are often all that's needed to get a slow labor moving and that membranes shouldn't be ruptured routinely.[6]
- *You may benefit from having your water broken if:*
  * Your labor is very difficult or slow to progress.

How to Avoid Unnecessary Use

- Discuss this intervention with your caregiver.
- Tell your caregiver that a longer labor is okay with you.
- Labor at home as long as possible.

How to Keep Labor as Safe as Possible If Your Membranes Are Ruptured Artificially

- Be prepared for stronger contractions.
- Continue to use all the support and comfort resources you have.
- Avoid having vaginal exams after your membranes have been ruptured.
- Keep moving and changing position often.
- Remember that your body knows how to birth your baby.

Directed Pushing

What to Know

- Research shows that pushing without an urge, breath holding, and limiting pushing during labor are not beneficial, and that prolonged breath holding may reduce fetal oxygenation.[7]
- The WHO recommends *not* directing laboring women to hold their breath or consciously sustain pushing.
- The American College of Nurse Midwives (ACNM) and the Association of Women's Health, Obstetric and Neonatal Nurses (AWHONN) recommend that a laboring woman follows her body's natural urge to push.

How to Avoid Unnecessary Use

- Remember that your body knows how to push your baby out.
- Listen to and follow your body's signals.
- Change position often while you're pushing.
- Ask your helpers to support your efforts to push naturally.
- Be patient with your body.
- Visualize your baby rotating and descending through your birth canal.
- Ask your helpers to keep comforting you while you push your baby out.
- If you have an epidural, "labor down"—that is, rest until you feel an urge to push. Your baby will gently move down the birth canal while you rest.

Starting or Speeding Up Labor Artificially with Pitocin

What to Know

- Pitocin increases stress on your baby and your uterus and makes contractions more difficult to manage.
- Pitocin use necessitates an IV and continuous EFM, restricts your mobility, and raises your risk of epidural and cesarean.
- The WHO believes that Pitocin induction and augmentation are often used inappropriately.
- The ACOG notes the risks of Pitocin use and recommends caution when deciding whether to use the drug.

You'll need induction if:

- * Your labor is slow and doesn't respond to movement, position change, and hydration.
- * You don't go into labor spontaneously by forty-two weeks gestation.

* You have a uterine infection.
* You have severe pregnancy-induced hypertension.
* Your baby has a growth problem.

How to Avoid Unnecessary Use

- Be patient waiting for labor to begin and to progress.
- Remember that your body knows how to give birth.
- Surround yourself with helpers who trust birth.
- Stay confident.
- Use all the comfort measures you've learned.
- Don't agree to be induced because your caregiver says your baby is getting too big.
- If your water breaks before contractions start, or if you're approaching forty-two weeks, discuss with your caregiver natural ways to stimulate contractions, such as drinking a bit of castor oil in juice, lovemaking, stimulating your nipples, acupuncture, and being active.
- Ask, "What if I wait?" if your caregiver is insistent about inducing labor.

How to Keep Induced Labor as Safe as Possible

- Make sure your helpers give you continuous emotional and physical support.
- Actively seek comfort in response to the pain of contractions.
- Remember that your body knows how to give birth.
- Visualize your baby rotating and descending through your birth canal.
- Keep moving and changing positions as much as possible.

Epidural

What to Know

- Seeking relief from labor pain without drugs protects your baby and your body from injury, helps labor progress, and facilitates breastfeeding, bonding, and other postpartum adjustments.
- Epidural use necessitates an IV, continuous EFM, and restricted mobility, and it over-relaxes vaginal muscles. All of these factors can prolong labor.[8]
- Epidural use increases the risk of instrument delivery and may increase the risk of cesarean.[9]
- Epidural use raises the risk of fever and postpartum separation to rule out infection.[10] Epidural drugs do reach your baby. Both of these factors can make breastfeeding initiation harder.

- *You may need an epidural if:*
  * Your labor is very long and difficult and you need to rest.
  * You have a cesarean.
  * Your blood pressure is very high.
  * You don't have good labor support.
  * Your birth site restricts your ability to find comfort in other ways.
  * You can't move beyond your fear of labor pain.

How to Avoid Unnecessary Use
- Labor at home as long as possible.
- Choose your caregiver and birth site carefully.
- Discuss your desires with your caregiver.
- Make sure you have excellent labor support.
- Use all the non-drug comfort measures you can.
- Be patient and remember that your body knows how to give birth.

How to Keep Labor as Safe as Possible If You Have an Epidural
- Use a wide variety of other comfort measures for as long as possible, so you don't need an epidural for your entire labor.
- Wait to push until you feel an urge to do so ("labor down").
- Ask your helpers to massage your hands and feet and help you stay as active as possible.
- Be patient with your breastfeeding baby and spend as much skin-to-skin time together as possible.
- If your baby doesn't latch well at first or you have other breast-feeding problems because of your epidural, ask hospital staff (preferably a lactation consultant) to help you express colostrum and feed it with a small cup or eyedropper.
- To avoid aggravating breastfeeding problems, tell the hospital staff not to feed your baby formula or use bottles or pacifiers.

Episiotomy

What to Know
- Research provides no evidence that an episiotomy reduces the risk of injury to the pelvic floor, improves healing, prevents birth injury to babies, or reduces the risk of future incontinence. Rather, the evidence shows that routine or liberal use of episiotomy is likely to be ineffective or harmful.[11]
- The WHO recommends eliminating routine or liberal episiotomy.
- *You may need an episiotomy if:*
  * You or your baby is in distress.
  * Your baby is very large or in an unusual position.

How to Avoid Unnecessary Use

- Ask potential caregivers their thoughts about episiotomy and choose your caregiver carefully.
- Push in upright positions that let your pelvic muscles stretch gently as your baby descends.
- Change positions often while you're pushing.
- Push spontaneously, according to your body's signals, not in a directed way.
- Remember that your body knows how to give birth.
- Be patient with your body.

What You Can Do If You Have an Episiotomy

- After birth, start doing Kegel exercises as soon as possible to help heal and strengthen your pelvic floor muscles. (See the box below.)
- After birth, take warm baths to increase circulation and decrease pain and apply ice to reduce swelling.

Kegel Exercises

Your perineal muscles support your uterus and other organs like a hammock. Kegel exercises strengthen these muscles and are important for all women to do. If you have an episiotomy, Kegels increase circulation, decrease swelling, and help healing. Here's how to do a Kegel:

1. Get in any position: sitting, standing, or lying down.
2. Focus on the muscles around your urethra and vagina, not the muscles of your buttocks, thighs, or abdomen.
3. Tighten (contract) your perineal muscles as if you were trying to stop urinating. It should feel like you're lifting them.
4. Hold this contraction as tightly as you can for a slow count of ten. Don't hold your breath. As you master this exercise, increase your count to twenty.
5. Repeat ten times throughout the day.

Cesarean Surgery

What to Know

- Though some obstetricians tout the safety of cesareans and their value in preventing pelvic floor damage, a systematic review of current research shows that vaginal birth is safer for mother and baby than a cesarean—unless there's a clear, compelling health reason for having the surgery.[12]

- The risk of pelvic floor damage in vaginal birth is extremely small if forceps, vacuum extractor, and episiotomy aren't used.
- Cesarean surgery increases your short-term risk of blood clots, stroke, surgical injury, infection, pain, separation from your baby, psychological trauma, longer hospital stay, emergency hysterectomy, and death. In the long term, it increases your risk of pelvic pain, bowel obstruction, infertility, and future pregnancy problems like ectopic pregnancy (pregnancy outside the uterus), placenta previa (placenta over the cervix), and uterine rupture.
- A cesarean raises your baby's risk of surgical injury, respiratory problems, and breastfeeding difficulties. It increases your future babies' risk of stillbirth, low birth weight, preterm birth, and central nervous system injury.
- If you've had a previous cesarean, there's a small chance your uterine scar could separate during labor and a small chance that the separation could endanger you or your baby. This is more likely if your labor is induced or if your scar is high and vertical.

You'll need a cesarean if:

* You are hemorrhaging.
* Your baby's oxygen supply is blocked.
* You have placenta previa.
* Your baby is in a transverse position (lying horizontally across your pelvis).
* You have poorly controlled diabetes or severe pregnancy-induced hypertension.
* You've had a previous cesarean, and your caregiver is unwilling to attend a VBAC or your hospital doesn't have round-the-clock anesthesia services.
* Your labor is not progressing at all, and either you or your baby is not doing well.
* Your baby is in a breech position (head up, feet or buttocks down) and your caregiver isn't skilled at assisting vaginal breech birth.
* Your baby's heart rate slows and doesn't improve when you change position, drink more fluids, breathe some oxygen, or turn your Pitocin down or off.
* You're carrying more than one baby, and one of your babies is in a transverse position or your caregiver isn't skilled at assisting vaginal multiple births.

How to Avoid Unnecessary Use

- Let your labor start and progress on its own unless there are clear, compelling health reasons to induce or speed up labor.
- Visit http://www.childbirthconnection.org to download the free booklet *What Every Pregnant Woman Needs to Know about Cesarean Section.* Also read Appendix D in this book.
- Choose a caregiver with a low cesarean rate.
- Discuss intermittent fetal monitoring with your caregiver.
- Remember that your body knows how to give birth.
- Plan for excellent labor support.
- Move and change positions often during labor.
- Labor at home for as long as possible.
- Work actively with your contractions.
- Keep up your energy by eating and drinking.
- Try lots of non-drug comfort measures before considering an epidural.
- If you have an epidural, let your baby move down the birth canal before pushing ("labor down"). Even with an epidural, your baby will slowly move down.
- If you've had a previous cesarean, visit http://www.childbirth connection.org/article.asp?ck=10212 to help you make the decision between a VBAC or repeat cesarean.
- Choose a caregiver who supports your decision to have a VBAC.
- Contact the International Cesarean Awareness Network (http://www.ican-online.org).
- If your baby is breech, discuss external version (manually turning your baby head-down) with your caregiver.

How to Keep Birth as Safe as Possible If You Have a Cesarean

- Have your partner and doula (or other helper) in the operating room.
- Hold your baby skin-to-skin as soon as possible after birth.
- Nurse your baby in the first hour after birth.
- Room in with your baby at the hospital.
- Have support from family and friends while you're in the hospital.
- Be patient with your baby as he or she learns to breastfeed.
- If your baby doesn't latch well at first or you have other breast-feeding problems, ask hospital staff to help you express colostrum and feed it with a small cup or eyedropper.
- To avoid aggravating breastfeeding problems, tell staff not to feed your baby formula or use bottles or pacifiers.

Learning from Experience

Sheila is planning for her second birth by examining what worked for her the first time and what didn't. She has more confidence this time, and she has a much clearer understanding of what *she* needs to cope with labor.

Sheila's Story

As my second birth approaches, my anticipation is dominated by the question *What can I do differently this time to make it better?*

My first birth was by no means bad. In fact, it went well in many ways: a vaginal delivery, a simple twenty-minute pushing stage, no episiotomy or tearing, and a beautiful, healthy, eight pound nine ounce baby girl. But labor was long: eighteen hours from the rupture of my membranes (8:00 A.M.) to my first contraction (2:00 A.M. the next day)—during which period I got very little rest—and nineteen hours from there to delivery (9:00 P.M.). This culminated in my choosing an epidural for pain relief late in labor, something I'd committed myself to avoiding.

I gave birth with a midwife in a hospital comparatively supportive of natural childbirth. A hospital, however, is a hospital, and the staff couldn't overlook the fact that my membranes had already been ruptured for twenty-four hours when we arrived at 7:30 A.M. (The evening before, I'd refused admission and sedation to help me recharge for the work ahead.) Intermittent EFM and IV antibiotics were required.

My contractions had been coming quite regularly five minutes apart for a full hour before we left for the hospital, but they became erratic once we got there. I was just one centimeter dilated. After a couple of hours of erratic contractions, my midwife recommended Pitocin to get things moving better. I was too busy doing the work of labor to argue, so my husband stepped in and insisted that since the baby was fine, we should wait awhile and give the contractions time to pick up. She agreed, and sure enough, contractions were close, regular, and progressing within an hour. It was now 11:30 A.M.

As my contractions escalated, I finally understood why I'd read so much about the need for freedom of movement. I found myself responding and adapting to the pain actively and unconsciously, guided by something beyond reason. For one series of contractions, what made sense was to push against the wall. Then suddenly I would shift to crouching on the ground. Then I'd rock in the rocking chair. This dance went on and on. I knew I was doing a "good job"—managing the pain, living through it. It was as bad as I'd imagined, but I still had fight within. This confidence was based on the assumption that my cervix was dilating quickly.

Sheila's Story cont.

But it wasn't. My midwife and nurses, to their credit, were reluctant to check my dilation often, but at this point they did so at my request. I was at three centimeters.

As the contractions grew more and more intense and coping with them became all-consuming, time flew by. I'd feel as though five minutes had passed, then look at the clock to find that more than an hour had. Day blurred into dusk, and I felt myself losing control, feeling frantic, tensing my entire body with each contraction, holding my breath.

There was room in my mind for almost nothing else but the unbelievable physicality of each moment. But in some pocket of mental clarity, I knew that my ability to handle the pain had changed because the pain itself had changed. It was stronger, sharper, faster, harder. That meant that I was making progress, opening up, getting closer to the end.

I knew that to keep going, I needed a shot of encouragement—not the kind I was already getting from my husband, midwife, and nurses, but evidence to support my conviction. I needed to hear that I was almost fully dilated, that all the work I'd been doing had helped. So I asked my midwife to check me. She was reluctant, but I prevailed.

I was so certain that she was going to announce, "You're at seven!" When she said, "Three and a half," I collapsed into bed. I looked at the clock: I'd dilated just a half-centimeter in four hours. Every ounce of will to go on seeped out of me.

At that moment, I realized, "I don't have to do this anymore." I decided I wanted and needed pain relief. No one had even suggested it; my nurses, midwife, and husband had been absolutely supportive of unmedicated labor. When I told my midwife I wanted to discuss pain relief, she discouraged having an epidural. But I knew my problem was sheer exhaustion. It was 4:30 P.M., and I'd been awake for over thirty-two hours.

My husband, knowing the snowball effect an epidural can have, said, "I know you can do this." But to me, it wasn't a question of my ability. I'd been doing it for an eternity, and it had gotten me almost nowhere. I'd reached the end of my rope. I decided to go ahead with the epidural. Moments later, the anesthesiologist came in. Almost immediately, the drugs took effect and I fell into a two-hour sleep. It was 5:00 P.M.

Contractions slowed during my nap. When I awoke at 7:00 P.M., my baby's head still wasn't engaged. My midwife suggested nipple stimulation and brought in a breast pump to help. After a while, she checked my dilation. Seven centimeters—progress! Then a nurse suggested emptying my bladder—perhaps that was obstructing the head. It seemed to do the trick. A few minutes later, my midwife checked me again: ten centimeters, and the baby's head was engaged.

It was 8:30 P.M. and time to push. After all that had come before, I anticipated a long pushing stage. But twenty minutes later, after only a few contractions, our daughter Maisie emerged into the world.

What will I do differently this time around? I can't predict how labor will start or how long it'll take. I can't will my water not to break eighteen hours before contractions start. But I now know what I can do, say, think, and hear that'll help me manage labor better, both physically and emotionally.

I now know, for example, that it's critical to get as much rest as I can while I can. I think this will be easier this time simply because I'm no longer anticipating the unknown. With Maisie I was so excited and afraid and antsy that I couldn't possibly sleep. It was like I was five years old, waiting for dawn on Christmas morning. This time, if events unfold in the same way, I know I'll be much calmer.

I also know for sure now that I *will* survive labor, that my body can handle it from start to finish, and that it really will end at some point. In the thick of my first labor, when the pain was at its worst, I was sure of none of these things.

I now know that I need to focus on relaxing as much of my body as possible during a contraction, rather than tensing as I did during the toughest contractions with Maisie. I knew that intellectually going into my first labor, but that knowledge was of no use without knowing exactly what contractions would feel like.

I now know what I need to hear when labor gets really hard. "You're *not* going to die." "This isn't going to last forever." "Your body can do this." "You've done this before." I've asked my husband to tell me these things.

I now know that being in a standard hospital maternity room affected my confidence. As supportive as my midwife and nurses all were, we were in the same room and with the same staff I'd have had if I'd gone in intending to have an epidural and lie in bed for the duration of my labor. This time I'll give birth in an alternative birth center within a hospital—entirely separate from the regular maternity ward—with suites that have birth tubs, birth balls, and queen-size family beds. I think being in an environment that promotes natural, normal childbirth will make a big difference in my confidence.

As I sit a month from my due date, I'm more anxious than I was in my first pregnancy because I know in a visceral way what labor entails. But it's a completely different kind of anxiety, one that has empowered me to prepare in a more practical way for the task ahead.

Postscript

All my planning and preparation—both physical and psychological—paid off in the birth of my second daughter. Ellen Virginia was born underwater,

Sheila's Story cont.

into an environment of absolute tranquility, after just five hours of labor and about ten minutes of pushing.

Throughout each stage, I was able to maintain control, stay on top of the pain, and take things one contraction at a time. The water provided tremendous physical relief and, I am convinced, sped up the process substantially: I was five centimeters when I got in the tub and was ready to push twenty minutes later. Transition was barely detectable.

The warm water's effect on my pain was instantaneous. The moment I sank in the tub, I felt transformed. Though the pain certainly didn't disappear, it became both muted and more focused. The isolation of the pain helped me manage it. Rather than tensing up when a contraction hit, and consequently feeling it everywhere, I could relax the rest of my body and just float through it.

My choice of location and caregivers turned out to be ideal as well. I was attended by one nurse and my midwife, who simply stood back and let me be in charge of the experience, offering words of support when warranted and periodically checking the baby's heart rate with a stethoscope—but nothing more.

All in all, it was an exhilarating, empowering, incredible experience. It was exactly what I'd hoped it would be.

PLANNING FOR LIFE WITH BABY

Your birth plan shouldn't end with your baby's entry into the world. The minutes, hours, days, and weeks after your baby's birth are just as important for both of you.

Around the world new mothers all need the same thing—we need to be mothered so we can mother our babies. Most cultures have customs that ensure this. But in the United States today, if you don't plan for it ahead of time, you may not have the care and support you need to help you learn how to be a mother.

You and your baby's most important goals after birth should be to recover, to get to know each other face to face, and to establish breastfeeding. Your "baby plan" should include ways to develop and maintain confidence in yourself and your baby, to have support, and to stay together as much as possible.

Recovering from Birth

The word *recover* means both "to regain health" and "to regain balance." You and your baby aren't sick, but you do both need to adjust physically, emotionally, and socially. Following are some strategies that may help.

In the First Days

- Make rest a top priority.
- Remember to eat and drink. Keep handy a variety of tasty, easy, nutritious snacks that you can eat with one hand.
- Make sure your support team is in place.
- Have someone hold your baby while you shower or bring your sleeping baby into the bathroom while you shower.

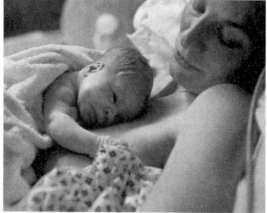

- Let others mother you.
- Stay active but don't get overtired.
- Eliminate nonessential work and activities.
- Talk about your birth.
- Keep your baby close.

In the First Weeks

- Ask for help with cooking, cleaning, shopping, laundry, and care of older children.
- Eat meals you made and froze before birth.
- Have takeout food during the first weeks to save your energy.
- Spend time night and day with your baby.
- Continue to limit nonessential work and activities.

Having Support

Who will be most helpful to you after your baby's birth? Your support people will be very important in the first days and weeks, so choose them carefully. They should value and support your breastfeeding and your work as a mother. They should make you feel comfortable and competent. At the very least, they should be willing to work hard. One hard-working full-time helper will do, or a number of helpers may share the load.

How to Plan for Support

- Ask your baby's grandmother to stay with you for the first week.
- Ask your partner to take vacation time or parental leave after your baby is born.
- Hire a teen to spend three hours every afternoon doing household chores.

- Interview and hire a professional postpartum doula. Unlike a baby nurse, who will only care for your baby, a postpartum doula cares for you, helps you with breastfeeding and baby care, and does simple but important household chores, such as light cleaning, cooking, and laundry.
- Interview potential health caregivers for your baby and choose one who listens well, respects your questions, encourages and supports breastfeeding, and makes you feel comfortable and competent.

Getting to Know Each Other

Before your baby's birth, you may find it helpful to learn about babies so you'll know generally what to expect. Your best teacher will be your baby. You'll learn the most important lessons about how to be a mother simply by watching and responding to your child.

- Before birth, read the book *Your Amazing Newborn*[13] and watch the related video *Amazing Talents of the Newborn*.[14] (For more information, see Recommended Resources.)
- Before birth, spend time with other mothers and babies.
- From the moment of birth, stay close to your baby. Spend time together skin-to-skin often in the first few days.
- If you give birth at a hospital, room in with your baby.
- At home, have your baby sleep in your bedroom—in your bed, in a "sidecar" sleeper, or in a cradle, bassinet, or crib close to your bed. (See page 215 for more information on safe cosleeping.)
- Wear your baby in a sling or other soft baby carrier as you move through your day.
- Postpone guests who expect to be waited on and who distract you from your baby's needs. Welcome guests who are eager to help, freeing you and your baby to rest and get to know each other.
- Look for early infant feeding cues (see page 202) and respond to them as quickly as possible.
- Learn what comforts your baby by experimenting with a variety of infant soothing techniques, like swaddling, rocking, cuddling, listening to music, or dancing.
- Attend a La Leche League meeting, where you can nurse your baby, learn about breastfeeding, and socialize with other mothers and babies in a relaxed and helpful atmosphere.
- Look for other mother-baby support groups at your neighborhood community center, church, or clinic.

Establishing Breastfeeding

Breastfeeding is nature's most powerful way of helping mothers recover from birth, learn mothering skills, and fall in love with their babies. It's also nature's way of ensuring that babies are well nourished, protected against disease, and allowed to develop optimally. The American Academy of Pediatrics (AAP) recommends that babies be exclusively breastfed (no water, juice, formula, other fluids, or solids) for six months and continue breastfeeding until at least one year.[15] Following are some ways you can get your breastfeeding relationship off to a good start. (For more information and advice on breastfeeding, see Chapter 12, pages 202–5, and Chapter 13, pages 216–17.)

Before Birth

- Talk to women who are breastfeeding or have breastfed babies.
- Watch babies at the breast.
- Attend a La Leche League meeting.
- Get the name of a lactation consultant.
- Read about breastfeeding in *Lamaze: Pregnancy, Birth & Beyond* (http://magazine.lamaze.org/).
- Buy a breastfeeding book like *The Ultimate Breastfeeding Book of Answers* by Jack Newman. (For more information, see Recommended Resources.)
- Remember that your body knows how to breastfeed your baby.
- Talk to your caregiver about delaying newborn testing and other routine procedures.

In the First Hours

- Keep your baby skin-to-skin with you.
- Watch for early infant feeding cues.
- Nurse your baby within the first hour after birth.
- Delay newborn tests and routine procedures until after the first breastfeeding.
- Remember that colostrum is nutrient-rich and that your baby doesn't need to eat much in the first hours and days of life.

In the First Days

- Sleep in the same room with your baby and be together as much as possible.
- Don't limit your baby's time at the breast or hold your baby off between feedings.

- Let your baby finish the first breast before offering the other.
- Learn how to tell if your baby is swallowing milk.
- Become a confident nurser by learning how to tell if your baby is getting enough milk and trusting that you will produce lots of milk.
- Learn how to position your baby for a good latch.
- Don't use bottles or pacifiers until breastfeeding is well established.
- Be patient with yourself and your baby as you both learn to breastfeed.
- If you choose to have your baby circumcised, wait at least twenty-four hours after birth and insist that he be given pain medication. Be prepared to provide extra soothing and wake your baby to breastfeed if necessary.
- If you need to be separated from your baby, pump your breasts and store your milk.
- Don't supplement your breast milk with formula unless there is a clear, compelling health reason.
- Remember that colostrum is nutrient-rich and that your baby doesn't need to eat much in the first hours and days of life.

In the First Weeks

- Remember that responding to your baby's needs does not spoil him; rather, it's the only way you can teach your baby to trust you.
- Sleep in the same room with your baby and be together as much as possible.
- Wear your baby in a sling or other soft baby carrier throughout the day.
- Nurse your baby whenever he or she shows signs of hunger (at least eight to twelve times every twenty-four hours).
- Learn to nurse lying down in bed so you don't need to wake fully to nurse at night.
- Remember that breastfeeding is a top priority.
- Be patient with yourself and your baby as you learn to breastfeed.
- Stay confident, even if your breastfeeding journey is bumpy.
- Call a lactation consultant, your local La Leche League leader, or the La Leche League hotline (847-519-7730) if you have breast-feeding problems or you're concerned about whether your baby is getting enough milk. *Don't delay.*
- Remember that breast milk is all the nutrition your baby needs for at least six months.

If You're Not Able to Breastfeed

Here are some tips to promote bonding and development even if you're not able to breastfeed your baby:

- Sleep in the same room with your baby and be together as much as possible.
- Wear your baby in a sling or other soft baby carrier throughout the day.
- Respond to your baby's needs before he or she cries.
- Hold your baby, make eye contact, and talk to your baby during feedings.
- Hold, look at, and talk to your baby even when you're not feeding.

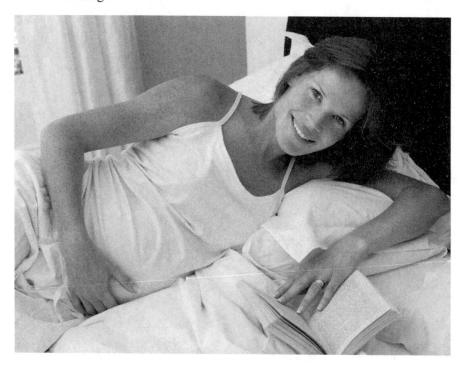

READY FOR THE JOURNEY

You've made your plans. You've folded and refolded all the tiny undershirts. You've organized your baby's layette a dozen times. The days may drag as you await your baby's arrival. But that special day will indeed arrive—and it's coming soon.

Relax and savor the last days of your pregnancy. Take a long walk. Enjoy a special food you crave. Rest and pamper yourself.

Have your hair trimmed or get a manicure. Window shop. Water your plants. Have a leisurely cup of tea with a friend. Lie down with a book and drift into a nap. Have a candlelight dinner with your partner and ignore the phone.

Even if you're at your job until labor begins, mental preparation can help you feel rested, calm, and well equipped. Place a flower at your workstation. Eat a tasty, healthy snack. Take a stroll on your lunch break. Spend a few minutes using relaxation techniques at your desk.

When labor finally starts, you'll be rested, relaxed, and ready for the journey. The passage from pregnancy to motherhood is the most exciting, life-changing journey you'll ever take.

Chapter 11

GETTING THE SAFE, HEALTHY BIRTH YOU WANT: COMMUNICATION, NEGOTIATION, AND DECISION-MAKING

Good plans shape good decisions.
That's why good planning helps to
make elusive dreams come true.
—Lester Bittel

Making important decisions is always challenging. Making a decision when pregnancy or labor isn't going as you'd hoped or making a decision that requires your caregiver to practice differently than usual can be especially hard.

If you want to have a safe, healthy birth, chances are at some point during pregnancy, labor, or postpartum you'll find yourself discussing and negotiating your care with a powerful, perhaps intimidating healthcare system. Even if you've chosen your caregiver and birth site carefully, you'll still face the reality that the typical birth in the United States is far from simple.

To make real-life decisions that you believe are best for *you* and *your baby* (as opposed to hypothetical decisions that are statistically best for mothers and babies collectively), you need complete, accurate, up-to-date information. You need confidence in your knowledge, your body, and your rights. You need to be aware of the potential obstacles so you're not caught by surprise. And of course, you need to be able to communicate clearly, honestly, and respectfully.

It's hard to be nonconformist, especially when you're in unfamiliar territory and feeling vulnerable. We hope this chapter will make your job a little easier by giving you some practical strategies for communicating and negotiating with the healthcare system. We also hope reading the following pages, which feature women's stories of informed decision making in action, will encourage and inspire you.

STRATEGIES

Be Alert

Getting caught off-guard can put you at an emotional and practical disadvantage. To avoid unpleasant surprises, be aware of the following issues that tend to pop up around pregnancy and birth. Many caregivers and hospitals today:

- assume all expectant mothers want a full range of prenatal tests;
- induce labor before forty-two weeks, sometimes as early as thirty-seven weeks;
- speed up labor when they think it's taking too long and sometimes as soon as you arrive in the hospital;
- routinely use continuous electronic fetal monitoring and intravenous fluids;
- separate mothers and babies after birth;
- restrict movement and position during labor;
- support and sometimes encourage elective cesarean surgery;
- do cesareans when they think labor has gone on too long;
- discourage or refuse to do vaginal birth after a cesarean (VBAC).

You should also be prepared for pressure to go along with the options presented to you. Your caregiver or hospital may use "safety" to persuade you, suggesting risks you incur if you don't go with the program. Or you may be promised less pain or a shorter labor. A powerful way some caregivers try to influence your decisions is by telling you, "I would never allow my wife to…."

Remember that the specific risk for you and your baby—and you *are* unique individuals in unique circumstances—is different from the statistical risk for all mothers and babies collectively. Remember, too, that usually the safest and healthiest way to give birth is with nature in the driver's seat. Make your decisions calmly and deliberately, according to best evidence and careful consideration of your situation and your values, not by reacting emotionally.

> Debra Bingham, former Director of Maternal Child Nursing at a large medical center, has this advice if your nurse tells you that the hospital rules won't allow something you want: "Don't tell her to check with your doctor. Ask her to call the nursing supervisor (her boss). Often what patients are told are strict rules really aren't."

Be Informed

You probably already know a great deal about safe, healthy birth from reading this book, talking to others, taking classes, and doing research of your own. If an unfamiliar issue arises, you can find out more about it. It's always a good idea to have a complete understanding of the issue at hand before making a decision.

You can quickly and easily find excellent, evidence-based, up-to-date information about pregnancy, birth, and baby care by checking out the many trustworthy books and videos listed in the Recommended Resources. If online research is more your style, visit the following informative, user-friendly websites.

- http://www.childbirth connection.org, especially http://www.childbirthconnection.org/article.asp?ck=10064 to view *Effective Care in Pregnancy and Childbirth: A Synopsis*
- http://www.cochrane.org
- http://www.lamaze.org
- http://www.acnm.org (American College of Nurse-Midwives)
- http://www.motherfriendly.org (Coalition for Improving Maternity Services)
- http://www.lalecheleague.com (La Leche League International)

Be Confident

Be confident in the knowledge you've worked so hard to acquire. If you don't feel confident in your knowledge, learn more until you do.

Be confident in your body and your baby. We hope this book has given you all the reasons you need to trust nature's plan for pregnancy and birth, as well as your ability to carry out that plan.

Be confident that no one cares more about your well-being and your baby's well-being than you do, and no one is better qualified to make decisions about you and your baby. Furthermore, it's your right and responsibility to make such decisions. Unless you're incapacitated or facing an emergency that puts your life or your baby's life in immediate peril, you have the right to decline practices that you feel aren't in your best interest.

Be a Good Communicator

When you're faced with a choice about your care in pregnancy or birth, it's critical to ask questions. Regardless of your circumstances, the following tips can encourage dialogue, help you get the information you need, and promote negotiation and understanding.

- Ask for more information about what's being recommended or offered. For example, ask, "Could you tell me more about this?" Or say, "I'd like a better understanding of why you recommend this for me."
- Inquire about alternatives. For example, ask, "Are there other things I could do?" Or ask, "What other options are there?" If you've heard of an alternative, ask about that.
- Ask, "What will happen if I wait?"
- Ask, "What are the risks of doing nothing?"
- Consider the response you get in the context of what you already know. Don't be afraid to point out what you know or mention that your knowledge differs from what you're now hearing.
- Try not to put your caregiver or hospital staff on the defensive. Use "I" statements to keep the focus on you and avoid pointing fingers. Remember that this is a conversation, not a debate. You don't need to change anyone else's beliefs; you're simply gathering information as part of the process of making a personal choice.

STORIES

Margaret

I didn't think I wanted a routine sonogram with my second baby, but at the last minute I thought, "Why not?" So I went ahead with it.

I was shocked when my midwife called and told me the sonogram showed "something strange in part of the brain."
I asked her what that meant, and she said she didn't know. She encouraged me to talk directly to the doctor who read the sonogram.

I called several times, and finally he returned my call. He said he'd only seen it once before, and that baby was fine. He said one option was to have a more sophisticated sonogram to get a better look. I asked what further information that would give. He said he didn't know. I asked what would happen if I did nothing, and he said that it would probably make no difference.

I was particularly concerned that if there were something seriously wrong with my baby, it might not be wise to give birth in the birth center I was planning to use. I asked about that. I also wanted to know if additional information would change the course of my pregnancy, since I planned to have my baby no matter what.

The doctor reassured me that what he saw was probably "clinically insignificant" and that it didn't have implications for where I gave birth or the course of my pregnancy. I told him that based on our discussion, I wouldn't have more testing.

He responded, "I think you are very wise."

Margaret's story is a good example of a thoughtful discussion in which both parties communicate honestly and openly. Margaret communicated her concerns clearly, and her doctor shared honestly what could be learned from additional testing without trying to sway her decision. Based on this discussion, Margaret was able to make an informed choice. Her decision was actually an informed refusal to do additional testing.

Robin

I had my first three babies in Haiti. I was shocked when I arrived at the hospital for the birth of my fourth baby (in the U.S.) and learned I was expected to stay in bed. I asked why. The nurse said that the hospital policy was that all laboring women had to stay in bed.

I said, "I've had three babies. I know how to labor. I walk and rock and moan. And I can't do that in bed." The nurse tried to convince me that it was important to be in bed.

I couldn't listen to her. I got out of bed, went out the door, and walked up and down the halls, moaning with the contractions. The nurse called my doctor, but I didn't care.

When he arrived, I told him, "I know how to be in labor." He shrugged his shoulders, and they let me keep walking.

When I felt the urge to push, I let the nurse know, went back to my room, and pushed my baby out.

Robin's first three births made her very confident that she knew just what she needed to do in labor. She wasn't the least bit intimidated by the hospital environment. Her determination was difficult for the hospital staff to fight. And her self-assurance was probably contagious!

Mary

I arrived at the birth center in hard labor at 7:00 A.M. I was already seven centimeters dilated. My midwife asked if I wanted her to break my water. I asked why.

My midwife said, "The baby's head is right there. If I break your water, you will have your baby very quickly. Otherwise, it will probably be an hour or so."

My labor was moving just about as fast as I could handle. A quicker labor was tempting, but I reminded myself that a fast labor isn't as important as being able to work with labor—which I was just barely able to do.

I told her I didn't want her to break my water, that I was okay with labor taking a bit longer. I went into the tub, stayed there about an hour, then got out and had my baby.

Even in hard labor, Mary was focused enough to ask the right question: Why? She could then figure out whether the option being offered made sense for her. She decided that a faster birth wasn't a benefit for her. She communicated her wishes effectively to her midwife, who listened to her.

Linda

I had a cesarean for my first birth. I labored on a stretcher in a hallway for six hours because there were no beds available in the labor suite. I was unable to move. In retrospect it's not surprising that I made no progress, and that my doctor then convinced me and my husband that I needed a cesarean.

With my second baby I found a doctor who told me I could try for a VBAC. I also attended Lamaze classes, and when we discussed birth plans and communicating with our doctors, my childbirth educator encouraged me to start asking questions.

So I did. My doctor kept insisting I could have a trial of labor, but as my due date came closer he began to talk about the advantages of another cesarean. I asked him how many of his patients actually gave birth vaginally after a cesarean. He evaded the question and then talked at length about the risks of VBAC.

My husband and I decided it was clear he wasn't supporting our plan for a trial of labor. We discovered later from a nurse at the hospital that he had never attended a VBAC.

I asked my childbirth educator to recommend a doctor who supported VBACs. Our insurance wouldn't pay for the new doctor, but a natural birth was important enough to us that we were willing to pay ourselves.

We changed doctors at thirty-seven weeks. Our families weren't supportive. They were sure our doctor was protecting us from ourselves and that it was safer to have another cesarean. But we were sure of our decision.

I gave birth to a nine-and-a-half-pound baby girl after four hours of labor. It was an incredible experience. We're so glad we asked questions, got the information we needed, and made the decision to change doctors.

Linda's questioning and her increasing awareness of her doctor's mixed messages compelled her to consider other options. It was hard to change doctors late in her pregnancy, and the pressure from family made it even harder. But Linda and her husband were well informed, and they knew what they wanted.

Jen

I developed gestational diabetes, and at thirty-seven weeks my doctor started talking about inducing if I didn't go into labor in the next week or so. I asked why, and she told me that she always worried about being late with gestational diabetes.

I looked at the information in The Cochrane Library *and talked to my aunt, who's a childbirth educator. I knew my baby wasn't in danger, and neither was I.*

But I felt so pressured by my doctor. I didn't want a medical induction. I wanted to go into labor naturally. I asked her what would happen if we just waited. She told me that my baby might be too big if we waited until my due date, and then I would need a cesarean.

Again, I researched and found this wasn't true. I asked my doula if she had ideas for encouraging labor to start naturally. At her suggestion, over the next two weeks I did visualization and went twice a week for acupuncture.

At thirty-nine weeks I went into labor on my own. I arrived at the hospital eight centimeters dilated after three hours of labor. And my baby was seven pounds!

Jen's story is a common one. Many women are tempted by induction—the last weeks of pregnancy are hard, and it's natural to want to hold one's baby at last. And in Jen's case, "safety" was offered as another reason for induction. But Jen knew that an unnecessary induction could make her labor more difficult and start a cascade of interventions. She wanted to increase her chances of having a normal birth. So she learned more about both gestational diabetes and induction, and as a result, she stopped worrying about nonexistent risks. She also found alternatives that helped her body go into labor naturally.

Sheila

A week before my due date, early in the morning, my water broke. When I called my midwife, she reassured me and said I should expect contractions to start soon.

Twelve hours later she called back to ask what was happening. Nothing. She wanted us to come to the hospital, to get started on antibiotics, to get some sleep. If there were still no contractions in the morning, she'd induce labor.

We didn't want to go to the hospital yet, or to be induced. We asked what the alternatives were and what would happen if we waited awhile.

Our midwife made it clear that although she believed labor would start in the next twelve hours if we stayed at home, she was mandated to follow hospital protocol, which was admission to the hospital and antibiotics after twelve hours from rupture of membranes.

I would've just gone to the hospital, but my husband reminded me of the cascade of interventions. We told the midwife we wanted to stay home, and if contractions hadn't started by morning (twenty-four hours after my water broke), we'd come to the hospital then.

The midwife agreed, but said she'd have to document our refusal to come to the hospital at twelve hours. We were fine with that.

At 3:00 A.M. contractions started. We arrived at the hospital in active labor at 11:00 A.M. But the pressure of waiting for labor to begin had taken its toll; I was exhausted when labor got intense. Still, I'm glad we did what we did. I did get antibiotics but avoided induction.

For our second baby, I chose a midwifery practice in a birth center that had less restrictive policies in hopes that my midwives wouldn't feel pressured and pass that pressure on to me.

Sheila's story is an example of hospital policy dictating caregiver practice. Sheila and her midwife were both in a bind. Based on best evidence, there was no reason to hurry labor just yet. Their compromise was to note Sheila's refusal on her chart. But the decision to stay at home didn't alleviate the pressure that Sheila felt to have labor start. Ultimately, labor did start on its own—and despite Sheila's exhaustion, she gave birth naturally and safely to a healthy baby girl.

Michelle

I started having contractions about 6:00 P.M., and at 7:30 my mother insisted I call my doctor. I refused, but she was insistent. She said she knew all the signs and that I was moving quickly.

She was right. When we arrived at the hospital at 8:15, I was nine centimeters dilated. By the time I got to my room, the nurse said to go ahead and push if I felt like it.

I didn't really, but I tried. Then I hung out and waited about an hour until I felt the urge. I was full of energy, but my baby just wasn't moving down. My doula and mother and husband encouraged me and helped me into lots of different positions. My baby was doing fine.

At midnight—after almost four hours of pushing—I was still at it. I still had energy, and my baby was still doing fine. But my team was discouraged, and I was needing a pep talk.

My doctor came in, and I asked what was happening. She said she didn't think I could push the baby out. I asked what would happen if we waited, since my baby and I were okay. Her answer? "You can push for another hour or two, but it won't make any difference. That baby isn't going anywhere. You're going to have a cesarean now or later."

I was terribly disappointed, but when she said that all my confidence went. I had no energy to keep going.

All Michelle needed to keep going was a boost of confidence. And since both she and her baby were doing well, it made sense to keep trying a bit longer. She asked the right questions, but was understandably vulnerable when her doctor told her that her hard work was futile. She'll never know if another hour would've made a difference. She now wishes she had insisted on pushing longer, and with her next baby she plans to use a midwife who won't give up on her so easily.

Elizabeth

I was a bit surprised when, early in my pregnancy, my doctor asked whether I was planning for a vaginal birth or a cesarean. I told him I thought I wanted a vaginal birth but didn't realize I had a choice. He described how safe cesareans are and told a few stories of his other patients, "all busy, smart women," who chose to have cesareans for their first babies. I left his office feeling strange but wondering if a cesarean just might be a lot easier all the way around.

Every visit he encouraged me to think about the cesarean. He also talked a lot about induction as soon as the baby was "big enough." When I told a friend I was considering a cesarean, she was aghast. She told me I needed to do some reading and talking with women who had had cesareans. It didn't take me long to find out that cesareans are risky for mothers and babies. I questioned my doctor, and he stood by his assessment that cesareans are safe. My husband and I talked about our options. On some level, I knew that even if I opted out of having a cesarean, I had lost confidence in my doctor. At twenty-eight weeks, I changed to a midwifery practice and had a baby boy, completely naturally. I am so grateful that my friend spoke up and that I took the time to research my options.

One part of Elizabeth's story is becoming more and more common. Some obstetricians are offering cesarean as an option (when there's no medical indication for the surgery) and leading women to believe it's a safe choice. Happily, the other part of Elizabeth's story is also becoming more common. When she realized she might be getting misleading information, she did her own research. What she discovered led her to change caregivers. In the end, she had the safe, healthy birth she wanted.

Jenne

Even before I reached my due date, a nurse-midwife recommended that I have routine labor induction, telling me that I was unlikely to go into labor on my own because I had a high body mass index (BMI). I was suspicious. I worked as an assistant to a medical researcher, which gave me access to PubMed (the U.S. National Library of Medicine search service) and allowed me to read articles about the relationship between high BMI and spontaneous labor.

After reviewing the medical literature, I found no evidence that I was at risk of post-term pregnancy or its consequences.

In addition, I contacted Henci Goer, an expert on obstetric research, about labor induction methods and learned that the drug misoprostol (Cytotec) was associated with adverse events and that, should labor induction become necessary, other methods were just as effective as misoprostol and were safer than the drug.

With the support of a doula and my partner, I refused the induction, went into labor at forty-one weeks, stayed home well into active labor, and had a healthy and exhilarating vaginal birth two hours after arriving at the hospital. After giving birth, I posted my story on a social networking website with thousands of regular visitors seeking pregnancy and birth information, and I contributed feedback about my midwives and hospital at http//www.thebirthsurvey.com.

Jenne not only accessed information herself, but she also made personal contact with Henci Goer through her forum on Lamaze's website (http://www.lamaze.org/OnlineCommunity/AskanExpert/tabid/363/Default.aspx). With Henci's additional information in hand, and with the support of her doula and partner, Jenne declined the induction. By posting her story on http//www.thebirthsurvey.com, she allowed other women to learn from her experience. Posting your story on the website will be an excellent way to share your birth experience, too!

Jill

A few days after an ultrasound at thirty-seven weeks estimated that my baby weighed ten pounds, my midwife called to say, "Sweetie, you need a c-section." She told me that I was at risk for shoulder dystocia, and ended our prenatal relationship with a referral to an obstetrician. At the insistence of a friend, I obtained a second opinion and accessed the medical library at the university where I worked, to read journal articles and clinical practice guidelines about safe vaginal birth.

After days of research, I was confident in my decision to plan for a vaginal birth. Just shy of thirty-nine weeks, I went into labor spontaneously, stayed home for as long as possible, and with the support of a doula, gave birth to a healthy ten-pound, three-ounce girl without incident. Two years later and again supported by a doula, I gave birth to an even bigger baby in a freestanding birth center with midwives.

Looking for a way to help at least one woman protect herself from the aggressive tactics of defensive medicine, I started a website, http://www.theunnecesarean.com. Less than a year after launching my site, I've received as many as fifty thousand visits each month, have thousands of followers on Facebook and Twitter, and have become a consumer voice for the right to informed refusal.

How many stories have you heard about women who were induced or had planned cesareans because their caregivers thought the baby was too big for a safe vaginal birth? Many times after such a diagnosis, the baby turns out to be small at birth; however, even if not, women can and do safely deliver very large babies vaginally, as Jill's experience demonstrates.

Jill increased her confidence by getting a second opinion and accessing the wealth of information on vaginal birth. She used her experience to help other women have access to information about unnecessary cesareans. As a result, Jill is making a substantial contribution to other women's abilities to make informed decisions as they plan for the safest births possible.

YOUR JOURNEY

The path of your pregnancy, labor, birth, and postpartum will be uniquely yours. Along the way you may encounter bumps that require interventions you hadn't anticipated or bumps that require you to steadfastly refuse interventions. All of the women featured in this chapter used the internet, books, childbirth classes, and other women's experiences to help them make informed decisions. Rather than passively following "doctor's orders," they accessed the wealth of information that's readily available and made decisions that protected their babies and themselves.

Only you can figure out what's best for you. You'll make good decisions if you have full, accurate information, if you communicate honestly and openly with your caregiver, and if you have confidence in yourself.

Chapter 12

GREETING YOUR NEWBORN

*A child is born, and for a moment the
wheeling planets seem to stop in their tracks,
as past, present and future meet.*
—Sheila Kitzinger

This chapter describes the events that should occur in the hours after giving birth as well as events that may occur in some birth settings.

It also discusses your newborn's appearance, abilities, and behavior and expands on the importance of breastfeeding.

Greeting your newborn should be a time to cherish. Prepare to protect that time by reading the following sections carefully, asking questions about your birth site's policies and protocol, and making your wishes known *before* you give birth.

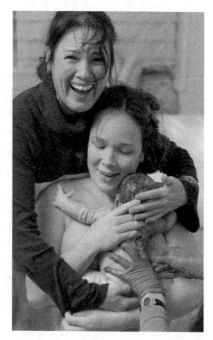

BABYMOON:
THE MAGICAL TIME FOLLOWING BIRTH

Nothing can describe the moments when you first gaze at your newborn's face and the following hours when you marvel at everything she does. Anthropologist Sheila Kitzinger calls this brief, precious period the "babymoon" and reminds parents that it's something more than a sequel to delivery.[1] The babymoon is another part of the beautiful, unique dance between mother and child. These first hours establish the foundation of your future together, allowing love, trust, and understanding to grow.

During the babymoon, a mother and her newborn need time that's unhurried by the clock. But depending on where the birth occurs, getting plenty of uninterrupted time may prove difficult. If you give birth in a hospital, standard protocol is designed to make every procedure efficient and identical for every patient—and this usually requires following a strict timetable. Your baby's umbilical cord may be clamped and cut within a minute or two after birth. You may be hurried to birth your placenta, rather than birthing it at your own pace. The staff may want to examine your baby in a warming bed, put medicine in her eyes, and dress her in a warmed gown and blanket. They may wish to further observe and treat your baby in the nursery.

If you give birth at home or in a birth center, your midwife knows that there's no reason to separate you and your baby during the first few hours. Someone can assess your baby's health without removing her from your arms (the safest place for your baby to be). Your baby's umbilical cord doesn't need to be cut immediately—in fact, it shouldn't be. You don't need to birth your placenta right away. Your midwife understands the importance of protecting the hours after birth, when you should have the quiet privacy to "learn" your baby while you're both alert, to hear her sounds and smell her newborn odors, to stretch out her little legs for a first diaper change, to gaze and to fall in love.

The hours after birth can be just as intense as those during labor, and the initial moments can be a real shock. You may find yourself holding your newborn and wondering, "Is this really happening to me?" Your body is exhausted from the hard work it's done. The rush of adrenalin during your final pushes may have left you trembling and your teeth chattering. These physical reactions may be accompanied by an emotional high unlike any other. You may weep or laugh uncontrollably. A warm blanket and a pair of socks will help control the trembling and chattering teeth—and undisturbed, uninterrupted time with your newborn will help focus your emotions.

During these first few hours, no one needs to show you how to bond with your baby. You both simply need the privacy, peace, patience, and confidence to do what your bodies, hearts, and minds already know how to do. If you're giving birth in a hospital, the staff's job is to create a quiet, intimate environment for you and your baby's first hours together, even if it's handling twenty other births at the same time. It's your job to diligently prepare for the event and discuss your wishes with caregivers and staff until you're satisfied with their responses and you're certain everyone understands your expectations for birth and beyond.

Some hospital midwives encourage their clients to write to hospital administrators about any grievances they have with outdated policies that separate them from their healthy babies. Hospital regulations get changed and brought up to date only after complaints and requests are repeatedly made. Don't be afraid to speak up.

> Navajo midwife Ursula Knoki-Wilson talks about the sacred moments after a baby's birth at her clinic. "It's a time of listening, of mutual respect, of dignity, and harmony. The mother and father shake the baby's hand at birth, honoring this little one as a separate individual. And then they formally name the baby: 'Hello, my baby, (Navajo name). You come into my hands riding on a beautiful white (or other color) horse.' "[2] The unhurried hours after the baby's birth are important ceremonial ones that build strong bonds between baby and parents.

THE IMPORTANCE OF BONDING

In the late 1960s two pediatricians, Marshall Klaus and John Kennell, noticed that hospital routines denied mothers and babies the opportunity to get to know each other after birth. Their subsequent research revealed a "sensitive period" in the first hours after birth and showed the importance of the intense connection (bonding) of mother and baby during that time. Their research demonstrated that spending this brief time together resulted in healthier children and stronger attachments between the babies and mothers.[3] It became the impetus for changing hospital routines to give mothers undisturbed time with their newborns.

> "You are never really prepared to witness this miracle, no matter how many times you have seen it happen. When mother and baby find each other for the first time, the world seems to stand still for a few moments, as if honoring mother and baby in this magical moment."
>
> —Elena

Skin-to-Skin: The Best Place to Be

Just as the best place for your baby to grow from conception was in your womb, the best place for him right after birth is on your skin, not in a warmer or another person's arms. This skin-to-skin contact is also called "kangaroo care," because the natural warmth, protection, and nutrition a mother's body offers her newborn is like the safe haven a baby kangaroo enjoys in its mother's pouch. Ina May Gaskin and her team of midwives at the Farm Midwifery Center designed their postpartum routines around this skin-to-skin time. They believe that mother and baby "are doing something more important than just lying together. They are falling in love."[4]

After you give birth, your deflated abdomen becomes a nest of loose skin for your baby. While in the nest, the skin-to-skin contact promotes the gentle, natural regulation of your baby's heart rate and body temperature. It also helps him establish regular breathing patterns and sustain high, stable blood sugar levels. Exposure to the natural bacteria on your skin during the first hours reduces his risk of illness from germs in the environment. Newborns who have skin-to-skin contact with their mothers cry very little, if at all—compare this reaction to the often upset babies who are examined and warmed in a warmer across the room or in the hospital nursery. It makes sense that babies respond well to touch. For forty weeks, a baby is in constant contact with his mother's body.

Skin-to skin contact can facilitate breastfeeding. Researchers in Sweden have discovered that when a newborn is placed on his mother's abdomen, in time he can make his way to his mother's breast and actually latch on by himself.[5] Baby is helped along by the familiar smell of amniotic fluid on his hands, the smell and warmth of his mother's skin, the sound of her voice, and the "target" of her darkened nipple.

Skin-to-skin contact can also benefit you by keeping oxytocin levels high. After giving birth, your uterus is the size of a grapefruit. In the hours and days that follow, contractions are needed to help shrink it to its normal pear size. Oxytocin levels are very high as your baby moves through your birth canal and remain high as you and your newborn first touch each other, stare into each other's eyes, and breastfeed together. The high levels of oxytocin keep your uterus contracted to reduce bleeding. Oxytocin is also partly responsible for the "falling in love" feeling you have when you first meet your newborn. Oxytocin helps you feel calm and responsive. In the days following birth, oxytocin helps ward off postpartum depression, continues to keep your uterus contracted, and speeds healing.

While against your skin, your baby's hand and head movements stimulate the release of additional oxytocin and endorphins, increasing milk production and keeping you and your baby calm and relaxed.[6] Endorphins have been called nature's narcotic. Research shows that when our bodies work hard, endorphin levels rise, especially when we feel secure, warm, and loved. Endorphins do more than block pain reception: in the initial moments after giving birth, endorphins help accelerate a mother's ability to bond with her baby. Endorphin levels are especially high within twenty minutes after the birth, and they're strongly present in her breast milk.

For all its physical and emotional benefits, skin-to-skin contact should be a carefully protected routine. During this intimate time, mothers become acutely aware of their newborn's needs—and who else is touching the baby and what's being done to him. Neither mother nor newborn misses a beat in the first hours when left together, and others should trust them to follow each other's lead. Baby and mother will know when it's time for a feeding, when it's time for comforting, when it's time for exploring.

To make sure you and your baby are given time for skin-to-skin contact, request that he's put on your bare abdomen or chest right after birth, with a warmed receiving blanket laid over you both and a hat on his damp head to help keep the warmth in. Also request that any examination of him is done while he's in your arms. Nothing should interrupt your baby's assurance that your body is a safe haven.

Kate found out hours after her daughter's birth that a staff member had drawn blood from the baby's foot in the hospital's nursery without her or her husband's consent. "She was a big baby—almost ten pounds—and she was healthy. They took her to the nursery while they finished up with me. I guess it was routine—they thought there was a chance my big baby might be diabetic. Later, I hated discovering that little prick hole in her heel, not knowing what her reaction might have been, or even how they did it." When a newborn stays with her mother, little goes undetected in the first hours after birth.

Rooming In: Keeping Baby and Mother Together

Before the twentieth century, when births occurred at home, mothers and babies stayed in the same room during the first days after birth. When births moved to hospitals, the medical community believed that mothers needed to rest alone and that babies were safer when kept in nurseries. As a result, mothers saw their babies only periodically during the day for feedings, following a strict schedule set by the hospital staff.

If you give birth in a hospital, protocol may lead staff to suggest that you let them care for your baby in the nursery so you can sleep better. Make no mistake—giving birth is hard work, and rest and sleep are important in the first days. Without rest, a mother's exhaustion may lead to sickness, sadness, or feeling overwhelmed. Her tired, stressed-out behavior may lead to a cranky baby, who picks up on her mother's signals. To be the calm, rested caregiver your baby needs, it's important that you sleep and rest, but that is actually easier in close physical contact with your baby. Studies show that mothers

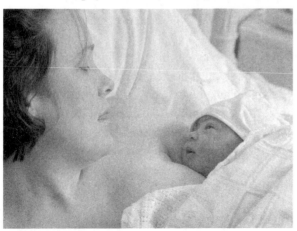

whose babies stay in nurseries don't necessarily sleep more or any better. In fact, mothers and babies who stay together without any separation rest better.[7] You may sleep more peacefully knowing that your baby is next to you. You're there to make sure she stays warm, and you can immediately respond to her cries. During breast-feeding, high levels of prolactin and oxytocin actually help you relax and sometimes even doze off during feedings.

Rabbi Harold Kushner talks about a woman giving birth as bringing a new living soul into the world, perhaps the most creative thing anyone could do. "Just as nurturing a child within her for nine months draws on the mother's physical resources, giving that child a soul draws on her spiritual resources. It would make sense for a new mother, despite all that a newborn infant demands of her, to take time to replenish her soul in the weeks after the birth."[8] Finding time to rest and be replenished (that is, to be repaired, refilled, restored) with a newborn is an important habit to form during the first hours after birth and beyond.

Rooming in allows baby and mother to rehearse the cues and responses that help with two important developments: The mother can learn her baby's cues and needs more quickly, which means the baby can trust that her messages will get responses. This means that breastfeeding gets off to a better start, too. When your newborn awakens hungry with you holding her or just a step away, she sends signals that you've learned to recognize, and you put her to the breast well before she cries.

"It makes sense that the more time two people spend together, the sooner they get to know each other," says nurse and Lamaze childbirth educator Jeannette Crenshaw,[9] who adds that babies who room in with their mothers gain more weight per day,[10] are less likely to be become jaundiced (have yellowish skin as the liver catches up to break down red blood cells),[11] and sleep more peacefully.[12] Studies show that mothers who room in with their babies for longer periods of time—including during the night—score higher on tests that measure the strength of attachment to their babies.[13]

One of Anne's fondest memories of her daughter's home birth was the pediatrician's visit. "She was born before dawn broke, and it was sunset when the doctor arrived and came upstairs to our bedroom to check her out. She and I hadn't left the warmth of that bedroom all day, we were so content. Jenny was sleeping on my stomach, her head turned toward him, her little mouth barely opened in a relaxed O. He was Welsh and stopped midway across our very softly lit room and whispered, 'Oh, father! Get a photo of this wee baby before I take a look.' We have that picture up on our wall, of Jenny sleeping peacefully on me that first night with us. She never left that spot all the time he quietly examined her and then said goodnight to us."

A Few Final Words on Bonding

Because research shows that being together is best for mother and baby, more hospitals need to protect and promote kangaroo care and rooming in. If you plan to give birth in a hospital, make sure you insist on being given the time and opportunity to get to know your baby—uninterrupted and undisturbed. But also remember that forming a strong attachment to your baby is not something done only during the first few hours and days of your baby's life. Bonding is a lifetime process.

> "I will absolutely never forget the pure delight and enormous smile your sister had that first time she saw you in my arms. What an amazing feeling it was for all of us to finally have our whole family together in one bed. It felt like a party after your birth. Everyone floated happily in and out of the room while I laid in the bed getting to know you, nursing, and eating homemade quiche that Grandma had brought."
>
> —Amy

PROCEDURES AFTER BIRTH

Cutting the Umbilical Cord

The umbilical cord is a tough, flexible rope of blood vessels that connects your baby to your womb and works with the placenta to nourish him. Considering the amount of tumbling and turning a baby does in the womb, it's not surprising that the cord can end up looped around the neck. Most often it's not a cause for alarm. The birth attendant gently slips the cord over the baby's head during the birth.

At birth, the cord protrudes from your baby's navel, often pulsating for many minutes after the birth. It continues to provide him oxygen and nourishment and ease his transition to the outside world. Although many doctors clamp and cut the cord within a minute or two after birth, a systematic review of the recent research found that immediate cord clamping was associated with a higher incidence of infant anemia that persisted for months; plus, in settings where lead poisoning is common, it's also a risk factor for lead poisoning (because lead competes with iron to bond with hemoglobin).[14]

By contrast, delaying cord cutting provides important benefits to mother and baby. For example, the "placental transfer" of blood after the birth plays a key role in healthy respiratory transition for the baby and decreases postpartum blood loss.[15] In addition, delaying the procedure ensures that you and your baby have uninterrupted time to get to know each other—as long as your baby is still connected to you, no one can separate you! Delaying the procedure also gives your baby the chance to adjust to his new surroundings more calmly.

Banking Cord Blood

Umbilical cord blood contains stem cells that may be able to treat many diseases. Stem cells divide to create red and white blood cells and platelets. They're the "building blocks" of the blood, the immune system, and body tissues. While the potential curative use of stem cells is promising, the development of stem cell research and cord blood banking is still in the early stages.

There are private and public companies that offer cord blood banking. For a fee that can range from several hundreds to thousands of dollars (depending on the company), parents can have their baby's cord blood frozen and stored, making stem cells available should the child develop a disease that these cells may be able to treat. Parents can also donate their baby's cord blood for research or for treatment. However, parents should know there's absolutely no guarantee that a cord blood transplant will offer appropriate treatment or that it'll provide a cure. There's also no guarantee that a company can successfully store the cells until they're needed—or that it'll stay in business.

There are other compelling reasons for not banking your baby's cord blood. The procedure usually involves immediate or early cord clamping, which is now considered more harmful to mother and baby than delayed cord cutting. Also, many have argued that the baby is intended to receive stem cells at birth, not at a later point in life. Last but not least, the procedure may interfere with the skin-to-skin contact between mother and baby during the critical first minutes after birth.

The American Academy of Pediatrics (AAP) believes that because there's a lack of evidence that an individual child would ever need stored umbilical cord blood, it's difficult to recommend that parents store their children's cord blood for future use. The AAP also expresses concern that families are especially vulnerable to emotional marketing at the time of birth.[16]

Birthing the Placenta

Your placenta grew with your baby in the womb from the cells of the fertilized egg. Through the umbilical cord, it nourished, maintained, and protected your baby throughout your pregnancy. The placenta is also called the afterbirth; however, birthing the placenta is an important part of the process of birth. Your uterus continues to contract after your baby's born, gently loosening and separating the placenta from the uterine wall. Keeping your baby skin-to-skin exerts gentle pressure on your uterus, and your baby's movements on your chest stimulate your body to release increasing amounts of oxytocin. This is nature's way of encouraging the placenta to separate and deliver.

How and when you birth your placenta depends on where the birth occurs. Many hospitals set a specific time limit on when you should birth the placenta (sometimes as soon as ten to fifteen minutes after your baby's birth). Hospital staff often hurry the birth of the placenta by tugging on the umbilical cord or by applying strong pressure to the top of your abdomen, and many doctors give intravenous (IV) Pitocin to stimulate the uterus to stay contracted and deliver the placenta quickly. All these practices are potentially harmful.

Other caregivers let you birth the placenta on your own and at your own pace. You're not rushed in any way. Instead, you spend the first minutes after the birth concentrating on your baby, holding and touching her as you get to know each other. Later on, your midwife or birth attendant might help you sit up or squat so gravity can help bring down the placenta. You might push it out, just as you pushed your baby out. Holding and nursing your baby encourages the uterus to contract and expel the placenta. This less aggressive process may take thirty minutes but may quite safely take longer—and you will have your baby in your arms the entire time.

The placenta is an amazing, life-giving organ that sometimes gets ignored in the rush of birth. Some women have no desire to see it. But some do. These women describe the placenta as beautiful—its network of blood vessels looking like a tree of life.

In his book *Childbirth without Fear*, Grantly Dick-Read said that in the past not many of his patients wanted to see the placenta. "Today, nearly every mother who watches her baby born asks me to show her the placenta. This I do, and I point out the bag in which the infant, now lying peacefully in her arms, developed and became a perfect little human being."[17]

More and more women attach symbolism to the placenta, recognizing it as an important life source for their babies. Many cultures around the world observe rituals that honor the placenta: a ceremonial planting of it in ancestral land (Maori); special preparation and use of its potential "life-source" power in certain medicines (Chinese); washing, wrapping, and burying it as a "sibling" of the newborn (Malaysian). Many women request to keep the placenta, then later plant it with a tree or shrub in honor of the newborn. If you give birth in a hospital, its policy may be to use the placenta for skin grafts and treatment of burn victims, or it may simply discard or incinerate the placenta.

Whatever you'd like done with your placenta, make the decision before birth and make your wishes known to everyone attending your birth. This way, its fate won't be decided without your input during the exciting moments when everyone's busy meeting your newborn.

> "I was helped out of the birth tub, and I carried my baby into bed. *My* bed. Everyone came into the room, marveling at the birth that had just been witnessed. The midwives took care of the umbilical cord and placenta, while the baby remained undisturbed with me. My mom poured the special sparkling juice that I'd bought for the birth, and we toasted the newest member of our family. Then slowly things wound down and eventually it was just the three of us, our new family. We were in our house, in our bed, and together we fell asleep."
>
> —Amanda

Checking the Apgar Score and Birth Weight and Length

At one minute and again at five minutes after birth, your midwife, a nurse, or another birth attendant will check your baby's breathing, heart rate, skin color, muscle tone, and reflexes. This procedure is called the Apgar score after Virginia Apgar, the anesthesiologist who first suggested compiling a score to assess a newborn's overall condition. The birth attendant observes the baby and gives points for how well the baby's adjusting to life outside the womb. The higher the score, the better the baby's adjustment.

These simple observations are visual only and are somewhat subjective. There's no reason why your baby needs to be taken from you while being observed. The birth attendant can check your baby quietly and as efficiently as possible—while he's still in your arms or on your chest.

Your baby's weight and length don't need to be measured immediately after birth. These assessments can wait until you and your
baby have had some uninterrupted time together.

Screenings and Other Routine Procedures

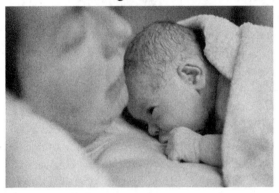

Healthcare officials, state
health agencies, researchers,
and parents will likely never
agree on what tests should
or should not be given to a
newborn. Individual states
may offer exemptions to
routine procedures for
medical, religious, or
philosophical reasons.

Before your baby's birth, learn all you can about the following
tests and procedures. Contact a local hospital or your state's public
health department to find out what other tests and procedures your
state mandates.

Vitamin K

Vitamin K helps the blood clot. Although babies are born with
extremely low levels of it, colostrum (the mother's first breast milk)
is rich in vitamin K. Although giving a newborn vitamin K (either
orally or by injection) is mandatory in many states, its necessity—and
risk—is controversial. Some medical reports claim that the mandatory
administration of vitamin K may not be based on sound science.[18]
Some studies recommend that hospitals change their policies so only
newborns at risk of blood clotting problems get vitamin K. These are
babies who were born prematurely or by cesarean section, whose
mothers' diets were low in vitamin K during pregnancy, or whose
mothers took drugs or antibiotics during pregnancy.

Administering vitamin K exemplifies how medical science can
create a problem that it must solve with yet another intervention.
After World War II, American research determined that formula was
superior to breast milk, and consequently more babies were formula-
fed than breastfed. However, formula doesn't contain the vitamin K
that's naturally present in breast milk, so the mandates to administer
vitamin K to newborns arose to remedy this problem.

A more natural, reasonable approach to providing newborns with vitamin K is to encourage mothers to eat adequate amounts of foods with vitamin K (such as leafy green vegetables) during pregnancy and after birth so their breast milk contains it. Breastfeeding your baby should give him enough vitamin K naturally if you're getting enough of the vitamin yourself, and, even more importantly, if you make sure that he receives plenty of hind milk (the last milk of each feeding) when he breastfeeds.

Well before your baby's birth, find out your state's laws about administering vitamin K to newborns. Make an informed decision about vitamin K and communicate your wishes to your birth attendants. If you can't opt out of the shot or oral dosage, ask that the treatment be delayed for at least an hour or until your baby has breastfed and adjusted to the surroundings.

Eye Drops or Ointment

To prevent gonorrhea and other infections from attacking a newborn's vision, many states mandate hospitals to administer antibiotic eye drops or ointment in the eyes of all infants, even if they have not been exposed to gonorrhea or other sexually transmitted diseases. These drops are gentler than they were in the past (none of them, however, catches all sexually transmitted diseases), but they still can irritate many babies' eyes. Although this procedure may be mandatory, parents can opt out of it. Check your state's mandates on eye treatment. If you can't opt out of it, delay the procedure for an hour or at least until after your baby has breastfed and adjusted to the surroundings. After all, he can't see when his eyes are covered in medicine.

Newborn Metabolic Screening Tests

Years ago all babies were screened for a very rare condition called phenylketonuria (PKU) with a blood test. Babies with PKU don't have the enzyme to process the proteins they eat, leading to possible mental and physical problems. Today, babies are routinely tested for a wide variety of rare but serious metabolic diseases with a simple blood test. Screenings for diseases vary among U.S. states, but many screen for cystic fibrosis, sickle cell anemia, congenital hypothyroidism, among others. Early detection and treatment of these diseases can improve outcomes dramatically.

The baby's heel is pricked to get the blood sample, a painful procedure. Breastfeeding during any painful procedure will decrease your baby's perception of pain dramatically.[19]

Glucose Screening

Hospitals give a glucose screening (blood sugar test) to babies who are under five pounds or over nine pounds at birth, or if mother is diabetic. These babies are at risk for developing low blood sugar in the first hours of life. Babies who show signs of low blood sugar (trembling or shaking) are also tested. The best way to prevent low blood sugar in your baby is hold him skin-to-skin and to nurse him soon and often. And if your baby does indeed develop low blood sugar, breastfeeding is the best medicine.[20]

Hepatitis B Vaccination

Hepatitis B is a serious disease caused by a virus that attacks the liver. It is a sexually transmitted disease, and can also be transmitted by blood. If you have active hepatitis or are a chronic carrier, your baby will be given the hepatitis B vaccine shortly after birth. The vaccine is mandatory for all newborns in many hospitals. The AAP recommends that infants receive a first dose either in the first days after birth, or at one month. Learn about the benefits and risks of the hepatitis B vaccine before your baby is born. Make sure the hospital staff knows your wishes about the vaccination.

Vaccinations

Healthcare providers, state health agencies, researchers, and parents will likely never agree on what vaccines a child should receive. And experts don't seem to agree on the number of vaccinations, when they should be given, and how the vaccines should be combined in a given injection. Before your baby is two years old, he may receive vaccinations for diphtheria, tetanus, pertussis (whooping cough), influenza, polio, measles, mumps, rubella, pneumococcal conjugate, and chicken pox. Some babies react to a vaccination with a fever, vomiting, or lethargy. It's worth learning about each vaccine beforehand so you can discuss its effectiveness and necessity with your baby's caregiver more knowledgeably. Some states offer exemptions to routine vaccinations for medical, religious, or philosophical reasons. Keep in mind that the first and most important "vaccine" your baby should receive is your breast milk. The immunities, antibodies, and countless other protections will benefit your baby for as long as you breastfeed him.

Deciding about Circumcision

One of the least agreed-upon procedures in the American medical community is circumcision. This procedure involves cutting off the foreskin from the tip of the penis. Once a routine procedure, questions about the necessity of circumcision have risen in the past few decades. A longtime belief that supports circumcision is its potential medical benefits, like its ability to lower the risk of urinary tract infections, penile cancer, and some sexually transmitted diseases.

The evidence, however, indicates that circumcised boys are only slightly more protected from these problems than intact (uncircumcised) boys and that other factors (like diet and behavior) better determine risk. Other reasons for circumcision are religious beliefs, social customs (for example, circumcision makes boys look like their fathers), and cultural beliefs (for example, the mistaken belief that circumcision makes hygiene easier). Until the 1970s, circumcision was so routine in hospitals that parents often weren't informed before their babies had the surgery.

> "I'm glad our first baby was a girl," Shawna recalls. "We hadn't really worked out the issues around whether to circumcise. Had we consented to what the hospital wanted to do, we would have said yes at the time." The couple's son was born two years later, and after finding out more information about the procedure, they decided against circumcision. "Our son's grandfather was not circumcised, his father was, and now this new boy is not. It was never an issue—their different appearance—between my husband and his father, and I'd guess it won't be one for our son."

Today, the American Academy of Pediatrics maintains that there are no compelling medical reasons to circumcise baby boys.[21] The United States is the only country in the world that routinely performs this surgery for secular reasons. Like the risks associated with any surgery, possible risks of this procedure include pain, infection, bleeding, mutilation, interference with breastfeeding, and even death. The procedure includes strapping the baby into a special constraint, and too often it's done without any anesthesia. Don't be fooled into believing your baby won't feel any pain.

If you decide to leave your baby intact, know that he won't be alone. In the U.S. today, less than 60 percent of newborn boys are circumcised, and this rate has declined steadily over the last few decades. In other countries around the world, intact boys greatly outnumber circumcised boys.

If you decide to have your baby circumcised, the AAP recommends that anesthesia be used—and something more than just a topical cream.[22] You may want to follow the guidelines based on Jewish tradition, even if you aren't of Jewish faith. The procedure is performed on the eighth day after birth, when vitamin K levels are at their peak and the blood's clotting ability has kicked in. Your baby is never out of your presence, and you can comfort him throughout the procedure.

YOUR NEWBORN'S APPEARANCE, ABILITIES, AND BEHAVIOR

Your baby will take her time to stretch out of the fetal position—a pose she was in for so long. There's much for you to see as your baby unfolds her fingers, arms, and numerous creases in her skin. Her beautiful tiny fingernails and toenails may bring you hours of contemplation.

The biggest part of your newborn's body is her head. Labor and birth may have temporarily changed its shape (molding), but it'll regain a normal shape within days. She may have a blister on her head (caput) that developed when her head pressed against your cervix during labor. It'll eventually disappear.

She has tiny ears; silky, slicked down hair (if she has hair); and if the lighting isn't too bright, wide-open eyes that seek you out. The puffiness in her face will decrease now that she's out of the watery womb. Increased hormone levels at birth have made her genitals swollen, but the swelling will decrease as the hormones level off.

Your newborn will probably keep her hands closed into little fists, even while asleep. Her grasping reflex is so strong, you can help her pull herself into a sitting position. Even her little feet—with toes lined up like peas in a pod—try to grasp like hands when touched.

The following sections describe your baby's appearance, abilities, and behavior in more detail.

Skin and Sense of Touch

While your baby was in the womb, your body made vernix (a creamy, white, lanolin-like substance) to cover and protect her skin. She'll be born covered in a little or a lot of vernix. (Some babies are born covered with more of it than others.) Your baby's body may also still have lanugo, the downy hair that covered her body while in the womb. It'll disappear within a couple of days.

Your baby spent the last forty weeks comfortably and safely immersed in amniotic fluid and covered in vernix. After birth, there's no reason to wash away the vernix or the scent of amniotic fluid. In fact, it's particularly important that the fluid's scent stay on your baby's hands so she can taste and smell it and connect the scent to the taste and scent of your skin. Once born, she can be patted dry with warm towels as she lies on your bare chest or abdomen. A lifetime of baths and showers, soaps and towels, awaits her, but the first precious moments should be spent touching and connecting with you.

In the first couple of days after birth, your baby's skin and the whites of her eyes may take on a yellowish tinge. This coloring, called jaundice, is related to bilirubin levels in her blood. Bilirubin is a pigment produced by the normal breakdown of red blood cells in the liver, and it's discarded in stool (poop). The normal process of eating and excreting prevents bilirubin levels from becoming dangerously high.

Jaundice is common in babies because their livers are still developing and removing extra red blood cells needed for fetal circulation. The yellowish color will fade away naturally within a week or two as your baby eats more and her liver matures. A breastfed baby sometimes stay yellow a bit longer, but this condition is absolutely normal. If your breastfed baby is nursing well and gaining weight, there's no cause for concern.

To treat jaundice, some hospitals routinely place newborns under a special ultraviolet light to help break down the bilirubin in the skin. However, this procedure is rarely necessary. In fact, some experts now believe that jaundice may be a normal phenomenon in newborns.[23] To prevent jaundice from becoming a problem, breastfeed your baby at least ten to twelve times a day. The extra feedings of breast milk will help your baby excrete extra bilirubin in stool. You might also expose your baby to sunlight. Its ultraviolet rays work the same way as the hospital's artificial "bili-lights."

The skin is the body's largest sense organ, and babies thrive and develop best when their skin is touched. Not only does immediate and constant touching stimulate the production of growth hormones and aid the immune system, but it also helps establish better sleep patterns and prevent distress.

In the weeks ahead, carry your baby against you or in a sling or front carrier as often as you can. The contact will let you both learn how to respond to each other's signals and needs. Consider giving your baby a daily massage to relax and quiet yourselves together.

Mouth, Voice, and Sense of Taste

Your baby's mouth may look like a beautiful little rosebud. She'll use it to yawn, sneeze, cough, hiccup, and coo—all responses to her new environment and little rehearsals for life ahead. But from this perfect tiny orifice, she'll emit a mighty cry. A newborn's cry is nature's call, a universal summons for attention, and it's vital to her survival. At birth, some babies cry more than others, and some babies will require more attention in response to their cries than others. You may have seen a mother insert her pinky finger into her baby's mouth to quickly settle down the little one. This action helped meet two important needs: the need to be held and the need to suck.

The sucking and rooting reflexes are your baby's most important survival tools. Immediately after birth, she may begin to nudge (the rooting reflex) toward your nipples, which throughout pregnancy have darkened into "targets" she can see more easily. Your baby sucks in response to stress or fear, as well as for comfort and nutrition. During the first hours, sucking your breasts brings colostrum (the rich, clear "first milk" that's loaded with antibodies) into her little body. Her continued sucking eventually brings in your milk and helps your uterus contract more efficiently in the hours and days after the birth. Some babies are born ready to breastfeed right away. Some may need a little more time, choosing to nurse a little more sedately. If your baby's a strong nurser, it's common for a little blister to form on the inside of her upper lip.

Your baby was born able to taste. In fact, her taste buds were already developing when she was just eight weeks or so into gestation.[24] While in the womb, she tasted the spices, flavorings, and chemicals that you ate and absorbed then passed on to her through the placenta. During the first few months, she'll respond positively to only sweet flavors—and your breast milk is indeed sweet to the taste.

Eyes and Sense of Sight

At birth, a newborn's eyes often appear red and puffy, and there may be broken blood vessels in the eyeballs, caused by pressure exerted on them during birth or by the drops or ointment she may have received after birth. Light-skinned babies usually have blue-gray eyes, and dark-skinned babies usually have brown eyes. Permanent color won't develop for about six months. Some babies can produce tears from birth, but most don't for six weeks or so.

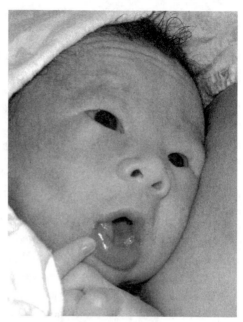

The dark, beautiful orbs peering out from your newborn's face can see objects at close range (within eight to ten inches). Research shows that babies can recognize their mothers' faces in as little as four hours after birth. Your baby can even respond to your facial expressions, especially when you're within eight to ten inches of his face. Studies confirm that movement attracts babies' sight and newborns prefer curved shapes over straight ones, patterns in contrasting colors over plain patterns, and ordered patterns over random patterns. And they find the human face the most attractive thing to look at.[25]

Your baby's alertness at birth allows for her first "reading lesson"—assuming that no drugs were given during the birth process to dull his responses. As you and your baby gaze at each other, you're reading each other's cues, sending each other messages, making contact. Your baby may stare at you intently for long periods as he sorts through the surrounding stimuli. Or he may close his eyes, desiring a little more time before entering the bright, stimulating new environment. These hours of alert gazing send parents this important message: Pay attention!

Ears and Sense of Hearing

Months before your baby's birth, she can hear your internal body sounds as well as the sounds of the outside world—voices (especially yours), rumbling vehicles, ringing bells, barking dogs, sounds that surround us every day. Within the first hours of life, her tiny ears channel a great deal of information, helping her analyze and categorize the new surroundings.

Studies show that newborns prefer a live human voice over a recorded or telecast voice and an animated voice over an emotionally flat one.[26] Babies also prefer to be looked at while spoken to. When you instinctively speak directly to your newborn in a gentle, high-pitched voice, she listens and responds in recognition. She turns her head to the sound source, opens and brightens her eyes, and moves her arms and legs.

Nose and Sense of Smell

At birth, your newborn's nose appears flat and broad. Her brain's olfactory (smell) center formed very early in fetal development, so she likely has a sense of smell at birth. Her sense of smell (and taste) helps her reach your breast and nurse. Studies show that within a few days of birth, your baby can distinguish among the scent of your milk and other skin odors.[27] Certainly, your scents are the most familiar and comforting to your newborn—yet another important reason to not wash away amniotic fluid or vernix from her skin right after birth. It's also a good idea to wrap your baby in soft clothing that you've worn so your scent will comfort her.

Behavior

At birth, reactions to the new environment vary from baby to baby. If your baby isn't separated from you, he'll likely pensively and inquisitively stare at his new surroundings for an hour or much longer. If he's separated from you, he'll probably become distressed as he seeks the comfort of your skin to reassure him that he can trust these new surroundings.

Your newborn may begin vocalizing right away, making little grunts or whimpering rhythmically while staring at his new world. It's as though he's waiting to hear some familiar, gentle, and reassuring words and sounds he can respond to. Or your baby may be more reserved, seeking the safety and comfort of your arms a bit longer before more actively engaging with his surroundings. He may prefer silence or hushed voices and may be startled by noise, brightness, chatter, and bustle.

Researchers have observed several states in newborn behavior. (See the following list.) Your baby's behavior will follow a pattern that'll develop at its own pace.[28]

- **Quiet alert state:** If any drugs given during the labor and birth haven't dulled her responses, your baby's first hour is one of attentiveness and quiet inquisitiveness. She focuses all her energy to look directly into your eyes and to listen to the surrounding voices. After this initial quiet alert state in the first hour of life, there are often few such prolonged periods over the next few days. Usually, briefer periods of curious, exploratory behavior occur around feeding time. In the first week of life, the normal baby spends only 10 percent of any twenty-four-hour period in this state.

- **Active alert state:** During this state baby is very different. He moves his arms and legs every two or three minutes (not continuously but rhythmically), makes small sounds, and looks around. These bursts of movements happen before feeding or when baby is fussy.

- **Crying state:** Crying is your baby's mode of communication. Her cry signals a need that you can learn to discern from other cries, such as recognizing "I'm hungry" from "I need a diaper change." Pediatrician Marshall Klaus and his wife, Phyllis, have lovingly studied newborn behavior and encourage parents to recognize their newborn's different cries: "Sometimes it takes many tries to figure it out…. Holding the baby close, murmuring soothing words, and especially keeping oneself calm can be helpful in reading the baby's signals." Picking up your baby will often stop her crying, and research suggests that babies whose cries get responses quickly are less likely to cry at one year of age.[29]

- **Drowsy state:** This state occurs right before your baby drifts to sleep or right after she wakes up. It's similar to how you feel right before you fall into a nap on the couch, or just as you crawl out of bed in the morning in search of that first cup of coffee. In this state, your baby may continue to move a little as well as smile and frown.

- **Quiet sleep state:** A baby often drifts into this state at his mother's breast. It's deep and peaceful, with regular breathing, closed eyes, and few body movements.

- **Active sleep state:** In this state, your baby moves her eyes under closed eyelids, moves her arms and legs, speeds up her breathing, and displays a variety of endearing funny faces—goofy smiles, grimaces, and frowns—sometimes in quick succession. She tends to move or root around, as though seeking to get close to an edge

Sarah remembers well the strong feeling of recognition that swept over her when her newborn son was placed in her arms: "He made these lovely little noises, and I had such an overwhelming desire to keep whispering to him, 'I know you! I know you!' It was as if we'd been together forever—like these wise little eyes staring into mine were familiar, and he recognized his father and me. I sort of assumed he expected to hear us welcoming him home."

or object. Babies will move toward the warmth, sound, and smell of their mothers' bodies in bed before they'll settle into quiet sleep.[30] When she wakes up, she's usually coming out of active sleep.

MORE ON BREASTFEEDING

It's in your baby's nature to find your breast and latch on to it himself. When he's hungry, he'll give you cues, the same ones he makes when he moves into the active sleep state. For example, he may appear asleep, but his eyes are moving beneath his lids and he moves his arms and hands to his mouth. He bobs his head from side to side and may even try to suck on your arm or face if you're holding him. He may make small noises. These actions are his natural way of alerting you that he's ready to find the breast, latch on, and suck. If you wait until he cries—which may be as long as thirty minutes after he starts giving you cues—he's no longer in a state to nurse easily. You'll have to settle him down before he's ready to feed.

In the first hours after birth it's easiest to let your baby position and latch on your breast himself. Hold him skin-to-skin vertically between your breasts, and let him bob his head and move until he finds your breast. Your baby will know your breast by feel and your nipple by smell, not by sight.

Or you can position your baby wrapped around you. Make sure he can move freely. Remove constricting blankets and uncover his hands. Snuggle your baby close, resting his head on your wrist or forearm, positioning him on his side facing you. He should be able to see your face with his top eye. His ear, shoulder, and hips should be in a straight line, and his nose—not his mouth—should be level with your nipple. If you use a pillow, make sure you (not the pillow) are supporting your baby's body. As your baby nurses, support his neck and shoulders with your hand, but don't hold the back of his head. Supporting him this way gives him the freedom to move his head. When he feels your breast against his chin and lower lip and smells your nipple, he'll open his mouth wide and move his upper lip up and over the nipple. This is an off-center (or asymmetric) latch, and it's the equivalent of you opening your mouth wide and placing the bottom of a very large hamburger on your lower lip, then moving your mouth up and over the top of the burger to stuff as much as possible into your mouth. If you approached the burger straight on, you couldn't fit nearly as much into your mouth, even if it's opened wide. The same logic holds true for your baby and the breast.

When eating that huge hamburger you also squeeze it to make it easier to bite. You can make your breast easier for your baby to latch onto by making a "breast sandwich." It helps to hold your breast with your index finger under your breast and your thumb on top. Then rotate your fingers so your breast rests in a U between your thumb and fingers. Your fingers and thumb are at three o'clock and nine o'clock. Now squeeze your breast to make a sandwich as your baby opens his mouth wide and latches on.

If your baby latches on properly, you shouldn't feel pain as he nurses, although most women experience some discomfort initially when their babies start sucking—just until their milk lets down. Whether your breasts feel full or not, your ducts release the milk only when your baby's sucking releases the hormone oxytocin. You'll know your milk has let down if your baby begins to suck differently (*suck, suck, suck* changes to *suck, swallow, suck, swallow*). You may relax, feel warm, or get thirsty. Or you may simply notice that your baby has settled down and is more 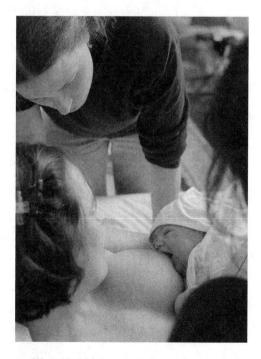 content. In the first days after birth, you'll notice your uterus contracting as you nurse. Oxytocin is doing double duty: allowing your milk to "let down" and keeping your uterus tight.

Your baby will nurse happily until he's full, at which time he'll spontaneously release the breast. He may be sleeping, or he may want to continue nursing from the other breast. (If he isn't interested in the second breast, that's okay.) The hind milk, the milk at the end of a feeding, is very high in fat. It's important that your baby get the hind milk so he'll get the calories he needs and gain weight faster. The only way you can be sure your baby's getting the hind milk is if he finishes a feeding himself. Don't limit his time on the breast or insist that he take both breasts.

How often should you feed your baby? Feed him whenever he gives any cues that he's hungry and at least eight to twelve times a day. The more your baby nurses, the more milk you make. Don't delay a nursing session, and don't limit how long he nurses.

How will you know your baby's getting milk at each feeding? You'll know by noticing the change in his sucking. He'll follow bursts of sucking with a pause as he swallows. You can also see his neck muscles move as he swallows.

At first, your baby gets colostrum from your breasts. His stomach is very small (the size of a walnut), and he doesn't need much of this very rich, clear liquid. Colostrum acts as a laxative, and your baby's first stool is the dark, tar-like meconium leaving his digestive system. Over the next two to four days, the color of his stool changes to a mustard yellow. The changing color of his stools is an important sign that he is getting your milk. Breastfed babies' stools are very watery, in part because there's so little waste—your baby's body can use almost everything in breast milk. Around the third day (sometimes sooner), your milk "comes in," and a feeling of fullness always accompanies it. Most women welcome this feeling as confirmation that they're actually making milk!

Ultimately, you'll know your baby's getting enough nutrition if he's gaining weight and wetting four to six disposable (or six to eight cloth) diapers and soiling at least three diapers in twenty-four hours. But it takes a few days for your baby to have this output. On day two he'll have two to three wet diapers and two stools, and over the next three days he'll work up to six wet diapers and at least three dirty diapers in a twenty-four–hour period.

Breastfeeding Help

We recommend several breastfeeding books and resources in Recommended Resources. For breastfeeding success, it's important that you have someone knowledgeable and experienced in the first weeks of nursing waiting in the wings in case you need help. The following are problems that are easily prevented and can be solved with simple solutions.

Engorgement

Engorgement is a painful condition in which the breasts become overly full with milk. Mothers whose babies are kept near so they can nurse frequently and efficiently in the first days don't become engorged. However, your breasts may become very engorged if your baby has had trouble latching and emptying your breasts in the first days, or if you've been separated from your baby. To prevent engorgement, keep your baby close and nurse frequently round the clock. To treat engorgement, have your baby nurse frequently. You may need to pump or hand-express some milk so your baby can latch on more easily. Or take a warm shower before nursing to help your milk begin dripping from your breasts and make your nipples softer. Once your baby's nursing, gently massage your breasts to encourage milk flow. Between feedings, ice may reduce swelling and pain. For more help, contact a lactation consultant.

Sore and Cracked Nipples

Your nipples shouldn't hurt when you nurse. If they do, it's almost always because your baby isn't latching on or sucking properly. It is important that you get help immediately. Don't wait. Contact a lactation consultant or someone knowledgeable about proper positioning and latch and have her watch you with your baby at the breast. She will help you with latch and position problems. As your nipples heal, once latch has been corrected, try changing your baby's position while nursing to move the pressure to an unaffected area. To help prevent cracked nipples, don't use soap to wash them—just use water and let them air-dry. Lanolin creams may help soothe sore nipples. Hydrogel pads (available from pharmacies) may also help relieve pain.

Baby Trouble

If your baby's sleepy because of medication you had in labor or is exhausted from the birth, he may not be interested in nursing during the first day or so, or he may have a lot of difficulty latching on and sucking. A lactation consultant can definitely help you. It's critical that your baby eat, and it's critical that milk is emptied from your breasts so you'll keep making more. If your baby hasn't had a successful nursing session in the first twelve hours, pump some colostrum and feed it to him with an eyedropper or small medicine cup. In most cases, there's no need to give him infant formula. Keep your baby skin-to-skin, pay attention to his feeding cues, and be patient—with yourself and with your baby.

BEYOND BABYMOON

The rush of your baby's birth is over, and now it's time to settle into being a family. At one time, women spent the days and weeks after giving birth lying in—an old term for that period of seclusion when a new mother concentrates on her newborn and is cared for by other women. Many traditional cultures have nurturing women who help care for the new mother and baby and manage the household. In traditional Jewish culture, for example, women care for a new mother entirely for the first thirty days after giving birth.

In our modern culture, in which so many women work outside the home and generations often don't live near one another, arranging a time for lying in can be difficult. Today's women expect (and are expected) to be independent and resilient, to jump back into prebirth routines in a slim, prebirth body, with every hair in place and appointments kept. This expectation makes women give the warped message *I'm back to normal! I'm good at this! Nothing has changed!* But becoming a mother does change a woman. Often a new mother doesn't realize that she needs nurturing just as much as her newborn does. She needs unrushed time and space to adjust to the transformation in her life.

"My first child was born at a home on a gloriously sunny morning in late September after a long night of hard and painful labor. One of my happiest memories of my daughter's birthday is of sitting on my bed that afternoon—after all the phone calls to astonished grandparents had been made, after the midwife had packed up and gone home to get some sleep, and after a ravenous hunger had set in—with my delicious, miraculous newborn swaddled on my lap as I devoured a pepperoni and onion pie that had been delivered from our favorite pizza joint. It was our second home delivery of the day."

—Betsy

To help make your time of adjustment easier, make some preparations before your baby's birth. Arrange for maternity leave, stock the freezer with premade meals, figure out what tasks you'll need help to do. These preparations can calm you and help you happily anticipate your baby's arrival. Once your baby's born, it's a time to relax obligations and rest. It's also a private, intimate, and emotional time that calls for protection and boundaries.

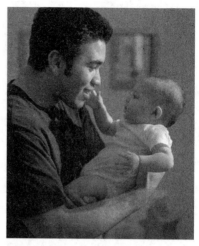

In a world where many feel isolated from one another, welcoming a new baby is a celebration friends and family long to attend. They're ready to admire the newborn, and encourage and congratulate the new parents. They're honored to arrange naming ceremonies, prepare special foods, take photographs, and give loads of gifts. Accept these gestures and encourage brief visits from well-wishers, but stay home and let them visit you—right in your bedroom, if necessary, where they can drink a cup of tea and admire you and your baby. Don't be shy asking visitors for help with dishes or laundry or any other task. Most will be eager to help. And don't worry about turning visitors away. Hang a "do not disturb" sign on your front door when you need to sleep and enjoy some privacy. Turn off your cell phones and land-line phones. Do whatever it takes to protect your quiet time with your new child.

During the first hours and days with your newborn, let yourself surrender to unhurried, undivided time so you can get to know this new person who has changed—and will continue to change—your life profoundly. Sharpen your listening and observation skills to learn how best to respond to your little one. The cues and clues are there—you just need to act on them confidently, like the good parent you are.

Brian's transition to fatherhood was like Alice's trip through the looking glass: "There was an exact moment when Jonathan came into my arms, and all of a sudden I was a father. You can talk about it all of those months beforehand, but the reality doesn't really hit until the moment you're holding him." He and his wife, Susan, had their quiet, regimented apartment life thrown into temporary chaos, with family and friends dropping in with food and gifts, people gathered in the bedroom hour after hour, the constant kitchen clean-up taken up by this visitor or that. "At the end of the partying, there we were, the three of us, and Susan and I were exhausted on just about every level. And we found ourselves speaking to each other not only as husband and wife, like we had been just days before, but also as mother and father. It was—I don't know—a weird transition."

Chapter 13

EARLY PARENTING

*Each day of our lives we make deposits
in the memory banks of our children.*
—Charles R. Swindoll, *The Strong Family*

LIFE WITH YOUR NEWBORN

When your new baby arrives, you spend more time listening and learning than you ever had before. You focus all your attention on

your little one, who has so much to teach you about caring for him. You learn more about parenting from each other than you ever could from any book or website. While with your baby, try to provide as quiet a setting as possible. It's difficult to learn his subtle behaviors in a setting with distractions.

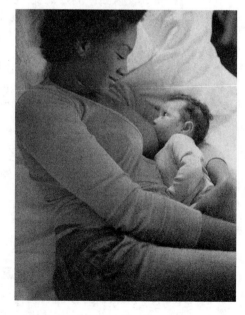

Speaking of distractions, you may notice that you're receiving advice as never before—advice from family, friends, professionals, even strangers. Most advice is well meaning. But much of it is uninvited, some of it may hurt your feelings, and some of it is just plain misinformation.

Your relationship with your baby is unique, and together you're charting unknown waters. So when a friend tells you her secret for getting a baby to stop crying, or when your mother suggests that you put your baby on sleeping and eating schedules, you may need to turn a deaf ear. What worked for Baby Susie or was the norm forty years ago may not apply to you and your baby.

This chapter describes a way to parent your new child so he feels safe and secure. It discusses sleeping and feeding: two activities central to your baby's well-being. It also discusses your emotional and physical health after giving birth and becoming a mother, as well as changes to your lifestyle and household now that your baby has arrived.

Getting advice often isn't easy, especially when the advice is about your ability to parent your child. When someone—particularly someone with whom you have an intense relationship, such as your mother or mother-in-law—gives you unsolicited advice on how to care for your baby, you may feel defensive, hurt, angry, judged, or inferior. The elevated levels of hormones in your postpartum body may keep you on edge for a while. A comment that you may have shrugged off before you got pregnant now stings.

To help you deal with unwelcome advice, repeat these affirmations to yourself:
- I have every reason to trust MYSELF to care for this baby.
- I know my baby, and my ears are tuned in a special way to my child.
- I am wise enough to learn the dance that's begun between this unique child and me.

At the same time, simply thank the person offering the advice and change the subject or, if the person is determined to expound on the advice, excuse yourself and leave the room.

PARENTING YOU BABY:
HOLD ME, FEED ME, LOVE ME

Nils Bergman, a public health physician, points out that although our babies are born with the skills and behaviors they need to grow and be well, they're the most immature of all mammals. As a result, they require a great deal of care, almost as if they were still in the womb. According to Dr. Bergman, the mantra our babies chant is *Hold me, feed me, love me.*[1] Keeping baby close and responding to baby's needs quickly builds trust, empathy, and affection. It also ensures baby will thrive physically and emotionally. Close, responsive, baby-led care is what nature intends for those first months of life. It might even be considered the golden rule of parenting.

Through your pregnancy when you caressed and spoke to your belly, you fostered loving attachments to your unborn baby. When you insisted that she stay with you once born, you continued to foster loving attachments to your newborn. And when your baby is at home, you have the opportunity to lovingly respond to her cues and signals, to her cries, and to things in her environment that might distress her. Just as your newborn thrives on touch in those first hours, your baby will continue to flourish when you stay

> "My mantra for those first few weeks of parenting was always *This too shall pass.* All the really hard stuff—the trifecta of physical pain when nursing: sore bottom, uterine cramping, and sore nipples; the sleep deprivation; the emotional roller coaster—all of that you just need to ride out, trusting that it won't go on forever. But so, too, the really delicious stuff—the smell of that little velveteen newborn head, those tiny little starfish hands, that amazing focused look in the baby's eyes, the sound of his breathing—all those things don't last. And you must constantly remind yourself that both the hard parts and the lovely parts will pass by so quickly. Don't stress the tough stuff; do cherish the precious bits. It's all so fleeting. All those hours I spent just gazing in wonderment at the baby I called 'watching baby TV.' "
>
> —Betsy

close and respond to her. This style of parenting will continue to decrease stress levels for you and your baby, helping him relax and sleep and grow and learn.

There's a lot to learn when your baby comes home, but letting your baby show you what he needs helps you learn these lessons naturally by keeping him close. The following two sections discuss how parenting that's responsive to baby needs can help your baby and you get the sleep and nutrition you both need.

Sleep

Nighttime Feedings

Just as your baby's development in the womb guides you through pregnancy and birth, his verbal and physical cues and responses guide you through early parenthood. During the early weeks, your baby nurses frequently to nourish his rapidly growing body and keep up your milk supply. These round-the-clock feedings help you and your baby communicate better, and they regulate sleeping and waking patterns for you both.

Nighttime feedings are extra important. At night, breast milk is richer in important fats that the baby needs. And round-the-clock feedings maintain prolactin levels. High prolactin levels ensure excellent milk supply and decrease fertility. Many women relish the richness of these quiet nighttime feedings, when nothing distracts mother or baby from this special bonding.

> Suzanne recalls those early weeks with her baby: "If I'd known how quickly those weeks would pass and how soon those times alone with my baby's dear little face looking up to me in the dimness of the night would end, I would have treasured the privilege even more. I would have whined less, I think, when I let tiredness bother me."

Sleep Schedules

Most parents of newborns and young babies long for a solid, uninterrupted night of sleep. Their own parents may advise, "Get that baby on a schedule so you can get some sleep!" But this advice is outdated and based on research done on formula-fed babies who had schedules imposed on them. Today, things are changing for the better. More and more babies are breastfed, and many share the same bed as their parents.

The research of James McKenna, PhD, director of the Mother-Baby Behavioral Sleep Laboratory at the University of Notre Dame, sheds light on the natural, typical sleep behaviors of babies and exposes the faulty research behind sleep schedules. Outside of North America, McKenna points out, parents don't consider their baby's unique sleep patterns as unusual or bothersome—they're normal for that baby. But in North America, parents are determined to get their babies to sleep, especially at night. Many see the baby's wakefulness as a problem, rather than a natural process. Some may even judge their parenting abilities by how well the baby sleeps in the early weeks and months.

McKenna concludes there's no universal answer when it comes to babies and sleep. A solution that works for one family may not work for another. Some babies are more easygoing and less demanding than others, and every family is different, with unique practices, challenges, and needs. Parents of sensitive babies or babies who are light sleepers might assume they're to blame if the babies don't sleep soundly. Any "expert" advice or programs often make these tired parents lose confidence, become frustrated, and mistrust their intuition and common sense.[2]

If you receive advice, criticism, or disapproval when your baby doesn't sleep at night, you may be tempted to try any "solution." Remember that your baby's wakefulness isn't a problem to fix. Instead, view the times he's awake as opportunities to get to know each other. By patiently accepting these early weeks and months of interrupted sleep—and understanding they're temporary—you reduce the pressure to get sleep at scheduled times. Babies usually sense when their parents (and environments) are more relaxed, so they relax more, too.

Cosleeping

Before the late 1700s, babies and mothers around the world slept together in the same bed. Around this time, in cultures affected by the Industrial Revolution (especially in Europe and North America), baby beds were introduced to families and soon become the norm. Today, the concept of cosleeping in a family bed is controversial. Some parents strongly feel their baby is safer and healthier when sleeping in a family bed. Others believe a family bed is unnatural, unsafe, and unhealthy.

Over the last two centuries, many cultures have forgotten the benefits of cosleeping—particularly North American culture, which has long stressed independent behavior in babies at earlier ages than in other cultures. But the popularity of cosleeping is growing, as medical and anthropological research shows that cosleeping promotes bonding and breastfeeding and perhaps prevents sudden infant death syndrome (SIDS).[3]

Just as skin-to-skin contact after birth benefits both newborn and mother, such close contact during the night also helps form stronger attachments between the two. Mother and baby sleep better because cries are met faster, which tends to make a baby cry less. Research shows that when mother and baby rest together, their sleep is less disturbed.[5]

La Leche League International, a well-known breastfeeding organization, recommends cosleeping as a healthy way to feed and care for babies. James McKenna believes that babies who sleep with their mothers enjoy greater natural immunization from breastfeeding because they're free to nurse more frequently. Plus, cosleeping increases the number of night feeds, keeping prolactin levels high and delaying the onset of ovulation. The decreased fertility of breastfeeding women is dependent on keeping prolactin levels high around the clock.

When scientific studies confirm that babies benefit psychologically and physically from cosleeping, writer Jennifer Coburn wonders, "Why do parents flock to [stores] to purchase dolls that have heartbeats, sing lullabies, and snore when they can do the same for free?" She goes on to speculate that sleep disorders—rather than being part of a baby's biology—are actually created by well-intended parents who've bought into the idea of isolating a baby in a baby bed in the nursery, letting him cry himself to sleep so he learns to sleep independently. "Making one's self available by intercom is simply not meeting the nighttime needs of an infant," she writes. "It's time Americans join the rest of the world and parent our babies twenty-four hours a day."[7]

When baby and mother sleep in the same bed, their body rhythms—including breathing patterns—synchronize. Some research shows that the shared sleep patterns and body rhythms may lower the risk of sudden infant death syndrome (SIDS).[6] A mother who's physically closer to her sleeping baby may sense when he's in trouble more quickly than if he were sleeping away from her.

Many cosleeping advocates believe that parents who sleep with their babies in the same bed are more confident and relaxed, eventually leading to more confident and relaxed children. Harvard University researcher Michael Commons found that babies who sleep alone might be more susceptible to stress disorders later on, with stress hormones actually causing physical changes in the brain.[8]

Despite the benefits of cosleeping, in 1999 the Consumer Product Safety Commission (CPSC) warned that putting a baby to sleep in an adult bed could be hazardous.[9] This warning, however, didn't explain that many deaths and accidents were the result of unsupervised babies who'd gotten trapped in the bed structure. The warning also failed to point out that some accidents and deaths were the result of an adult who'd used alcohol or drugs and rolled onto or smothered the baby. Furthermore, the warning was one-sided: it didn't mention the number of deaths or accidents that occurred in babies who slept alone and away from their parents.

Pediatrician and writer William Sears says, "On one hand, it is important to remind the parents who share a bed with their babies—and there are many—that they need to take certain precautions. On the other, these reports have unnecessarily frightened the millions of parents who safely and responsibly sleep with their babies." He concludes that when science and common sense don't match, perhaps faulty science and scientific reporting is to blame.[10]

Sleeping in the same bed may not be right for every family, but there are other ways to reap the benefits of cosleeping. Bedside co-sleepers or compact infant beds are perfect alternatives when sharing the same bed doesn't work. Some bedside co-sleepers can convert into freestanding bassinets, changing tables, and play yards.

If you choose to sleep with your baby in a family bed, follow these safety guidelines:[4]

- Sleep on a flat, firm, and smooth mattress that's large enough to accommodate everyone comfortably. Don't sleep on a pillow-top mattress, waterbed, beanbag chair, or sofa.
- Make sure there isn't any space between the mattress and the bed frame or wall.
- Remove all pillows and heavy blankets during the early months. Use only a thin blanket for cover. Be very careful when adding pillows or blankets as your baby gets older.
- Don't allow pets to sleep in the family bed with your baby.
- Put your baby on her back to sleep.
- Be wary of putting your baby in a family bed if you or anyone else is physically large. If there's a large dip in the mattress or if gravity makes your baby roll toward you while lying on the bed together, consider another sleeping arrangement.
- Do not put a baby in the family bed if you or anyone has used drugs or alcohol, is seriously sleep-deprived, or is smoking in the bed.

CONTINUED BREASTFEEDING SUCCESS

Ideally, you and your baby are happily breastfeeding during the first days and weeks. However, it's not unusual for you to have some breastfeeding trouble—especially if you had a particularly rough labor and birth that led to the separation of you and your baby, who was fed formula or from a bottle.

For breastfeeding success, the instructions are simple: Keep your baby with you, respond to her feeding cues, position her so she comes "up and over" your nipple and areola, feed her at least eight to twelve times a day, and don't discourage her from feeding during the night. See pages 202–5 for more information.

Avoid giving your baby a bottle or a pacifier until breastfeeding is well established. Bottle nipples and pacifiers can cause problems with your baby's ability to suck at your breast. Plus, pacifiers can mask her early feeding cues, so she spends less time at the breast. Remember, the more time your baby spends at the breast in the first weeks, the more milk you produce.

While your body's making breast milk, remember you can eat and drink normally. There's no need to avoid spicy foods, foods that produce gas, or chocolate. Drinking caffeine and alcohol in moderation is usually just fine. You don't need to drink cow's milk to produce breast milk, and you don't need to drink gallons of water. Drink when you're thirsty and just enough to quench your thirst. It was once thought that breastfeeding women needed to drink large amounts of fluids to maintain milk supply. It was discovered, however, that women who drank fluids in excess when they weren't thirsty actually *decreased* milk production.[11]

Breast milk is the only food your baby should have for at least

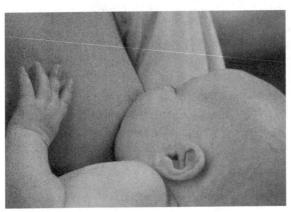

the first six months.[11] It's designed to provide all the nutrition she needs until she's ready to eat solid foods. Feeding her solids too soon only fills her with nutritionally inferior foods. Before they're six months old, most babies' digestive systems aren't developed enough to process solids effectively and safely, and many babies can't control their tongue and mouth muscles well enough to swallow solid foods safely.

Once your baby starts eating solid foods, breast milk should continue to be her main source of nutrition. The American Academy of Pediatrics recommends that babies consume breast milk for at least the first year,[13] and the World Health Organization extends this recommendation to the first two years.[14] The benefits of breastfeeding continue well beyond these recommended ages, and how long you continue to breastfeed your baby is a personal decision—one that's best made as your nursing relationship evolves. There's no need to decide early on how long you'll continue breastfeeding your child.

YOUR HEALTH

Symptoms of Emotional Distress

You've made it through forty weeks of pregnancy, with its nausea and weight gain. You've made it through the waiting and hard work of labor and birth. You now have a beautiful baby living with you—and you may be sad or depressed.

After giving birth, you'll experience emotional ups and downs. For some women, these emotional fluctuations are mild and subside within a few weeks. For others, they're overwhelming, long-lasting, and may require treatment. See page 219 to learn what's considered "normal" baby blues and what the symptoms are of postpartum mood disorders (PPMDs) and postpartum psychosis.

There's no clear scientific explanation for emotional distress after giving birth, although hormones, the environment, fatigue, and modern society have all been

> Writer Anne Lamott writes about her journey into single motherhood in her memoir *Operating Instructions: A Journal of My Son's First Year.* In it, she chronicles the familiar emotional roller coaster she rode from day to day, and night to night, as a first-time parent groping her way through the challenges of caring for her infant son. "I'm crazy tired. I feel as stressed out by exhaustion as someone who spent time in Viet Nam." Every woman has her own, specific reasons for feeling as she does, especially in the weeks after birth. Mothering magazine editor Peggy O'Mara reminds us that depression needs to be acknowledged. "Don't allow anyone, including yourself, to downplay your emotional experience."

Mothers Speak Out: What Postpartum Depression Feels Like

- *I felt overwhelmed by guilt because I wasn't happy. How could I be so sad and ungrateful with such a healthy, beautiful baby?*
- *Everything felt hopeless. I simply was not the mother that I had hoped to be for my baby.*
- *I should not be crying every day...but I am.*
- *Becoming a mother is a wonderful, amazing gift. It was terribly embarrassing for me to not feel so wonderful after having my baby.*
- *Expectations for being a new fabulous mom are high. I felt like I failed immediately and had to just keep it a secret.*
- *No one wants to admit that they have postpartum depression. I didn't. How could I actually say out loud the dark thoughts that were going on in my head about my baby, my partner, my life?*

Mothers Speak Out: What Helps

- *Finding out that how I was feeling...that postpartum depression... was normal.*
- *My husband helped to point out the signs of depression even though acknowledging it made me feel like a bad mom.*
- *I'm not sure. Other women empathized with me but no one ever really called it postpartum depression.*
- *Eventually, I sought help through counseling but I think that I waited six months too long by trying to manage it on my own. My marriage suffered because of it.*

blamed. New mothers who've experienced clinical depression before pregnancy may be more vulnerable to emotional distress. Some suggest the routine separation of newborns and mothers is a possible factor in the onset of emotional distress.

Just as having excellent support during labor can help a woman give birth confidently, having excellent postpartum support can help prevent a new mother from feeling overwhelmed and inadequate—emotions that can trigger sadness and depression if left unchecked. In many traditional cultures, family and friends care for and honor new mothers in the weeks and months after the babies' births. During this time, a new mother's only tasks are to nurse and get to know the baby. Before your baby's birth, try to find people you trust who can care for you during the days or weeks after your baby's birth. The support will better allow you to care for your baby—and better your chances of not slipping into a deep depression.

If you're feeling sad or depressed as a new mother, rather than carrying these emotions by yourself amid raging hormones and

Baby Blues

Affecting 60 to 80 percent of new mothers, baby blues are temporary and rarely last longer than a week. Signs may include:

- Crying easily
- Feeling overwhelmed
- Feeling a loss of control
- Feeling exhausted, anxious, or sad about being a parent
- Feeling a lack of confidence

Postpartum Mood Disorders (PPMDs)

PPMDs occur within the first year after giving birth and can be long-lasting and require treatment. There are four different emotional conditions with their own signs:

Postpartum Anxiety and Panic Disorder

- Shortness of breath
- Sensations of choking
- Lightheadedness
- Faintness
- Rapid heart rate
- Chest pain
- Immobilizing fear of being alone, of dying, of baby dying
- Fear of leaving home

Postpartum Obsessive-Compulsive Disorder

- Repeated, uncontrollable thoughts, speech, and rituals that interfere with normal daily living

Postpartum Depression

- Affects about 10 to 20 percent of new mothers
- Fear of leaving home inadequacy, and low self-esteem
- Loss of interest in everything
- Angry outbursts
- Thoughts of harming self or baby
- Sleeplessness
- Forgetting to eat or overeating
- Constant crying

Postpartum Posttraumatic Stress Disorder

- Flashbacks
- Recurrent nightmares
- Rage
- Extreme protectiveness
- Anxiety
- Panic attacks

Postpartum Psychosis

Postpartum psychosis is rare but serious. Its signs may include:

- Severe agitation
- Mood swings
- Depression
- Delusion

demanding newborn care, ask your midwife, doula, or caregiver for help. He or she can suggest ways to help you move into a better state of mind and body. Here's what else you can do when you feel you're headed into sadness and depression:

- Share your feelings with others.
- Eat well and don't push yourself too hard. Find some peaceful moments, perhaps on a walk by yourself or in a warm bath.
- Sleep is important and hard to come by. Think of how you can get both rest and sleep over a 24-hour period.
- Get some fresh air and sun, even if for just five or ten minutes.
- Relax your expectations. The laundry and dishes can wait. You can return phone calls and e-mails later. You need to concentrate on you and your baby now.
- Release your emotions rather than bottle them up. At times, being strong and staying controlled can do more psychological damage than letting go.
- Do something you enjoy at least once a day, even if it' just curling up with a magazine and a cup of tea. Anything you do for yourself, you're doing for your baby.
- Remember that you are not to blame if you're sad and depressed. These feelings can happen to anyone.

If your feelings of sadness and depression are not subsiding, or if you are experiencing any symptoms that point to more serious conditions, don't wait to get help. Get the help you deserve quickly.

Kathy McGrath, a social worker and childbirth educator who works with mothers with postpartum depression, has this to say about the condition: "It's real. But it doesn't reflect on your mothering ability. You are much more than this depression, but it might not feel like it. It will get better but it will take time and work."

Your Body

Many women have described their postpartum bodies with honor, humor, or horror—for example, "Earth Mother," "Mama Bod," the "meltdown." You may have heard other terms, or even thought up some of your own after seeing a woman shortly after she's given birth.

The time it takes a new mother to settle into her true postpartum shape and weight varies greatly from woman to woman. To help keep your body healthy and energized and to help keep up milk production, continue to eat a healthy, balanced diet. Keep in mind that much of your pregnancy weight will slowly but surely disappear as you breastfeed over the next several months.

Seek balance and moderation as you resume your prepregnancy activities. Don't rush your body into its postpartum shape and weight. Remember, it took

> Author Kristin Beck found that she loved her body more after her baby's birth than before she became pregnant. "Yes, I'm bigger and stretchier and jigglier...but in the meantime I made a whole other person! I stand taller now and walk with greater purpose. I'm proud of my baby body, knowing that it gave my son a comfy vessel in which to gestate and [has been] the source of all his nourishment since birth."[15]

forty weeks for your body to change during pregnancy—it'll likely take at least that long to change completely once again. Before starting a high-exertion exercise program, wait until your postpartum bleeding has stopped. Meanwhile, walk as much as you can. This gentle, invigorating activity is one that you can do with your baby, that gets you out of the house, and that helps you get back in shape.

Contrary to the messages our culture conveys to us through different media, no one body type defines beauty. Beautiful women come in all shapes and sizes. In your postpartum journey, trust your body to find its true shape and size as mother of your baby.

Your Sex Life

When, where, and how a new mother resumes her sex life varies greatly from woman to woman. Some women are physically and emotionally ready to have sex within weeks after giving birth, and some need more time. Some women and their partners may be so tired or focused on parenting a newborn that lovemaking is the last thing on their minds. Others may have trouble meshing their sexual roles with their new roles as parents. Still others may have difficulty adapting to the woman's changed body.

> Breastfeeding can decrease fertility. If you breastfeed exclusively and nurse at least once at night, you likely won't ovulate. Exclusive, round-the-clock breastfeeding is 98 percent effective in preventing pregnancy during the first six months. When your baby begins to eat solid foods, your fertility gradually returns—slowly, if you introduce solids slowly. Keep in mind, though, that breastfeeding doesn't guarantee you won't ovulate. If you're not ready for another pregnancy (and your body needs a rest between pregnancies), use common sense when having sex after your baby arrives.

Becoming lovers again after becoming parents can take time. Talk to each other, share your concerns and questions, be patient and understanding of each other, and don't hurry to resume the sexual activity you had before you became pregnant. Words and caresses can be empowering and healing—and sexy.

To help your sex life adjust to your life as a new mother, remember to eat well, get rest, and look after your physical, emotional, and relationship needs.

OTHER CONCERNS AFTER THE BABY ARRIVES

Managing Your Household

Was your kitchen counter clutter-free before the baby arrived? Is there a layer of grime on top of your refrigerator? Is your laundry piling up? Does your partner apparently not see—or care about—the stack of junk that's been growing on the coffee table for so long?

If you're someone whose home was in perfect order before your baby's birth, it probably isn't after his arrival—and that's okay. Like many, many new mothers, your priorities have shifted. Vacuuming the rug and dusting the furniture become less important. Instead, taking care of your baby's needs is first on your priority list. And this is the way it should be, as you welcome your little one into your family.

During the first few weeks, friends and relatives may give you advice or criticism on the state of your home. Their comments may make you question your ability to keep on top of things. If you can't keep a tidy home now, when your baby is small, how will you ever manage when he's older? Like unwanted advice, self-criticism can make you expend too much energy and wear yourself out over the wrong stuff, which makes you lose valuable learning and loving time with your baby.

Flash forward in your mind to a time when your newborn is now grown and moving out of your home to start adult life. Would you lament, "If only I'd kept my home cleaner and spent less time with him when he was a newborn"? Of course you wouldn't. This time with your new baby is fleeting, and it'll never be repeated. If you have to choose between getting the house in shape for Aunt Harriet's visit or rocking your baby as you listen to his sweet sounds, Aunt Harriet will just have to push aside the pile of towels to sit on your sofa. The time with your newborn is just too precious to waste, especially on housework.

However, at the very time when you least want to think about housework—and have little energy to do it—a disorganized household can overwhelm you. The best way to reduce stress in this area is to lower your expectations. Remember that you just can't do it all, and that caring for your baby, yourself, and the rest of your family is more important than having a spotless home. Another useful strategy: Analyze your household needs before your baby's birth and plan ahead to meet those needs. Putting a system in place can prevent arguments, keep your household running smoothly, and save you from managing all the details.

Deciding Whether to Return to Work

The decision of whether to return to work after having a baby is a difficult one for many new mothers. Women's decisions are driven by a wide array of financial, intellectual, and social factors. For some women, financial concerns make it impossible to stay at home and care for their babies. Other women are committed to the work that they do and look forward to combining work outside the home with mothering. Other women would prefer to stay at home but feel pressured to return to work by those who believe they should. Before your baby arrives, you may think you know your decision. But once your baby's born, you may have a change of heart. Writer and publisher Peggy O'Mara points out that a woman who's eight months pregnant can't imagine how she'll feel once the baby is born: "Some women simply never expect to be so in love with their babies."

Regardless of whether women return to work because they need to or because they want to, leaving their babies is difficult. Thanks to the Family and Medical Leave Act of 1993 (FMLA), many parents can stay home for at least a short time when they have

> **Making Stay-at-Home Parenting Work**
>
> If you (or your partner) decide to stay at home with the baby, talk to other stay-at-home parents so you know what to expect. Analyze your financial situation to see whether your family's budget can support having a stay-at-home parent. If stay-at-home parenting is possible for you, make adult interactions part of your daily schedule. Network with other stay-at-home parents, or parents who work part-time. Keep in mind that it's essential for your baby's development—and your sanity—to get out of the house and let the world stimulate you both.

Some parents balance childcare and household management with income-producing work by staggering their schedules or working at home or part-time. Here are some flexible employment options you may want to investigate:
- Sharing a full-time job with another employee (job-sharing)
- Working at a job that's designed to be part-time
- Working weekends, nights, and/or evenings
- Working flexible hours (according to your employer's and family's needs)
- Working a compressed workweek
- Seasonal work
- Substitute or backup employment
- Working odd jobs
- Working someplace where your child can accompany you
- Working at home

a new child without losing ground at work. The FMLA requires certain employers to grant an eligible employee a twelve-week unpaid leave upon the birth or adoption of a child and to restore the employee to the same or an equivalent job at the end of the leave. For more information on the FMLA, contact the nearest office of the Wage and Hour Division, listed in most directories under *U.S. Government, Department of Labor*, or visit http://www.dol.gov/esa/whd/fmla.

You may decide that when it comes to your baby's care, no one can replace you. Contrary to what you may be hearing, staying at home with your baby can be rewarding, fulfilling, exciting, and even fun, but it's definitely not easy (see page 223). The daily baby- and house-related chores and errands can be difficult to manage, as can the loss of income.

As you analyze your family's budget to see whether stay-at-home parenting is possible for you, include not only the cost of childcare, but also the cost of transportation to and from work, work clothing costs, and food costs while at work. These costs may make returning to work less cost-efficient than caring for your baby yourself. Organizations like Alternatives for Simple Living offer ways to live on less, and there are many books and websites on the subject as well. As writer Josh Hinds says, "Wealth comes in many forms, certainly not just monetary ones."

With this said, however, it may just be impossible financially for you or your partner to care for your baby full-time. You may want to consider flexible employment options (see sidebar below for more information). If both of you return to work, find and arrange suitable childcare well before your baby's birth. Formal daycare (daycare centers and home daycares) as well as informal daycare (nanny, au pair, babysitter, or a friend or relative) come with a host of challenges and concerns for you to consider, including certification documentation, safety procedures and record, and care styles, to name just a few.

Whatever childcare provider you decide to use, prepare your own interview questions, including ones that ask how the provider handles problems with sickness or behavior. Ask for references and follow up on them. Visit the sites a few times to observe how the provider and any staff members interact with children. Make at least one visit unannounced.

Each type of childcare has advantages and disadvantages. You must weigh the pros and cons of each before choosing the childcare that best ensures your baby's safety and well-being, meets your family's needs and budget, and gives you peace of mind. If you do return to work, many women find that waiting to do so until three to four months after the birth makes the transition for themselves and their babies easier.

When she became pregnant, Amy Bowan was young and just starting to climb the ranks as a technical writer for a software company. She planned to hire a nanny to care for her baby after a twelve-week maternity leave so she could return to work. "I brought home half the bacon in the family, and my career aspirations were just as important as my husband's," she said. She made all the necessary preparations for her absence at work.

After the birth, she began her nanny search, but "every time I looked at my baby, grief washed over me. The idea of leaving her, even for only twenty-four hours a week as I planned, sent me into a spiral of depression." A nanny was eventually hired, and Amy started back to work. She quickly learned that her husband would have to hand the baby over to the nanny in the mornings; she simply didn't have the heart to do it.

At work, Amy couldn't talk to others about her baby because it made her too sad. It took only a couple of weeks for her to make the choice to quit her job and care for her baby. "Didn't my baby deserve to wake up every morning knowing that someone who thought the world of her was going to spend the next twelve hours doing nothing but soak up every smile?" When she finds herself thinking about putting her career goals on hold, she's quick to respond, "I am grateful every day that I made the decision I did."

Pumping Breast Milk

If you're breastfeeding your baby, at some point you may want to have someone else feed him—whether so you can enjoy an evening on the town with your partner or so you can return to work. This means that you'll need to be able to pump your breast milk and store it. It's a challenge to continue to breastfeed when you and your baby are apart, but many women do it and do it successfully.

The longer you can put off starting to pump your milk, the better your milk supply will establish itself. Try to allow yourself at least four months before starting to pump, to get to know your baby and develop confidence in your ability to parent him. When you return to work, try to arrange for a part-time schedule for the first few weeks, if possible.

Don't even think about pumping and storing your breast milk until about two weeks before returning to work. Until then, just enjoy your baby and work on making a good milk supply. This means nursing frequently around the clock. Two weeks before your return to work, start pumping after one daytime feeding and store the milk. As the week progresses, increase pumping to after two daytime feedings. The week before your return, leave your baby with someone you trust for a short time and have that person give your baby a bottle of your breast milk.

> "Although I never liked pumping, I came to think of my trusty breast pump as the device that enabled me to return to work and stay connected to my baby. The truth is, it's hard to combine work and breastfeeding, but it can be done. And women who do so should be regarded as heroes."
>
> —Betsy

A baby almost always drinks from a bottle more willingly if someone other than his mother gives him the bottle.

When you return to work, your employer should know that women employees who continue to breastfeed take less time off because their babies get sick less often. Investigate your company's policy and attitudes, as well as your legal rights, regarding breast-feeding. Make arrangements for expressing milk during the workday, including break time; privacy; a pump (manual or electric; borrowed, rented, or bought), collection kit, and storage supplies; and a safe storage place for milk. The more comfortable the setting is where you pump, the more easily your milk can let down. Express milk a couple of times during the day at preset times, taking extra care to keep the pump and bottles clean and the milk cold.

Breastfeeding organizations like La Leche League International (see Recommended Resources) provide wonderful information for nursing mothers to help with breastfeeding problems or questions—and for employers to learn the importance of pumping breast milk at work. Most breastfeeding books offer guidelines for working and breast-feeding. Talk to women who have successfully combined working and breastfeeding. Giving your baby breast milk while separated from him helps maintain all the benefits breast milk provides—even when you're not there to give it to him.

Handling Sibling Rivalry

If you have other children, know that no two children respond the same way to the arrival of a new brother or sister. Some may find the new baby exciting and want to help with baby care. Others want nothing to do with this strange interloper. Sibling rivalry is not sur-prising, especially when an older sibling is still very young. At this age, the child won't want to share your time and affection with another child.

When your baby first comes home, your older child may suddenly demand that you hold, carry, or feed her, especially when you're busy attending to the baby. Or your child may regress to baby behavior— sucking her thumb, wetting herself, speaking baby talk. She may even act aggressively, handling the baby roughly or striking at you.

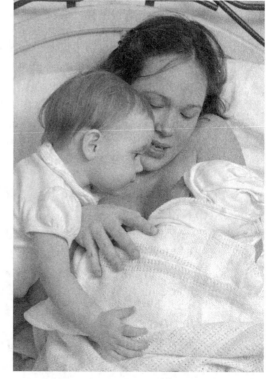

Can you prevent sibling rivalry? Preparing your child before the baby's birth is a good start. Talk about your pregnancy to your child, involving her in the birth preparations as much as possible. Read together a children's book about being a big sister or brother. Arrange to spend some time around other babies. Share photos of your child's birth and infancy so she knows how you celebrated and treasured her own first year.

When the baby comes home, here are some suggestions for keeping your older child on an even keel:

- Introduce your child to the baby as soon as possible, preferably with no other visitors present.
- Spend (and see that your partner spends) some uninterrupted one-on-one time with your child every day.
- Change your child's routine as little as possible. Make any big changes (a new bed or bedroom, a new play group, a new babysitter) several months before or after the birth.
- Listen carefully to your child's feelings about the baby and the changes in your family. Help your child put his or her feelings into words if necessary. Acknowledge negative feelings—never deny or discount them.
- Make sure your child understands that absolutely no hurting is allowed. Give your child safe ways to express negative feelings, like drawing angry pictures, acting out with dolls, or roaring like a lion.
- Baby your child if she seems to need it. Don't worry about regression, which is likely to be short-lived. Expect less independence, and you're likely to get more.
- Make sure your child has some private space and things that she doesn't have to share with the baby.
- Give your child special jobs to help the family and the baby, but don't overdo it—take your cues from your child.
- Point out the benefits of being an older child, like choosing what to eat, being able to go the park and play, and having friends.

Despite all the preparations to avoid sibling rivalry, your older child will probably act out at least once if she feels her baby sibling is hogging the limelight. You may find it difficult at times to find the flexibility and calmness to handle her, but she needs a good long hug and some loving words from you to let her know you love her just as much as ever.

Your Baby, Yourself

In the weeks and months after giving birth, you'll find yourself dealing with many firsts with your baby. His first sickness, first teething, first baffling behavior you don't feel quite equipped to handle. You'll have to make decisions on issues that you've never thought about. You'll have to figure out how to integrate your prebaby life into your postbaby life—if that's even possible.

There'll be times when you won't find answers to a pressing question or concern about your baby—not in a book or a website, not from a friend or relative. There'll be sleepless nights and times when you feel as though you're not a good enough parent.

Parenthood can be one of life's greatest challenges and, at the same time, one of life's greatest blessings. It has the potential to make you a more complete person. Parenthood helps you learn to trust your instincts and believe in your strengths.

Fred Rogers—that wise, gentle parent and TV personality who modeled a deep trust and respect for children of all ages—once said: "Please think of the children first. If you ever have anything to do with their entertainment, their food, their toys, their custody, their day or night care, their health care, their education—listen to the children, learn about them, learn from them. Think of the children first."[16]

Remember that your baby is always teaching you new things about yourself. Your role as a parent will grow and change daily—sometimes subtly; other times, dramatically. There'll be times when you feel elated, as though you're doing everything right. And there'll be times when your baby has frustrated or exhausted you beyond reason.

Be kind to yourself, especially when your parenting skills disappoint you, when you feel as if you simply have nothing more to give, or when you find yourself judging or shaming yourself. Remember that you and your baby are learning the steps of a new dance together, and you will make mistakes.

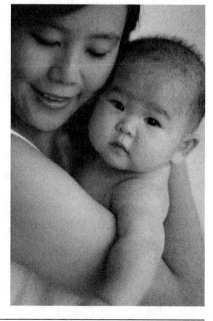

Parenting is an intense, intimate business, full of responsibilities and hard work. It's a crucial job that our world depends on for the development of confident, conscientious children who will one day follow in our footsteps. May the journey ahead with your new child be one of gentle discovery, patient giving, and boundless joy.

AFTERWORD

A baby is God's opinion
that the world should go on.
—Carl Sandburg

Charlotte's Account of Angela's Water Birth

This was Angela's first baby, and maybe because she had been a dancer in college, she simply trusted her body throughout pregnancy and birth. Angela chose midwife care, and after the reading she'd done, she decided she'd like to do a water birth.

Her due date came and went, and Angela and her midwife trusted that the baby knew when things should get started. On Sunday, a few spots of blood appeared, and that night she went to bed and slept well, despite occasional contractions and the sense of anticipation that her time was drawing near. On Monday, she felt out of sorts, contractions were coming a little more regularly, and her stomach was upset. And still she waited. Again, that night she went to bed, sleeping for a couple of hours before awakening to regular contractions a few minutes apart.

Angela and her husband packed themselves up to travel to the next town, where the hospital offered water births and her midwives practiced. She had asked a friend and me to be her doulas—women friends who would help, support, serve, and encourage her in her journey to motherhood. And so we answered the midnight call to come.

When the couple arrived in their hospital room, Angela undressed and the attending nurses asked them a few questions, checked the baby's heartbeat, and then stepped back out of the way to allow Angela to do her work.

By the time we doulas arrived in her darkened, quiet space, Angela had already stepped into the warm water of the tub. It was 3:00 A.M. and her contractions were a couple of minutes apart and regular. The midwife had been called and would make her way to the hospital in due time. Angela was in good spirits, quiet and centered and ready for the work that lay ahead. Her face was relaxed and her body buoyant in the water that protected and comforted her, so much like the amniotic fluid her baby had rocked, turned, and rested in over the past months.

By the time the midwife arrived, contractions had grown even closer and more regular. Angela moved about in the water this way and that—first on her knees, then onto her bottom, changing positions to get more comfortable as each new labor pain directed her to. She asked for drinks and an occasional cold cloth to her head as she rested in her husband's arms. We doulas kept in the background, yet close enough to offer encouragement and whatever support we were asked to give. The music that Angela had brought with her for labor played softly in the dark room. There were few questions, no references to the clock on the wall across the room, and all the while Angela shifted and breathed slowly and deeply with each contraction. A couple of times, a nurse slipped her little ultrasound instrument underwater to put it against Angela's contracting stomach and check the baby's heart rate. Angela continued her steady work uninterrupted, almost dozing between labor pains.

When she climbed out of the tub to use the toilet, the midwife did her first and only vaginal check and found that Angela was almost fully dilated. Soon after, when she was back in the water, Angela turned to me and asked, "Do you think it's time for me to begin pushing?" I knew the answer to this question! "You'll know when it's time to push," I reassured her as I put a spoonful of ice chips to her mouth, and back to her quiet work she went.

The dawn broke outside the room's windows, the shades were drawn to keep the room darkened and to protect the feeling of a safe haven. The music played on in the background, and then in the middle of a contraction Angela's breathing signaled to us that she was pushing. She knew it was time.

I slipped alongside her husband when Angela wanted another hand to grip. My friend shined a flashlight into the water, the only light in the room. The midwife stood watching the birth unfold and saw how well Angela's body was opening up with each push. "Do you want to feel your baby's head?" she asked. Angela's hand slipped out of mine, down into the water, to where the baby was beginning to crown.

There was a quiet shift change in the nursing staff, and the night nurse (very pregnant herself) asked to stay for the birth. Angela's pushing took on added strength, as she finished a contraction and announced, "This is so hard!" And we all agreed. "Yes! And you're doing such a beautiful job."

When the baby's head started to crown into the water, the midwife reached in to catch it. Angela pushed again, and the head was out; she pushed again, and the shoulders followed. The baby came into the midwife's hands, then was gently guided up through the water onto Angela's chest.

After a moment, mother and father were pleased to find out that this was the little one they planned to call Nora. The nurse checked over baby Nora as she stared up into her parents' faces.

In the days prior to her birth, Angela and I had spoken by telephone. I reminded her to think of flowers opening up and rivers flowing, and to get her arms around her husband's shoulders a lot in the days ahead. And she had. She'd been listening to one of the songs she would bring with her for the birth, a song with these wonderful words: ...*like a flower waiting to bloom, I'm waiting...*.

Angela's experience was one of patient waiting, trusting, and believing. She entered into her birth experience like a flower, just as she was designed to do. In that darkened room, there was no hint of drama, trauma, or a medical event. In that darkened room, a family event unfolded as gently as rain, as slowly and strongly as falling in love, as naturally as birth is designed to be.

Choosing the Road Less Traveled

If you're pregnant as you read these words, you're a privileged woman. *Privilege* is defined as a special right or an opportunity to do something regarded as a special honor. No matter what your income, your education, your social status, your appearance, or your circumstances, you're privileged when you do the work of growing and birthing a baby.

For you, the hard work that lies ahead isn't just coping with labor pain or pushing a baby out. The hard work is resisting the inertia of "what is" in modern birth. When you choose a natural birth because it is the safest and healthiest for you and your baby, you're choosing the road less traveled.

But it's not an untraveled road. Countless women have come to trust their bodies as they made choices about the *where, who, when,* and *what* of their births. Seek out their stories and find what you can learn from them. Midwife Ina May Gaskin says that birth stories like these share a world of wisdom, inspiration, and information: "Positive stories shared by women who have had wonderful childbirth experiences are an irreplaceable way to transmit knowledge of a woman's true capacities in pregnancy and birth."

Your own story will add to the history of strong, confident women who have approached birth as a normal, natural part of who they are. We hope the basic information we've shared in these pages has awakened your awareness of your own strength and wisdom—the strength and wisdom every woman carries.

You know what to do. You are beautifully and perfectly designed to give birth. You are not alone. May your choices, your story, your capabilities, and your strengths be an inspiration to other birthing women.

APPENDIX A

SAFE, HEALTHY BIRTH: WHAT EVERY PREGNANT WOMAN NEEDS TO KNOW

Judith A. Lothian, PhD, RN, LCCE, FACCE

Editor's Note

This article appears in The Journal of Perinatal Education, *18(3), 48–54, doi: 10.1624/105812409X461225. The author, Judith A. Lothian, is a childbirth educator in Brooklyn, New York, a member of the Lamaze International Certification Council, and the associate editor of* The Journal of Perinatal Education. *She is also an associate professor in the College of Nursing at Seton Hall University in South Orange, New Jersey.*

Abstract

In spite of technology and medical science's ability to manage complex health problems, the current maternity care environment has increased risks for healthy women and their babies. It comes as a surprise to most women that standard maternity care does not reflect best scientific evidence. In this column, evidence-based maternity care practices are discussed with an emphasis on the practices that increase safety for mother and baby, and what pregnant women need to know in order to have safe, healthy births is described.

Keywords

evidence-based maternity care, childbirth education, safe birth, healthy birth, healthy birth practices, induction, cesarean, movement in labor, labor support, routine interventions, epidural, episiotomy, intravenous in labor, nutrition during labor, maternal-infant interaction, breastfeeding, birth positions, normal birth, electronic fetal monitoring, informed decision making, choice in childbirth

Hygiene, better overall health, and antibiotics were responsible for the dramatic drop in maternal morbidity and mortality in the 20th century (Rooks, 1997). In the last half of the 20th century, advances in medicine made birth safer for high-risk women and for women with pre-existing medical conditions or serious complications in their current pregnancy. There is no scientific evidence to support that moving birth to the hospital or primary maternity care provided by obstetricians has made birth safer for healthy women with no pre-existing medical conditions (Enkin et al., 2000). Increasing evidence shows that the routine use of technology during labor and birth and the use of other routine interventions without a clear medical indication have contributed to the dramatic rise in the cesarean rate and other maternal and newborn complications, including a rise in maternal mortality in the United States (Goer, Leslie,& Romano, 2007). Each intervention interferes in often powerful ways with the process of labor and birth and increases risks for mother and baby.

A recent report published by the Milbank Memorial Fund, *Evidence-Based Maternity Care: What It Is and What It Can Achieve* (Sakala & Corry, 2008), highlights two key things: We know what makes birth safe for mothers and babies, and standard maternity care does not reflect this knowledge. The result is that birth is less safe for mothers and babies than it should be, causing harm where it could be avoided.[1]

What Every Pregnant Woman Needs to Know

Every pregnant woman needs to know that birth is intended to happen simply and easily and that six key birth practices make birth safer for mothers and babies. Every pregnant woman also needs to know that the standard maternity care is not evidence- based and, therefore, the health-care provider and place of birth will influence the care that she receives in powerful ways. Childbirth education can help women simplify pregnancy and birth and be a resource for understanding how decisions about maternity care influence the health and safety of mothers and babies.

Birth Is Intended to Happen Simply, Without Worry or Trouble

The physiologic process of birth is simply and carefully designed. Women's bodies are designed to grow, birth, and nourish babies. In the last weeks of pregnancy, a series of physiologic changes occur, mostly, as evidence suggests, orchestrated by the baby. The cervix softens and may begin to dilate and efface. The uterine muscle becomes increasingly responsive to oxytocin. At first, oxytocin levels rise gradually and, when labor starts, more quickly. The pain associated with strong uterine contractions (the result of higher levels of oxytocin) sends a signal to the brain that stimulates the ongoing release of the large amounts of oxytocin required for strong, effective contractions. Coping with the increasingly strong contractions (by movement, relaxation, and other comfort measures) insures the continued release of oxytocin.

Pain plays an important role in helping labor progress by insuring that increasing amounts of oxytocin are released. When oxytocin levels are high (and the contractions are painful), beta-endorphins ("nature's narcotic") are released. Endorphins help women manage the pain of contractions by inducing an almost dream-like state and decreasing pain perception. In a very real sense, nature does not abandon women during labor.

Stress hormones, however, disrupt the process. Especially in early labor, stress and anxiety can stop labor; in active labor, stress can slow progress. Privacy and feeling safe and protected emotionally as well as physically help keep catecholamine levels low and labor progressing.

Women begin to have an instinctive urge to push as the baby moves down the birth canal. Following the urge, quite naturally, and changing positions in response to what the woman is feeling not only helps the baby descend and rotate but also protects the baby and the birth canal. When the baby is just ready to be born, if oxytocin and endorphin levels are high, a natural release of catecholamines gives women a surge of strength to push the baby out.

The baby is born with high levels of catecholamines and endorphins and is alert and calm. Placed skin-to-skin with his mother, the baby will find the breast and self attach. Even the small movements of the baby, when skin-to-skin with his mother, stimulate the release of maternal oxytocin. Oxytocin facilitates the separation and delivery of the placenta, decreasing the risk of maternal hemorrhage, and sets the stage for efficient milk let down and successful breastfeeding. Babies kept skin-to-skin stay warmer, are less likely to become hypoglycemic, cry less, have more stable heart rates, and breastfeed for a longer duration than babies who are separated from their mother (Moore, Anderson, & Bergman, 2007).

Every pregnant woman needs to know that labor and birth are simply and beautifully designed. In order to keep labor and birth as safe as possible, and to minimize the risk of complications, it is essential to respect the simple, natural, physiologic process of labor and birth and not interfere in any way, unless there is a clear medical indication. There is an optimal way to give birth, and this is it.

Standard U.S. Maternity Care Is Not Evidence-Based

Standard maternity care in the United States is intervention intensive (Declercq, Sakala, Corry, & Applebaum, 2006), expects trouble (Strong, 2002), and does not promote, support, or protect physiologic birth (Sakala & Corry, 2008). Standard care in a hospital includes the routine use of intravenous lines, continuous electronic monitoring, epidurals, and restrictions on eating and drinking and movement (Declercq et al., 2006). Women give birth on their backs, and directed pushing is the norm (Declercq et al., 2006). None of these practices reflects the best available research (Coalition for Improving Maternity Services, 2007; Enkin et al., 2000). These interventions and restrictions make labor and birth more difficult for women by increasing stress, disrupting the hormonal orchestration of labor, and interfering with the natural, physiologic process of labor and birth. The result is unintended complications, including cesarean. The cesarean rate is now almost 32% in the United States and has been rising steadily. In some hospitals, the cesarean rate is over 50%. Most women do not know that cesarean surgery involves substantial shortterm risks for the mother and baby and long-term risks for the mother (Childbirth Connection, 2006; Coalition for Improving Maternity Services, 2007).

Every pregnant woman needs to know that maternity care that "expects trouble" actually creates trouble. Interfering in the natural, physiologic process of birth without compelling medical indication increases risks and complications for mothers and babies. What is often best for hospitals and maternity staff is not what is best for women and their babies (Sakala & Corry, 2008).

Evidence-Based Birth Practices Make Birth Healthier and Safer for Mothers and Babies

The World Health Organization identifies four care practices that promote, support, and protect normal birth (Chalmers & Porter, 2001). Lamaze International identifies two additional practices.

Together, these six practices are supported by research, including systematic reviews from The Cochrane Library and the Coalition for Improving Maternity Services (2007). Romano and Lothian (2008) provide a detailed overview of the research that supports these six care practices. Written for women and their families, the Lamaze Healthy Birth Practice papers describe the importance of each of the six practices for a healthy, safe birth and provide a synopsis of the evidence that supports each practice.[2] Every pregnant woman needs to know that these six evidence-based birth practices make birth healthier and safer for mothers and babies. Every pregnant woman needs to know that these six evidence based birth practices make birth healthier and safer for mothers and babies.

Healthy Birth Practice #1: Let Labor Begin on Its Own (Amis, 2009)

In most cases, the best way to insure that the baby is ready to be born and the mother's body is ready to birth her baby is to let labor begin on its own. In the last weeks of pregnancy, the baby moves down into the pelvis, the cervix softens, and the uterine muscle becomes more receptive to oxytocin. The baby's lungs mature, and he puts on a protective layer of fat. Every day makes a difference in how mature the baby is and how well he is able to make the transition to life outside the womb (Kamath, Todd, Glazner, Lezotte, & Lynch, 2009).

Elective labor induction not only increases the use of analgesia and epidural anesthesia but also the incidence of nonreassuring fetal heart rate patterns, shoulder dystocia, instrument delivery, and cesarean surgery (Goer et al., 2007). It isnot without risk for the baby either, increasing the need for neonatal resuscitation and increasing the likelihood of low birth weight and admission to the neonatal intensive care unit (Goer et al., 2007). Although women are told that if a baby is thought to be large it is safer to induce labor early, this is not true. Suspected macrosomia is not an indication for induction, and induction for suspected macrosomia does not reduce the incidence of shoulder dystocia and is associated with an increased risk of cesarean (Sanchez-Ramos, Bernstein, & Kaunitz, 2002).

Every pregnant woman needs to know that it is healthier and safer for both mother and baby to let labor begin on its own.

Healthy Birth Practice #2: Walk, Move Around, and Change Positions Throughout Labor (Shilling, 2009)

Moving in labor helps women cope with strong and painful contractions while gently moving the baby into the pelvis and through the birth canal. The pain of contractions can be a guide to the laboring woman as she moves in response to what she feels, trying to find comfort as the contractions become increasingly strong. Finding comfort in a variety of ways, including movement, helps labor progress. When women are able to cope with increasingly strong contractions, increasing amounts of oxytocin are released, and this keeps labor progressing. Movement in response to pain also protects the baby and the birth canal, especially during pushing. Research supports that walking, movement, and changing positions may shorten labor, are effective forms of pain relief, and are associated with fewer nonreassuring fetal heart rate patterns, fewer perineal injuries, and less blood loss. Walking during the first stage of labor decreases the likelihood of cesarean surgery and forceps and vacuum extraction deliveries (Storton, 2007).

Every pregnant woman needs to know that walking, movement, and changing positions during labor help labor progress, enhance comfort, and decrease the risk of complications

Healthy Birth Practice #3: Bring a Loved One, Friend, or Doula for Continuous Support (Green & Hotelling, 2009)

In labor, women feel better when cared for and encouraged by people they know and trust. For most women, that means family or close friends. Family and friends support the laboring woman in simple but important ways: protecting her privacy, helping her get comfortable, creating a cocoon that helps her feel safe and protected. This is especially important in the unfamiliar and often overwhelming hospital environment.

In recent years, doulas have provided continuous emotional and physical support for laboring women and their families. Doulas have the advantage of knowing labor and birth well and knowing countless ways of helping women find comfort and feel protected and safe in labor. This experience is a big advantage, especially in restrictive hospital environments. Research findings demonstrate that labor support reduces the likelihood of requesting pain medication, reduces the likelihood of having severe postpartum pain, and increases the likelihood of having a spontaneous vaginal birth. Women who have continuous labor support are more satisfied with the birth experience, have fewer cesareans, and are less likely to use Pitocin during labor (Hodnett, Gates, Hofmeyr, & Sakala, 2007; Leslie & Storton, 2007).

Every pregnant woman needs to know that continuous emotional and physical support in labor makes birth safer and healthier for mother and baby.

Healthy Birth Practice #4: Avoid Interventions That Are Not Medically Necessary (Lothian, 2009)

In most hospitals, women routinely have an intravenous line, continuous electronic fetal monitoring, and an epidural. Most hospitals also restrict eating and drinking in labor. Each of these practices has the potential to interfere with the process of labor and birth and create complications.

Intravenous lines and electronic fetal monitoring restrict women's ability to walk, change positions, and find comfort as the contractions become increasingly painful. Food and fluids are typically restricted to prevent the extraordinarily rare occurrence of aspiration if general anesthesia is required. If women are able to eat and drink in labor, there is no need for intravenous lines. No research suggests that labor and birth are safer if food and fluids are restricted and intravenous lines are in place. In fact, increasing evidence indicates that the routine use of intravenous lines may contribute to fluid overload in labor (Goer et al., 2007).

The routine use of continuous electronic fetal monitoring compared with intermittent auscultation increases the likelihood of instrument vaginal delivery and cesarean surgery but does not reduce the incidence of cerebral palsy, stillbirth, low Apgar scores, newborn death rates, or admission to the neonatal intensive care unit. In essence, the routine use of electronic fetal monitoring increases the risk of the mother having a cesarean with no difference in outcome for the baby (Goer et al., 2007).

Epidurals interfere in the process of labor and birth in important ways. Because there is no pain, the brain does not get the message to keep releasing oxytocin. Consequently, contractions need to be stimulated with Pitocin. Pitocin does not pass the blood brain barrier; therefore, the body does not know to release endorphins. Women miss out on the valuable effects of endorphins during labor. Epidural use is associated with longer labors, increased likelihood of instrument delivery, more malpositioned babies, more tearing, and an increased risk of cesarean surgery, especially if the epidural is given early in labor (Goer et al., 2007; Lieberman & O'Donoghue, 2002).

Every pregnant woman needs to know that each of these interventions has unintended effects. When interventions are used routinely, they set the stage for a cascade of other interventions, the physiologic process of labor and birth is disrupted, and women and babies are exposed to unnecessary risks.

Healthy Birth Practice #5: Avoid Giving Birth on the Back, and Follow the Body's Urges to Push (DiFranco, Romano, & Keen, 2009)

Upright positions—including squatting, sitting, or lying on the side—make it easier for the baby to descend and move through the birth canal. Changing positions helps wiggle the baby through the pelvis by enlarging pelvic diameters. It is also more comfortable to give birth in positions other than on the back. The use of upright or side-lying positions during second-stage labor is associated with a shorter duration of second-stage labor, fewer forceps or vacuum births, fewer episiotomies, fewer abnormal fetal heart rate patterns, and less chance of having severe pain during pushing (Gupta, Hofmeyr, & Smyth, 2004).

Directed pushing is more stressful for the baby and is associated with increased risk of pelvic floor dysfunction (Schaffer et al., 2006). The alternative is to wait for and follow the instinctive urges to push that happen as the baby moves down the birth canal. Even with an epidural, it is safer to wait until the baby moves through the mother's pelvis on his own. Every pregnant woman needs to know that it is safer and healthier for mother and baby when the laboring mother pushes in positions other than on her back and follows her own urges to push rather than pushing in a directed way.

Healthy Birth Practice #6: Keep Mother and Baby Together – It's Best for Mother, Baby, and Breastfeeding (Crenshaw, 2009)

Physiologically, mothers and babies are meant to be together. Mothers are less likely to hemorrhage and are more satisfied. Babies stay warmer, their heart rates are more stable, and their respirations are more regular. They are less likely to become hypoglycemic or have breastfeeding difficulties (Moore et al., 2007). The benefits are so clear that it is considered a harmful practice to separate mothers and babies unless there is a serious medical indication (Enkin et al., 2000). All the routine care of the baby right after birth can be done with the baby placed skin-to-skin with his mother.

Every pregnant woman needs to know that keeping her baby with her is not just a nice option, but keeping her baby close makes the early hours and days after birth safer for mothers and babies.

The Health-care Provider and Place of Birth Make a Difference

If the health-care provider and place of birth do not provide care that is evidence-based, healthy women are less likely to have optimal, safe, healthy births. Women need to be cared for in a place where they have privacy and feel protected and safe emotionally (not just medically). They need to be cared for by providers who respect the physiologic process of labor and birth and do not interfere unless there is a clear medical indication to do so. Women need to know that hospital and obstetrician care may not be the best way to achieve an optimal birth, and that planned out-of-hospital births (home or free-standing birthing center) are a safe option for healthy women (Enkin et al., 2000; Leslie & Romano, 2007).

Women also need to know that midwifery care is associated with longer prenatal visits, more education and prenatal counseling, and fewer hospital admissions. Women cared for by midwives are less likely to need pain medication, have more freedom of movement, and are more likely to eat and drink in labor. Women cared for by midwives are less likely to have routine interventions of any kind, have fewer complications, and are less likely to have a cesarean. In addition, there are fewer babies born preterm, with low birth weight, or with birth-related injuries when midwives provide primary care to pregnant women (Enkin et al., 2000; Leslie & Storton, 2007).

The Birth Survey[3] is a grassroots activist project of the Coalition for Improving Maternity Services. In an attempt to increase transparency in maternity care, *The Birth Survey* provides a forum for sharing information about hospitals and care providers. It is an excellent resource for information about hospital and provider intervention rates as well as women's personal experiences with individual hospitals and providers. It is an important resource that every pregnant woman should know about and use when making decisions about place of birth and provider.

Every pregnant woman needs to know that the most important way to insure a healthy, safe birth is to choose a provider and place of birth that provide evidence-based maternity care and do not interfere in the natural, physiologic process of birth unless there is a compelling medical indication to do so.

Childbirth Education Can Help Simplify Pregnancy, Birth, and Maternity Care Decisions

Childbirth education can simplify pregnancy and birth and help women navigate the maze of modern obstetrics in order to have a safe, healthy birth. Pregnancy is complex and fraught with potential for worry and confusion. It is easy to fall into the trap of thinking that things can go terribly wrong. Excellent childbirth education can help women learn how simple birth can and should be, how to stay confident in their ability to grow and birth their babies, and how to avoid "spoiling the pregnancy" with worry and fear.

Preparation for birth and mothering starts at the beginning of pregnancy (Lothian, 2008). It takes 9 months to grow a baby and to prepare emotionally and physically for birth and being a mother. Over the course of the pregnancy, women slowly attach to their babies, getting to know them through kicks and periods of rest and through changes to their own bodies as the pregnancy progresses. The physical growth of the baby happens simply and easily from one day to the next throughout pregnancy, but the emotional and psychological changes of pregnancy can easily be disrupted. Standard prenatal care and medicalized labor and birth interfere in powerful ways with nature's plan, creating fear and uncertainty when nature intends confidence and competence to develop.

Childbirth education, right from the beginning of pregnancy, can help women choose health-care providers and places of birth that provide evidence- based maternity care, make thoughtful but sometimes difficult decisions about prenatal testing, and deal with fears for themselves and their babies. And, over the course of the pregnancy, childbirth education can help women develop plans for labor so that labor and birth can unfold optimally in the safest, healthiest way possible.

Childbirth education can help women connect with excellent resources and research to help them make decisions about their pregnancies and births that ultimately will make birth healthier and safer for them and their babies. Some of those resources include Lamaze's weekly pregnancy e-mails (*Lamaze. . .Building Confidence Week by Week*[4]) and the six Lamaze Healthy Birth Practice papers. Other resources include information provided by the organizations Childbirth Connection, the Coalition for Improving Maternity Services, and Choices in Childbirth.[5]

Childbirth education provides a forum for discussing options, helping women to choose wisely and communicate effectively with care providers and hospitals. Knowing where and when there are choices, and where and when there are no realistic choices, is vital information for women wanting to have safe, healthy births. Childbirth educators can help untangle the issues and help women get a full understanding of their rights, not just to informed consent but also to informed refusal.

Evidence-Based Maternity Care: What It Is and What It Can Achieve (Sakala & Corry, 2008) is a call to action. If evidence-based maternity care is to become a reality, every pregnant woman needs to know how to have a safe, healthy birth and make decisions that reflect this knowledge. Childbirth educators, nurses, midwives, obstetricians, and hospital administrators need to "rock the boat," to speak boldly and bluntly, to honestly tell pregnant women what they need to know in order to have safe, healthy births.

Notes

1. To download or order a copy of *Evidence-Based Maternity Care: What It Is and What It Can Achieve* and to view additional resources on planning for pregnancy, labor and birth, and the postpartum period, visit the Childbirth Connection Web site (www.childbirthconnection.org).
2. To view and download each of the six Lamaze Healthy Birth Practice papers, visit the Lamaze Web site (www.lamaze.org).
3. *The Birth Survey* is structured around the Coalition for Improving Maternity Service's evidence-based 10 Steps to Mother-Friendly Care and other quality of care indicators. The purpose of *The Birth Survey* is to provide women with a venue to give feedback about their birth experiences with specific doctors, midwives, hospitals, and birth centers, and to make this feedback available on the

survey's Web site as searchable reports. For more information about *The Birth Survey*, visit http://www.thebirthsurvey.com.

4. Log on to Lamaze's Web site (www.lamaze.org) to sign up for the weekly pregnancy e-mails, *Lamaze...Building Confidence Week by Week.*

5. To learn more about making informed maternity care decisions, visit the following organizations' Web sites: Childbirth Connection (www.childbirthconnection.org), the Coalition for Improving Maternity Services (www.motherfriendly.org), Choices in Childbirth (www.choicesinchildbirth.org), and Lamaze International (www.lamaze.org).

References

Amis, D. (2009). Healthy birth practice #1: Let labor begin on its own. Washington, DC: Lamaze International.

Chalmers, B., & Porter, R. (2001). Assessing effective care in normal birth: The Bologna Score. *Birth* (Berkeley, Calif.), 28(2), 79–83.

Childbirth Connection. (2006). *What every pregnant woman needs to know about cesarean section* (2nd revised ed.). New York: Childbirth Connection. Retrieved June 13, 2009, from http://www.childbirth connection.org/article.asp?ck1/410164

Coalition for Improving Maternity Services. (2007). Evidence basis for the ten steps of mother-friendly care [Supplement issue]. *The Journal of Perinatal Education*, 16(Suppl. 1).

Crenshaw, J. (2009). Healthy birth practice #6: Keep mother and baby together – It's best for mother, baby, and breastfeeding. Washington, DC: Lamaze International.

Declercq, E. R., Sakala, C., Corry, M. P., & Applebaum, S. (2006). Listening to mothers II: Report of the second national U.S. survey of women's childbearing experiences. New York: Childbirth Connection.

DiFranco, J., Romano, A. M., & Keen, R. (2009). Healthy birth practice #5: Avoid giving birth on the back, and follow the body's urges to push. Washington, DC: Lamaze International.

Enkin, M., Keirse, M., Neilson, J., Crowther, C., Duley, L., Hodnett, E. , et al. (2000). *A Guide to Effective Care in Pregnancy and Childbirth.* New York: Oxford University Press.

Goer, H., Leslie, M. S., & Romano, A. (2007). The Coalition for Improving Maternity Services: Evidence basis for the ten steps of mother-friendly care. Step 6: Does not routinely employ practices, procedures unsupported by scientific evidence. *The Journal of Perinatal Education*, 16(Suppl.1), 32S–64S.

Green, J., & Hotelling, B. A. (2009). Healthy birth practice #3: Bring a loved one, friend, or doula for continuous support. Washington, DC: Lamaze International.

Gupta, J. K., Hofmeyr, G. J., & Smyth, R. (2004). Position in the second stage of labour for women without epidural anaesthesia. *Cochrane Database of Systematic Reviews*, Issue 4, Art. No.: CD002006.

Hodnett, E. D., Gates, S., Hofmeyr, G. J., & Sakala, C. (2007). Continuous support for women during childbirth. *Cochrane Database of Systematic Reviews*, Issue 3, Art. No.: CD003766.

Kamath, B. D., Todd, J. K., Glazner, J. E., Lezotte, D., & Lynch, A. M. (2009). Neonatal outcomes after elective cesarean delivery. *Obstetrics and Gynecology*, 113(6), 1231–1238.

Leslie, M. S., & Romano, A. (2007). The Coalition for Improving Maternity Services: Evidence basis for the ten steps of mother-friendly care. Appendix: Birth can safely take place at home and in birthing centers. *The Journal of Perinatal Education*, 16(Suppl. 1), 81S–88S.

Leslie, M. S., & Storton, S. (2007). The Coalition for Improving Maternity Services: Evidence basis for the ten steps of mother-friendly care. Step 1: Offers all birthing mothers unrestricted access to birth companions, labor support, professional midwifery care. *The Journal of Perinatal Education*, 16(Suppl. 1), 10S–19S.

Lieberman, E., & O'Donoghue, C. (2002). Unintended effects of epidural analgesia during labor: A systematic review. *American Journal of Obstetrics and Gynecology*, 186(Suppl. 5), S31–S68.

Lothian, J. A. (2008). Navigating the maze: The journey of becoming a mother. *The Journal of Perinatal Education*, 17(4), 43–47.

Lothian, J. A. (2009). Healthy birth practice #4: Avoid interventions that are not medically necessary. Washington, DC: Lamaze International.

Moore, E. R., Anderson, G. C., & Bergman, N. (2007). Early skin-to-skin contact for mothers and their healthy newborn infants. *Cochrane Database of Systematic Reviews*, Issue 3, Art. No.: CD003519.

Romano, A. M., & Lothian, J. A. (2008). Promoting, protecting and supporting normal birth: A look at the evidence. *Journal of Obstetric, Gynecologic, and Neonatal Nursing*, 37(1), 94–105.

Rooks, J. (1997). *Midwifery and Childbirth in America*. Philadelphia: Temple University Press.

Sakala, C., & Corry, M. P. (2008). *Evidence-based maternity care: What it is and what it can achieve.* New York: Milbank Memorial Fund. Retrieved June 14, 2009, from http://www.childbirthconnection.com/pdfs/ evidence-based-maternity-care.pdf

Sanchez-Ramos, L., Bernstein, S., & Kaunitz, A. M. (2002). Expectant management versus labor induction for suspected fetal macrosomia: A systematic review. *Obstetrics and Gynecology*, 100(5), 997–1002.

Schaffer, J., Bloom, S., Casey, B., McIntire, D., Nihira, M., & Leveno, K. (2006). A randomized trial of the effects of coached vs. uncoached maternal pushing during the second stage of labor on postpartum pelvic floor structure and function. *American Journal of Obstetrics and Gynecology*, 192(5), 1692–1696.

Shilling, T. (2009). Healthy birth practice #2: Walk, move around, and change positions throughout labor. Washington, DC: Lamaze International.

Storton, S. (2007). The Coalition for Improving Maternity Services: Evidence basis for the ten steps of mother-friendly care. Step 4: Provides the birthing woman with freedom of movement to walk, move, assume positions of her choice. *The Journal of Perinatal Education*, 16(Suppl. 1), 25S–27S.

Strong, T. H., Jr. (2002). *Expecting trouble: The myth of prenatal care in America.* New York: NYU Press.

APPENDIX B

THE MOTHER-FRIENDLY CHILDBIRTH INITIATIVE: THE FIRST CONSENSUS INITIATIVE OF THE COALITION FOR IMPROVING MATERNITY SERVICES

Mission

The Coalition for Improving Maternity Services (CIMS) is a coalition of individuals and national organizations with concern for the care and well-being of mothers, babies, and families. Our mission is to promote a wellness model of maternity care that will improve birth outcomes and substantially reduce costs. This evidence-based mother-, baby-, and family-friendly model focuses on prevention and wellness as the alternatives to high-cost screening, diagnosis, and treatment programs.

---

*Glossary
- *birth center*: Free-standing maternity center
- *doula*: A woman who gives continuous physical, emotional, and informational support during labor and birth—may also provide postpartum care in the home.
- *episiotomy*: Surgically cutting to widen the vaginal opening for birth.
- *induction*: Artificially starting labor.
- *morbidity*: Disease or injury.
- *perinatal*: Around the time of birth.
- *rupture of membranes*: Breaking the "bag of waters."

Preamble

Whereas:

- In spite of spending far more money per capita on maternity and newborn care than any other country, the United States falls behind most industrialized countries in perinatal* morbidity* and mortality, and maternal mortality is four times greater for African-American women than for Euro-American women;
- Midwives attend the vast majority of births in those industrialized countries with the best perinatal outcomes, yet in the United States, midwives are the principal attendants at only a small percentage of births;
- Current maternity and newborn practices that contribute to high costs and inferior outcomes include the inappropriate application of technology and routine procedures that are not based on scientific evidence;
- Increased dependence on technology has diminished confidence in women's innate ability to give birth without intervention;
- The integrity of the mother-child relationship, which begins in pregnancy, is compromised by the obstetrical treatment of mother and baby as if they were separate units with conflicting needs;
- Although breastfeeding has been scientifically shown to provide optimum health, nutritional, and developmental benefits to newborns and their mothers, only a fraction of U.S. mothers are fully breastfeeding their babies by the age of six weeks;
- The current maternity care system in the United States does not provide equal access to health care resources for women from disadvantaged population groups, women without insurance, and women whose insurance dictates caregivers or place of birth;

Therefore,

We, the undersigned members of CIMS, hereby resolve to define and promote mother-friendly maternity services in accordance with the following principles:

Principles

We believe the philosophical cornerstones of mother-friendly care to be as follows:

Normalcy of the Birthing Process

- Birth is a normal, natural, and healthy process.
- Women and babies have the inherent wisdom necessary for birth.
- Babies are aware, sensitive human beings at the time of birth, and should be acknowledged and treated as such.
- Breastfeeding provides the optimum nourishment for newborns and infants.
- Birth can safely take place in hospitals, birth centers, and homes.
- The midwifery model of care, which supports and protects the normal birth process, is the most appropriate for the majority of women during pregnancy and birth.

Empowerment

- A woman's confidence and ability to give birth and to care for her baby are enhanced or diminished by every person who gives her care, and by the environment in which she gives birth.
- A mother and baby are distinct yet interdependent during pregnancy, birth, and infancy. Their interconnectedness is vital and must be respected.
- Pregnancy, birth, and the postpartum period are milestone events in the continuum of life. These experiences profoundly affect women, babies, fathers, and families, and have important and long-lasting effects on society.

Autonomy

Every woman should have the opportunity to:
- Have a healthy and joyous birth experience for herself and her family, regardless of her age or circumstances;
- Give birth as she wishes in an environment in which she feels nurtured and secure, and her emotional well-being, privacy, and personal preferences are respected;
- Have access to the full range of options for pregnancy, birth, and nurturing her baby, and to accurate information on all available birthing sites, caregivers, and practices;
- Receive accurate and up-to-date information about the benefits and risks of all procedures, drugs, and tests suggested for use

during pregnancy, birth, and the postpartum period, with the rights to informed consent and informed refusal;

- Receive support for making informed choices about what is best for her and her baby based on her individual values and beliefs.

Do No Harm

- Interventions should not be applied routinely during pregnancy, birth, or the postpartum period. Many standard medical tests, procedures, technologies, and drugs carry risks to both mother and baby, and should be avoided in the absence of specific scientific indications for their use.
- If complications arise during pregnancy, birth, or the postpartum period, medical treatments should be evidence-based.

Responsibility

- Each caregiver is responsible for the quality of care she or he provides.
- Maternity care practice should be based not on the needs of the caregiver or provider, but solely on the needs of the mother and child.
- Each hospital and birth center is responsible for the periodic review and evaluation, according to current scientific evidence, of the effectiveness, risks, and rates of use of its medical procedures for mothers and babies.
- Society, through both its government and the public health establishment, is responsible for ensuring access to maternity services for all women, and for monitoring the quality of those services.
- Individuals are ultimately responsible for making informed choices about the health care they and their babies receive.

These principles give rise to the following steps which support, protect, and promote mother-friendly maternity services:

TEN STEPS OF THE MOTHER-FRIENDLY CHILDBIRTH INITIATIVE FOR MOTHER-FRIENDLY HOSPITALS, BIRTH CENTERS,* AND HOME BIRTH SERVICES

To receive CIMS designation as Mother-Friendly, a hospital, birth center, or home birth service must carry out the above philosophical principles by fulfilling the Ten Steps of Mother-Friendly Care:

A mother-friendly hospital, birth center, or home birth service:

1. Offers all birthing mothers:
   - Unrestricted access to the birth companions of her choice, including fathers, partners, children, family members, and friends;
   - Unrestricted access to continuous emotional and physical support from a skilled woman—for example, a doula* or labor-support professional;
   - Access to professional midwifery care.

2. Provides accurate descriptive and statistical information to the public about its practices and procedures for birth care, including measures of interventions and outcomes.

3. Provides culturally competent care—that is, care that is sensitive and responsive to the specific beliefs, values, and customs of the mother's ethnicity and religion.

4. Provides the birthing woman with the freedom to walk, move about, and assume the positions of her choice during labor and birth (unless restriction is specifically required to correct a complication), and discourages the use of the lithotomy (flat on back with legs elevated) position.

5. Has clearly defined policies and procedures for:
   - collaborating and consulting throughout the perinatal period with other maternity services, including communicating with the original caregiver when transfer from one birth site to another is necessary;
   - linking the mother and baby to appropriate community resources, including prenatal and postdischarge follow-up and breastfeeding support.

6. Does not routinely employ practices and procedures that are unsupported by scientific evidence, including but not limited to the following:
   - shaving;
   - enemas;
   - IVs (intravenous drip);
   - withholding nourishment or water;
   - early rupture of membranes*;
   - electronic fetal monitoring.

Other interventions are limited as follows:

- Has an induction* rate of 10% or less;
- Has an episiotomy* rate of 20% or less, with a goal of 5% or less;
- Has a total cesarean rate of 10% or less in community hospitals, and 15% or less in tertiary care (high-risk) hospitals;
- Has a VBAC (vaginal birth after cesarean) rate of 60% or more with a goal of 75% or more.

7. Educates staff in non-drug methods of pain relief, and does not promote the use of analgesic or anesthetic drugs not specifically required to correct a complication.

8. Encourages all mothers and families, including those with sick or premature newborns or infants with congenital problems, to touch, hold, breastfeed, and care for their babies to the extent compatible with their conditions.

9. Discourages non-religious circumcision of the newborn.

10. Strives to achieve the WHO-UNICEF "Ten Steps of the Baby-Friendly Hospital Initiative" to promote successful breastfeeding:

   1. *Have a written breastfeeding policy that is routinely communicated to all health care staff;*
   2. *Train all health care staff in skills necessary to implement this policy;*
   3. *Inform all pregnant women about the benefits and management of breastfeeding;*
   4. *Help mothers initiate breastfeeding within a half-hour of birth;*
   5. *Show mothers how to breastfeed and how to maintain lactation even if they should be separated from their infants;*
   6. *Give newborn infants no food or drink other than breast milk unless medically indicated;*
   7. *Practice rooming in: allow mothers and infants to remain together 24 hours a day;*
   8. *Encourage breastfeeding on demand;*
   9. *Give no artificial teat or pacifiers (also called dummies or soothers) to breastfeeding infants;*
   10. *Foster the establishment of breastfeeding support groups and refer mothers to them on discharge from hospitals or clinics.*

Bibliography

American Congress of Obstetricians and Gynecologists. Fetal heart rate patterns: monitoring, interpretation, and management. *Technical Bulletin* No. 207, July 1995.

—. Guidelines for vaginal delivery after a previous cesarean birth. *ACOG Committee Opinion* 1988; No 64.

Canadian Paediatric Soc, Fetus, and Newborn Committee. Neonatal circumcision revisited. *Can Med Assoc* J 1996;154(6):769-780.

Enkin M, et al. *A Guide to Effective Care in Pregnancy and Childbirth* 2nd rev ed. Oxford: Oxford University Press, 1995. (Data from this book come from the Cochrane Database of Perinatal Trials.)

Goer H. *Obstetric Myths Versus Research Realities: A Guide to the Medical Literature*. Westport, CT: Bergin and Garvey, 1995.

Bureau of Maternal and Child Health. Unity through diversity: a report on the Healthy Mothers Healthy Babies Coalition Communities of Color Leadership Roundtable. Healthy Mothers Healthy Babies, 1993. (A copy may obtained by calling (202) 821-8993 ext. 254. Dr. Marsden Wagner also provided maternal mortality statistics from official state health data.)

International Lactation Consultant Association. Position paper on infant feeding. rev 1994. Chicago: ILCA, 1994.

Klaus M, Kennell JH, and Klaus PH. *Mothering the Mother*. Menlo Park, CA: Addison-Wesley, 1993.

—. *Bonding: Building the Foundations of Secure Attachment and Independence*. Menlo Park, CA: Addison-Wesley, 1995.

Wagner M. *Pursuing the Birth Machine: The Search for Appropriate Birth Technology*. Australia: ACE Graphics, 1994. (Dr. Wagner's book has the "General Recommendations" of The WHO Fortaleza, Brazil, April, 1985 and the "Summary Report" of *The WHO Consensus Conference on Appropriate Technology Following Birth* Trieste, October, 1986.)

Ratified by these members of the Coalition for Improving Maternity Services (CIMS), July, 1996

Organizations

(Names of organizations' officers may have changed since ratification.)

Academy of Certified Birth Educators (Olathe, KS), Linda M. Herrick, RNC, BSN, CCE, CD; and Sally Riley, BSEd, CCE, CD, & Judie C. Wika, RNC, MSN, CNM, CCE, Co-Directors

American Academy of Husband-Coached Childbirth (The Bradley Method™), (Sherman Oaks, CA), Jay and Marjie Hathaway, Executive Directors

American College of Nurse-Midwives (Washington, DC), Joyce Roberts, CNM, PhD, FACNM, President

American College of Domiciliary Midwives (Palo Alto, CA), Faith Gibson, CPM, Executive Director

Association of Labor Assistants and Childbirth Educators (Cambridge, MA), Jessica L. Porter, President

Association for Pre- & Perinatal Psychology and Health (Geyserville, CA), David B. Chamberlain, PhD, President

Association of Women's Health, Obstetric, and Neonatal Nurses (Washington, DC), Joy Grohar, RNC, MS, President

Attachment Parenting International, (Nashville, TN), Lysa Parker, BS, & Barbara Nicholson, MEd, Co-Founders

Birthworks, Inc. (Medford, NJ), Cathy E. W. Daub, RPT, CCE, President

Center for Perinatal Research & Family Support (River Vale, NJ), Debra Pascali-Bonaro, Executive Director

Doulas of North America (Seattle, WA), Barbara A. Hotelling, RN, BSN, CD, FACCE, President

The Farm (Summertown, TN), Ina May Gaskin, President

Global Maternal/Child Health Association (Wilsonville, OR), Barbara Harper, RN, President

Informed Home Birth/Informed Birth & Parenting (Fair Oaks, CA), Rahima Baldwin Dancy, CPM, President

International Association of Infant Massage (Oak View, CA), Ellen Kerr, RN, BSN, MST, CIMI, President

International Childbirth Education Association (Minneapolis, MN), Cheryl Coleman, RN, BSN, ICCE, President

International Lactation Consultant Association (Raleigh, NC), Karen Kerkhoff Gromada, MSN, RN, IBCLC, President

La Leche League International (Schaumburg, IL), Carol Kolar, RN, Director of Education & Outreach
Lamaze International (formerly ASPO/Lamaze), (Washington, DC), Deborah Woolley, CNM, PhD,
    FACCE, President
Midwifery Today (Eugene, OR), Jan Tritten, TMME, Editor
Midwives Alliance of North America (Newton, KS), Ina May Gaskin, President
Midwives of Santa Cruz (Santa Cruz, CA), Roxanne Potter, CNM, Kate Bowland, CNM, Co-Directors
National Association of Childbearing Centers (Perkiomenville, PA), Susan Stapleton, MSN, CNM, President
National Association of Postpartum Care Services (Denver, CO), Gerri Levrini, RN, MSN, CNAA, President
North American Registry of Midwives (Nashville, TN), Sharon Wells, MS, LM,CPM, Coordinator
Wellness Assoc. (Ashville, NC), John W. Travis, MD, MPH, & Meryn G. Callander, ME, BSW, Co-Directors

Individuals

Sondra Abdulla-Zaimah, RN, CNM, CPM, Senegal, W. Africa
Shannon Anton, CPM, San Francisco, CA
Susanne Arms, Bayfield, CO, *Immaculate Deception*
Gini Baker, RN, MPH, IBCLC, FACCE, Escondido, CA
Maggie Bennett, LM, CPM, Seaside, CA
Brian Berman, Bainbridge Island, WA
Mary Brucker, CNM, DNSc, Dallas, TX
Raymond Castellino, DC, RPP, Santa Barbara, CA
Elena Carrillo, LCCE, FACCE, CD, Mexico City, Mexico
Robbie Davis-Floyd, PhD, Austin, TX, *Birth as an American Rite of Passage*
Henci Goer, ACCE, Sunnyvale, CA, *The Thinking Woman's Guide to a Better Birth*
Dorothy Harrison, IBCLC, Edmunds WA
Jack Heinowitz, PhD, San Diego, CA, *Pregnant Fathers*
Tina Kimmel, MSW, MPH, Berkeley, CA
Marshall Klaus, MD, Berkeley, CA, *Bonding—Building the Foundation for Secure Attachment
    and Independence*
Phyllis Klaus, CSW, MFCC, Berkeley, CA, *The Amazing Newborn*
Judith Lothian, RN, PhD, FACC, Brooklyn, NY
Susan Sobin Pease, MBA, CIMI, CMT, San Francisco, CA
Paulina G. Perez, RN, BSN, FACCE, Johnson, VT *Special Women*
James W. Prescott, PhD, San Diego, CA, *Brain Function and Malnutrition*
Mayri Sagady, RN, CNM, MSN, San Diego, CA
Karen N. Salt, CCE, Coconino Community College, Flagstaff, AZ
Irene Sandvold, DrPH, CNM, Rockville, MD
Roberta M. Scaer, MSS, Boulder, CO, *A Good Birth, A Safe Birth*
Betsy K. Schwartz, MMHS, Coconut Creek, FL
Penny Simkin, PT, Seattle, WA, *Pregnancy, Childbirth, and the Newborn*
Linda J. Smith, BSE, FACCE, Bright Future Lactation Resource Ctr., Dayton, OH
Suzanne Suarez, JD, RN, Tampa, FL
Sandy Szalay, ARNP, CCE, Seattle, WA
Marsden Wagner, MD, MSPH, Washington, DC, *Pursuing the Birth Machine*
Diony Young, Geneseo, NY

A partial list of organizations and individuals endorsing this Initiative
(for current list, see http://www.motherfriendly.org)

Organizations

Academy for Guided Imagery, Mill Valley, CA
American Holistic Nurses Association
Birth Network of Santa Cruz County, CA
The Boston Women's Health Book Collective, Boston, MA

C/Sec, Inc., Ocean City, NJ
Canadian Society for the Prevention of Cruelty to Children, Midland, Ontario
Citizens for Midwifery, Athens, GA
The Compleat Mother, Minot, ND
Doctors Opposing Circumcision, Seattle, WA
International Cesarean Awareness Network, Redondo Beach, CA
The Massachusetts Friends of Midwives, Boston, MA
Mothering Magazine, Santa Fe, NM
National Association of Parents and Professionals for Safe Alternatives in Childbirth, Marble Hill, MO
National Center for Violence Prevention, Ashland, OR
The Nurturing Parent Journal Online, Prescott, AZ
Nurses for the Rights of the Child, Santa Fe, NM
Physicians for Midwifery, Lafayette, LA
Touch the Future, Nevada City, CA

Individuals

Patch Adams, MD, *Geshundeit!*
Thomas Armstrong, PhD, *The Radiant Child*
Elizabeth N. Baldwin, JD, North Miami Beach, FL
Elisabeth Bing, RPT, FACCE, *Six Practical Lessons for an Easy Childbirth*
David Bresler, PhD, Associate Clinical Professor of Anesthesiology, UCLA School of Medicine
Elliott E. Dacher, MD, *Whole Healing*
Rae Davies, BSH, The Birth Company
Larry Dossey, MD, *Prayer is Good Medicine*
Murray W. Enkin, MD, FRCS(C), Prof. Emeritus, Depts of Ob/Gyn, Clin. Epid., & Biostatistics, McMaster Univ., *A Guide to Effective Care in Pregnancy and Childbirth*
Eunice K. M. Ernst, CNM, MPH, Mary Breckinridge Chair of Midwifery Perkiomenville, PA
Sharron S. Humenick, PhD, RN, FAAN, Editor, *Journal of Perinatal Education*
Laura Huxley, *Children Are Our Ultimate Investment*
Dorothy J. Jongeward, PhD, *Born to Win*
Risa Kaparo, PhD, California Inst. of Integral Studies
John H. Kennell, MD, *Mothering the Mother*
George Leonard, Mastery
Jean Liedloff, *The Continuum Concept*
Ashley Montagu, PhD, *Touching*
Michel Odent, MD, *Birth Reborn*
Kathy Oriel, MD, Asst. Prof, Dept Family Medicine, U. of Wisc, Madison
Jeffery J. Patterson, DO, Prof, Dept Family Medicine, U. of Wisc, Madison
Joseph Chilton Pearce, *Magical Child*
Kent Peterson, MD, *Handbook of Health Assessment Tools*
Jane Pincus, *Our Bodies, Ourselves*
Judith Rooks, CNM, MPH, MS, FACNM, *Midwifery and Childbirth in America*
Martin F. Rubin, MD, Clinical Faculty, UC San Francisco, School of Medicine, Medical Director, Sonoma County (CA) Dept of Mental Health
Regina Sara Ryan, MA, *Wellness Workbook*
Linda J. Smith, BSE, FACCE, IBCLC, Bright Future Lactation Resource Centre
Patty Stuart-Macadam, PhD, Dept. Anthropology, U. of Toronto

Help Circulate this Initiative

CIMS (pronounced "kims") is a coalition of individuals and organizations volunteering their time to make childbirth a safer, more natural experience. Please help disseminate this Initiative by giving out copies, reprinting it in newsletters, sending it to local newspapers and government representatives, mentioning it on talk shows, etc. (with complete attribution). We urge you to mail copies (or forward the

Web address) to appropriate friends and acquaintances along with a personal note requesting that they similarly forward it.

Get Free Copies of Our Publications

Copies of this document (as well as a simpler version for the general public—Having a Baby? Ten Questions to Ask) in both English and Spanish, can be downloaded at <www.motherfriendly.org>. Both are available in Acrobat Reader files (pdf) that print out compactly, as well as in "rich text format" (rtf) files that open in most word processors.

© 1996 by The Coalition for Improving Maternity Services (CIMS). Permission granted to freely reproduce in whole or in part along with complete attribution to: CIMS <www.mother-friendly.org>, <info@motherfriendly.org>

APPENDIX C

THE RIGHTS OF CHILDBEARING WOMEN (REVISED, 2004)

Childbirth Connection is a not-for-profit organization that has been dedicated to improving maternity care in the United States since 1918. This statement outlines a set of basic rights that Childbirth Connection has identified and promotes for all childbearing women. It applies widely accepted human rights to the specific situation of maternity care. Although most of these rights are granted to women in the United States by law, many women do not have knowledge of their rights.

Fundamental Problems with Maternity Care in the United States

This statement was developed in response to serious and continuing problems with maternity care in the United States, including:

- The United States is the only wealthy industrialized nation that does not guarantee access to essential health care for all pregnant women and infants. Many women, especially those with low incomes, lack access to adequate maternity care.
- A large body of scientific research shows that many widely used maternity care practices that involve risk and discomfort are of no benefit to low-risk women and infants. On the other hand, some practices that clearly offer important benefits are not widely available in U.S. hospitals.
- Many women do not receive adequate information about benefits and risks of specific procedures, drugs, tests, and treatments, or about alternatives.
- Childbearing women frequently are not aware of their legal right to make health care choices on behalf of themselves and their babies, and do not exercise this right.

We must ensure that all childbearing women have access to information and care that is based on the best scientific evidence now available, and that they understand and have opportunities to exercise their right to make health care decisions. Women whose rights are violated need access to legal or other recourse to address their grievances.

Every Woman's Rights

Consideration and respect for every woman under all circumstances is the foundation of this statement of rights.

1. Every woman has the right to health care before, during, and after pregnancy and childbirth.

2. Every woman and infant has the right to receive care that is consistent with current scientific evidence about benefits and risks.* Practices that have been found to be safe and beneficial should be used when indicated. Harmful, ineffective, or unnecessary practices should be avoided. Unproven interventions should be used only in the context of research to evaluate their effects.

3. Every woman has the right to choose a midwife or a physician as her maternity care provider. Both caregivers skilled in normal childbearing and caregivers skilled in complications are needed to ensure quality care for all.

4. Every woman has the right to choose her birth setting from the full range of safe options available in her community, on the basis of complete, objective information about benefits, risks and costs of these options.*

5. Every woman has the right to receive all or most of her maternity care from a single caregiver or a small group of caregivers, with whom she can establish a relationship. Every woman has the right to leave her maternity caregiver and select another if she becomes dissatisfied with her care.* (Only second sentence is a legal right.)

6. Every woman has the right to information about the professional identity and qualifications of those involved with her care, and to know when those involved are trainees.*

7. Every woman has the right to communicate with caregivers and receive all care in privacy, which may involve excluding nonessential personnel. She also has the right to have all personal information treated according to standards of confidentiality.*

8. Every woman has the right to receive maternity care that identifies and addresses social and behavioral factors that affect her health and that of her baby.** She should receive information to

help her take the best care of herself and her baby and have access to social services and behavioral change programs that could contribute to their health.

9. Every woman has the right to full and clear information about benefits, risks, and costs of the procedures, drugs, tests and treatments offered to her, and of all other reasonable options, including no intervention.* She should receive this information about all interventions that are likely to be offered during labor and birth well before the onset of labor.

10. Every woman has the right to accept or refuse procedures, drugs, tests and treatments, and to have her choices honored. She has the right to change her mind.* (Please note that this established legal right has been challenged in a number of recent cases.)

11. Every woman has the right to be informed if her caregivers wish to enroll her or her infant in a research study. She should receive full information about all known and possible benefits and risks of participation, and she has the right to decide whether to participate, free from coercion and without negative consequences.*

12. Every woman has the right to unrestricted access to all available records about her pregnancy, her labor, and her infant; to obtain a full copy of these records; and to receive help in understanding them, if necessary.*

13. Every woman has the right to receive maternity care that is appropriate to her cultural and religious background, and to receive information in a language in which she can communicate.*

14. Every woman has the right to have family members and friends of her choice present during all aspects of her maternity care.**

15. Every woman has the right to receive continuous social, emotional, and physical support during labor and birth from a caregiver who has been trained in labor support.**

16. Every woman has the right to receive full advance information about risks and benefits of all reasonably available methods for relieving pain during labor and birth, including methods that do not require the use of drugs. She has the right to choose which methods will be used and to change her mind at any time.*

17. Every woman has the right to freedom of movement during labor, unencumbered by tubes, wires, or other apparatus. She also has the right to give birth in the position of her choice.*

18. Every woman has the right to virtually uninterrupted contact with her newborn from the moment of birth, as long as she and her baby are healthy and do not need care that requires separation.**

19. Every woman has the right to receive complete information about the benefits of breastfeeding well in advance of labor, to refuse supplemental bottles and other actions that interfere with breastfeeding, and to have access to skilled lactation support for as long as she chooses to breastfeed.**

20. Every woman has the right to decide collaboratively with care-givers when she and her baby will leave the birth site for home, based on their condition and circumstances.**

(At this time in the United States, childbearing women are legally entitled to those rights marked with *. The legal system would probably uphold those rights marked with **.)

© 2010 Childbirth Connection

Our Sources

The following sources have helped guide the development of this statement of rights:

American Hospital Association. A Patient's Bill of Rights, revised edition approved by the AHA Board of Trustees on October 21, 1992.

Annas, G. J. A national bill of patients' rights. New England Journal of Medicine 338, (10) 695-699, 1998.

Annas, G. J. The Rights of Patients, second edition. Carbondale, IL; Southern Illinois University Press, 1989.

Boston Women's Health Book Collective. Section on "Child-bearing" and chapter on "The politics of women's health and medical care." In: Our Bodies, Ourselves for the New Century. New York: Simon & Schuster, 1998, pp. 433-543, 680-722.

Coalition for Improving Maternity Services (CIMS). The Mother-Friendly Childbirth Initiative,1996. Available at: www.motherfriendly.org

Enkin, M., Keirse, M. J. N. C., Neilson, J., Crowther, C., Duley, L., Hodnett, E., and Hofmeyr, J. A Guide to Effective Care in Pregnancy and Childbirth, third edition. New York: Oxford University Press, 2000. Available at: www.childbirthconnection.org/guide/

International Childbirth Education Association, Inc. The Pregnant Patient's Bill of Rights. Minneapolis: ICEA, 1975.

President's Advisory Commission on Consumer Protection and Quality in the Health Care Industry. Appendix A: Consumer Bill of Rights and Responsibilities.In its Final Report: Quality First: Better Health Care for All Americans. Available at: www.hcqualitycommission.gov/final/append_a.html

United Nations. Universal Declaration of Human Rights. Published by the United Nations, 1948.

Thank you to George Annas, professor and chair of Health Law at the Boston University School of Public Health, for clarifying the legal status of the individual rights.

To Order a Printed Brochure:

For a single complimentary copy of *The Rights of Childbearing Women*, please send a self-addressed stamped envelope to: Childbirth Connection, 260 Madison Avenue, 8th Floor, New York, New York 10016. For multiple copies, consult www.childbirthconnection.org/bookstore/

Appendix D

Lamaze International Position Papers

Breastfeeding is Priceless: No Substitute for Human Milk

The World Health Organization (WHO), health care associations, and government health agencies affirm the scientific evidence of the clear superiority of human milk and of the hazards of artificial milk products. The WHO and the American Academy of Pediatrics recommend that mothers exclusively breastfeed their infants for the first six months, and continue for at least a year and as long thereafter as mother and baby wish.[1]

Human milk provides optimal benefits for infants, including premature and sick newborns. Human milk is unique. Superior nutrients and beneficial substances found in human milk cannot be duplicated. Breastfeeding provides optimum health, nutritional, immunologic and developmental benefits to newborns as well as protection from postpartum complications and future disease for mothers.

A U.S. Healthy People 2010 goal is to have three-quarters of mothers initiate breastfeeding at birth, with half of them breastfeeding until at least the 5th or 6th month, and one-fourth to breastfeed their babies through the end of the first year.[2] In 2007 only four states met all five Healthy People 2010 targets for breastfeeding.[3]

Maternity Care Practices Greatly Affect Breastfeeding

Labor, birth, and postpartum practices can facilitate or discourage the initiation, establishment, and continuation of breastfeeding.[4,5,6,7]

According to the U.S. Centers for Disease Control and Prevention (CDC), many birth facilities have policies and practices that are not evidence-based and are known to interfere with breastfeeding in the early postpartum period and after discharge.[8] The World Health Organization,[9] the American Academy of Pediatrics,[10] the American Academy of Family Physicians,[11] and the Academy of Breastfeeding Medicine[12] recommend that maternity health professionals provide birth and postpartum care that is supportive of breastfeeding.

The World Health Organization has identified the following intrapartum mother-friendly childbirth practices as supportive of breastfeeding:

- minimizing routine procedures that are not supported by scientific evidence;
- minimizing invasive procedures and medications;
- providing emotional and physical support in labor;
- freedom of movement and choice of positions during labor and birth;
- staff trained in non-drug methods of pain relief and who do not promote the use of analgesics or anesthetic drugs unless required by a medical condition;
- no unnecessary induction or augmentation of labor, instrumental delivery, and cesarean section.[13]

The quality of care provided in the first 24 hours after birth is critical to the successful initiation and continuation of breastfeeding. Hospitals and birth centers which encourage and support breast-feeding are more likely to care for mothers and newborns in the following ways:

- Provide mothers with comprehensive, accurate, and culturally appropriate breastfeeding education and counseling.
- Encourage skin-to-skin contact for at least thirty minutes between mother and baby within one hour of an uncomplicated vaginal birth or within two hours for an uncomplicated cesarean birth.
- Give mothers the opportunity to breastfeed within one hour of uncomplicated vaginal birth and two hours of an uncomplicated cesarean birth.
- Encourage newborns to receive breast milk as their first feeding after both uncomplicated vaginal birth and cesarean birth.
- Perform routine newborn procedures while keeping mother and baby skin-to-skin.

- Help mothers with breastfeeding and teach parents how to recognize and respond to their baby's feeding cues.
- Encourage rooming in and help the mother to be comfortable with baby care in her own room.
- Avoid separations of healthy mothers and babies, and encourage continuous skin to skin contact. Promote as much skin to skin contact of sick babies with mothers as possible.
- Do not give pacifiers to breastfeeding newborns, or any other supplements, formula, water or glucose water to healthy babies.
- Do not give mothers discharge gift bags with formula samples or formula discount coupons.
- Provide mothers with breastfeeding support after hospital or birth center discharge. Support may include: a home visit or hospital postpartum visit, referral to local community resources, follow-up telephone contact, a breastfeeding support group, or an outpatient clinic.[14]

Benefits of Breastfeeding for Children

Enhanced Immune System and Resistance to Infections
- The infant's immune system is not fully mature until about 2 years of age. Human milk contains an abundance of white blood cells that are transferred to the child, acting to fight infections from viruses, bacteria, and intestinal parasites.
- Human milk contains factors that enhance the immune response to inoculations against polio, tetanus, diphtheria, and influenza.[15]
- Breastfeeding reduces the incidence and/or severity of several infectious diseases including respiratory tract infections, ear infections, bacterial meningitis, pneumonia, urinary tract infections, and greatly reduces the incidence of infant diarrhea.
- After the first month of life, rates of infant mortality in the U.S. are reduced by 21% in breastfed infants.
- Breastfed infants are at lower risk for sudden infant death syndrome (SIDS).[16]

Protection Against Chronic Disease

- Exclusive breastfeeding for a minimum of four months decreases the risk of Type I diabetes (insulin-dependent diabetes mellitus) for children with a family history of diabetes, and may reduce the incidence of Type 2 diabetes later in life.

- Breastfed children are less likely to suffer from some forms of childhood cancer such as Hodgkin's disease, and leukemia.
- Breastfeeding reduces the risk for obesity, high blood pressure, and high cholesterol levels later in life.[17]
- Human milk contains anti–inflammatory factors that lower the incidence of bowel diseases such as Crohn's disease and ulcerative colitis.[18]
- The incidence of asthma and eczema are lower for infants who are exclusively breastfed for at least 4 months, especially in families at high risk for allergies.[19]

Breastfeeding Premature and High-Risk Infants

- Breastfeeding and banked human milk are protective and beneficial for preterm infants.
- Hospitals and physicians should recommend human milk for premature and other high risk infants.[20]
- Breast milk lowers the premature infant's risk for gastrointestinal and infectious disease and reduces the incidence of necrotizing enterocolitis (inflammation with possible tissue death and perforation of the small intestines and colon).[21]
- Human milk enhances brainstem maturation. Compared to premature babies who receive formula, preterm infants who receive breast milk score higher on future I.Q. tests.
- Breastfeeding the premature infant reduces hospital costs and the length of hospital stay significantly.[22]

Benefits of Breastfeeding for the Mother

- Women who breastfeed benefit from an increased level of oxytocin, a hormone that stimulates uterine contractions lowering the risk for postpartum bleeding. Women recover better with less blood loss at birth.
- Exclusive breastfeeding frequently but not always delays the return of a woman's ovulation and menstruation for a variable 20 to 30 weeks or more. This provides a natural means of child spacing for many.
- Breastfeeding may enhance feelings of attachment between mother and baby.
- Breastfeeding lowers a mother's risk for developing ovarian and pre-menopausal breast cancer and heart disease, and may

decrease the risk of osteoporosis later in life. The benefits increase the longer she breastfeeds.[23]

- Breastfeeding women without a history of gestational diabetes are less likely to develop Type 2 diabetes later in life.[24]

The Cost of Not Breastfeeding

- Private and government insurers spend a minimum of $3.6 billion dollars a year to treat medical conditions and diseases that are preventable by breastfeeding.[25]
- Since children who are not breastfed have more illnesses, employers incur additional costs for increased health claims, and mothers lose more time from work to care for sick children.[26]

References

1. American Academy of Pediatrics, Committee on Breastfeeding, Breastfeeding and the Use of Human Milk, Revised, Pediatrics 115 (2005): 496-506.
2. Office of Disease Prevention and Health Promotion, U.S. Department of Health and Human Services, (2000). Healthy People 2010, Maternal, Infant, and Child Health, 16-30. Washington, D.C. Healthy People, http://www.healthypeople.gov/Document/pdf/Volume2/16MICH.pdf
3. U.S. Centers for Disease Control and Prevention, Breastfeeding-Related Maternity Practices at Hospitals and Birth Centers-United States, 2007. Morbidity and Mortality Weekly Report, (June 13, 2008): 621-625. http://www.cdc.gov/mmwr/preview/mmwrhtml/mm5723al.htm
4. U.S. Department of Health and Human Services. Office on Women's Health, (2000). HHS Blueprint for Action on Breastfeeding. Washington, D.C. Office of Women's Health
5. American Academy of Pediatrics, 2005.
6. U.S. Centers for Disease Control and Prevention. Morbidity and Mortality Weekly Report, June 13, 2008
7. World Health Organization (2003). Infant and Young Child Feeding. A Tool for assessing National Practices, Policies and Programs. Geneva: WHO. http://www.who.int/nutrition/publications/infant-feeding/inf_assess_nnpp_eng.pdf
8. U.S. Centers for Disease Control and Prevention, Morbidity and Mortality Weekly Report, June 13, 2008.
9. World Health Organization, 2003.
10. American Academy of Pediatrics, 2005.
11. American Academy of Family Physicians (2007). Family Physicians Supporting Breastfeeding, Position Paper, http://www.aafp.org/online/en/home/policy/policies/b/breastfeedingpositionpaper.printerview.html
12. Academy of Breastfeeding Medicine, ABM Protocols, (2006). Protocol 15: Analgesia and Anesthesia for the Breastfeeding Mother. http://www.bfmed.org/Resources/Protocols.aspx
13. World Health Organization, 2003.
14. U.S. Centers for Disease Control and Prevention. Scoring Explanation for the 2007 CDC Maternity Practices in Infant Nutrition and Care (mPINC) Survey. http://www.cdc.gov/breastfeeding/pdf/mPINC_Scoring_Explanation.pdf
15. U.S. Department of Health and Human Services. Office of Women's Health, (2000).
16. American Academy of Pediatrics, 2005.
17. American Academy of Pediatrics, 2005.
18. United States Breastfeeding Committee, (2002). Benefits of Breastfeeding. http://www.usbreastfeeding.org/Issue-Papers/Benefits.pdf
19. Greer FR, Sicherer SH, Burks AW, and the Committee on Nutrition and Section on Allergy and Immunology. Effects of Early Nutritional Interventions on the Development of Atopic Disease in

Infants and Children: The Role of Maternal Dietary Restriction, Breastfeeding, Timing of Introduction of Complementary Foods, and Hydrolyzed Formulas. Pediatrics 2008;121:183-191.

20. American Academy of Pediatrics, 2005.
21. Agency for Healthcare Research and Quality, Evidence Reports and Summaries, 2007.
22. United States Breastfeeding Committee, 2002.
23. United States Breastfeeding Committee, 2002.
24. Agency for Healthcare Research and Quality, Evidence Reports and Summaries, 2007.
25. U.S. Breastfeeding Committee (2002). Economics of Breastfeeding.
   http://www.usbreastfeeding.org/Issue-Papers/Economics.pdf
26. Washington Business Group on Health (March 2000). Breastfeeding Support At The Workplace, Best Practices to Promote Health and Productivity, Family Health in Brief, Issue No. 2.
   http://www.businessgrouphealth.org/pdfs/wbgh_breastfeeding_brief.pdf

For more references on breastfeeding, visit:
- US Breastfeeding Committee: www.usbreastfeeding.org
- Centers for Disease Control: www.cdc.gov/breastfeeding
- La Leche League International: www.llli.org
- International Lactation Consultant Association: www.ilca.org

This fact sheet was co-authored by Nicette Jukelevics, MA, ICCE, and Ruth Wilf, CNM, PhD.

Lamaze International Position Papers

The Risks of Cesarean Section for Mother and Baby

The information provided in this position paper has been adopted from The Coalition for Improving Maternity Services (CIMS). The Coalition for Improving Maternity Services, a United Nations recognized NGO, is a collaborative effort of numerous individuals, leading researchers, and more than 50 organizations representing over 90,000 members. Promoting a wellness model of maternity care that will improve birth outcomes and substantially reduce costs, CIMS developed the Mother-Friendly Childbirth Initiative in 1996. A consensus document that has been recognized as an important model for improving the healthcare and well being of children beginning at birth, the Mother-Friendly Childbirth Initiative has been translated into several languages and is gaining support around the world.

Introduction

Cesarean section is the most common major surgical procedure performed in the United States. Lamaze International is concerned about the dramatic increase and ongoing overuse of cesarean section. The surgical procedure poses short- and long-term health risks to mothers and infants, and a scarred uterus poses risks to all future pregnancies and deliveries. For these reasons, Lamaze International recommends that cesarean surgery be reserved for situations when potential benefits clearly outweigh potential harms. The cesarean rate can safely be less than 15 percent[84] and 11 percent or less in low-risk women giving birth for the first time,[28] yet, in 2007 the U.S. cesarean rate was 32 percent.[30] When cesarean surgery rates rise above 15 percent health outcomes for mothers and babies worsen,[5] and increasing numbers of scheduled cesareans are contributing to the rising number of late-preterm births.[2,6]

Cesarean rates have been rising for all women in the United States regardless of medical condition, age, race, or gestational age,[52] and while the number of first cesareans performed without medical indication is increasing, no evidence supports the beliefs that these elective cesareans represent maternal request cesareans or that the rise in elective first cesareans has contributed significantly to the overall increase in cesarean rates.[52] Elective first cesarean at physician request may, however, play a significant role,[39] and the rise in elective repeat surgeries, which has climbed by more than 40 percent in the last ten years, certainly does.[64] Although 70 percent of women or more who plan a vaginal birth after cesarean (VBAC) can birth vaginally and avoid the complications of repeat cesarean surgeries,[28] almost all women today have a repeat operation because most doctors and many hospitals refuse to allow VBAC.[20,35,54]

A cesarean can be a life-saving operation, and some babies would not be born vaginally under any circumstances; however, it is still major surgery. Women have a legal right to know the risks associated with their treatment and the right to accept or refuse it.[14] Lamaze International encourages childbearing women to take advantage of their rights and to find out more about the risks of cesarean section so they can make informed decisions about how they want to give birth.

What are the potential harms of cesarean surgery compared with vaginal birth? Health outcomes after a cesarean may be worse because medical problems may lead to surgery. This fact sheet, however, is based on research that determined excess harms arising from the surgery itself. In other words, women with a healthy pregnancy who have a cesarean rather than a vaginal birth are at increased risk for the following complications as are their babies:

Potential Harms to the Mother

Compared with vaginal birth, women who have a cesarean are more likely to experience:

- Accidental surgical cuts to internal organs.[53,60,72]
- Major infection.[43,48]
- Emergency hysterectomy (because of uncontrollable bleeding).[38,48,83]
- Complications from anesthesia.[28]
- Deep venous clots that can travel to the lungs (pulmonary embolism) and brain (stroke).[28,48]
- Admission to intensive care.[58]

- Readmission to the hospital for complications related to the surgery.[18,28]
- Pain that may last six months or longer after the delivery.[19] More women report problems with pain from the cesarean incision than report pain in the genital area after vaginal birth.[19]
- Adhesions, thick internal scar tissue that may cause future chronic pain, in rare cases a twisted bowel, and can complicate future abdominal or pelvic surgeries.[19]
- Endometriosis (cells from the uterine lining that grow outside of the womb) causing pain, bleeding, or both severe enough to require major surgery to remove the abnormal cells.[27]
- Appendicitis, stroke, or gallstones in the ensuing year.[18,46,47,50] Gall bladder problems and stroke may be because high-weight women and women with high blood pressure are more likely to have cesareans.
- Negative psychological consequences with unplanned cesarean. These include:
  * Poor birth experience, overall impaired mental health, and/or self-esteem.[12]
  * Feelings of being overwhelmed, frightened, or helpless during the birth.[20]
  * A sense of loss, grief, personal failure, acute trauma symptoms, posttraumatic stress, and clinical depression.[37]
  * Death.[12,22]

Potential Harms to the Baby

Compared with vaginal birth, babies born by cesarean section are more likely to experience:

- Accidental surgical cuts, sometimes severe enough to require suturing.[1,28]
- Being born late-preterm (34 to 36 weeks of pregnancy) as a result of scheduled surgery.[6]
- Complications from prematurity, including difficulties with respiration, digestion, liver function, jaundice, dehydration, infection, feeding, and regulating blood sugar levels and body temperature.[25,26] Late-preterm babies also have more immature brains,[63] and they are more likely to have learning and behavior problems at school age.[25,26]
- Respiratory complications, sometimes severe enough to require admission to a special care nursery, even in infants born at early

term (37 to 39 weeks of pregnancy).[28] Scheduling surgery after 39 completed weeks minimizes, but does not eliminate, the risk.[31,32]

- Readmission to the hospital.[25]
- Childhood development of asthma,[3,78] sensitivity to allergens,[61] or Type 1 diabetes.[11]
- Death in the first 28 days after birth.[51]

Potential Harms to Maternal Attachment and Breastfeeding

Failure to breastfeed has adverse health consequences for mothers and babies. Breastfeeding helps protect mothers against postpartum depression, Type 2 diabetes, high blood pressure, heart disease, ovarian and pre-menopausal breast cancer, and osteoporosis later in life.[36,71] Breastfeeding helps protect babies against ear infections, stomach infections, severe respiratory infections, allergies, asthma, obesity, Type 1 and Type 2 diabetes, childhood leukemia, sudden infant death syndrome (SIDS), and necrotizing enterocolitis (a severe, life-threatening intestinal infection).[15,36]

- Women who have unplanned cesareans are more likely to have difficulties forming an attachment to their babies.[23]
- Women who have cesareans are less likely to have their infants with them skin-to-skin (cradled naked against their bare chest) after the delivery.[20] Babies who have skin-to-skin contact interact more with their mothers, stay warmer, and cry less. When skin-to-skin, babies are more likely to be breastfed early and well, and to be breastfed for longer. They may also be more likely to have a good early relationship with their mothers, but the evidence for this is not as strong.[16,57]
- Women are less likely to breastfeed.[21,44]

Potential Harms to Future Pregnancies

With prior cesarean, women and their babies are more likely to experience serious complications during subsequent pregnancy and birth regardless of whether they plan repeat cesarean or vaginal birth. The likelihood of serious complications increases with each additional operation.[28]

Compared with prior vaginal birth, prior cesarean puts women at increased risk of:

- Uterine scar rupture. Planning repeat cesarean reduces the excess risk, but it is not completely protective.[8,49,55,75]
- Infertility, either voluntary (doesn't want more children) or involuntary (can't have more children).[7,12,56,70,74,79,80]
- Cesarean scar ectopic pregnancy (implantation within the cesarean scar), a condition that is life-threatening to the mother and always fatal for the embryo.[67]
- Placenta previa (placenta covers the cervix, the opening to the womb), placental abruption (placenta detaches partially or completely before the birth), and placenta accreta, (placenta grows into the uterine muscle and sometimes through the uterus, invading other organs), all of which increase the risk for severe hemorrhage and are potentially life-threatening complications for mother and baby.[17,28,85]
- Emergency hysterectomy.[42,53]
- Preterm birth and low birth weight.[6,40,65,73,76]
- A baby with congenital malformation or central nervous system injury[12] due to a poorly functioning placenta.
- Stillbirth.[28,29,40,65,76]

Cesarean Surgery and Pelvic Floor Dysfunction

Cesarean proponents claim that cesarean surgery will prevent pelvic floor dysfunction, but it offers little or no protection once healing is complete and no protection in later life.[12] Moreover, risk-free measures such as engaging in exercises to strengthen the pelvic floor or losing weight can often improve or relieve stress urinary incontinence (loss of urine with pressure on the pelvic floor such as with exercise, laughing, sneezing, or coughing).[9,12]

- Cesarean surgery does not protect against sexual problems,[4,33,41] gas or stool incontinence,[10,59] or urge urinary incontinence (loss of urine after sudden need to void).[10,13,24,62,82]
- Cesarean surgery does not protect against severe stress urinary incontinence.[62,82] As many as one more woman in six having vaginal birth may experience stress urinary incontinence of some degree, mostly minor, at six months or more after birth.[10,13,24,62,82]
- Perhaps one more woman in twenty having vaginal birth will experience symptomatic pelvic floor prolapse (muscle weakness causes the internal organs to sag downwards).[45,66,77,81] With three or more vaginal births, this number may be as high as one more woman in ten.[66] However, many other factors, including smoking,

hysterectomy, hormone replacement therapy, constipation, irritable bowel syndrome, and urinary tract infections are also associated with pelvic floor prolapse.

Cesarean Section, Care Providers and Place of Birth

To reduce the risk of cesarean surgery, Lamaze International encourages women to seek providers and hospitals with low cesarean rates (15% or less) and those that support VBAC. Women can access this data from their state health departments. They can also access hospital-specific cesarean rates and rates for other birth interventions for several states at www.thebirthsurvey.com and a listing of hospitals that do or do not support VBAC from the International Cesarean Network at http://ican-online.org/vac-ban-info.

Healthy women at low risk for complications should also know that choosing midwifery care or giving birth in a birth center or at home can lower their risk for cesarean section.[68,69] Having a doula reduces the likelihood of a cesarean as well.[34]

This fact sheet was co-authored by Henci Goer, BA and Nicette Jukelevics, MA, ICCE.
© 2010 Coalition for Improving Maternity Services. Permission granted to freely reproduce with attribution.

This fact sheet is endorsed by the following organizations (as of Feb. 2010). Academy of Certified Birth Educators, Birth Matters Virginia, BirthNet of Albany NY, BirthNetwork National, Birth Network of Santa Cruz, Birth Works International, Childbirth Connection, Choices in Childbirth, Citizens for Midwifery, DONA International, International Childbirth Education Association, Lamaze International, The Lawton and Rhea Chiles Center for Healthy Mothers and Babies, Midwives Alliance of North America, National Association of Certified Professional Midwives, North American Registry of Midwives, Perinatal Education Associates, Reading Birth and Women's Center, The Tatia Oden-French Memorial Foundation, toLabor: The Organization of Labor Assistants for Birth Options and Resources.

References:

1. Alexander, J. M., Leveno, K. J., Hauth, J., Landon, M. B., Thom, E., Spong, C. Y., et al. (2006). Fetal injury associated with cesarean delivery. Obstet Gynecol, 108(4), 885-890.
2. Analysis shows possible link between rise in c-sections and increase in late preterm birth. (12/16/08). Retrieved 11/12/09, from http://www.marchofdimes.com/aboutus/22684_48910.asp
3. Bager, P., Wohlfahrt, J., & Westergaard, T. (2008). Caesarean delivery and risk of atopy and allergic disease: Meta-analyses. Clin Exp Allergy, 38(4), 634-642.
4. Barrett, G., Peacock, J., Victor, C. R., & Manyonda, I. (2005). Cesarean section and postnatal sexual health. Birth, 32(4), 306-311.
5. Betran, A. P., Merialdi, M., Lauer, J. A., Bing-Shun, W., Thomas, J., Van Look, P., et al. (2007). Rates of caesarean section: Analysis of global, regional and national estimates. Paediatr Perinat Epidemiol, 21(2), 98-113.
6. Bettegowda, V. R., Dias, T., Davidoff, M. J., Damus, K., Callaghan, W. M., & Petrini, J. R. (2008). The relationship between cesarean delivery and gestational age among us singleton births. Clin Perinatol, 35(2), 309-323, v-vi.
7. Bhattacharya, S., Porter, M., Harrild, K., Naji, A., Mollison, J., van Teijlingen, E., et al. (2006). Absence of conception after caesarean section: Voluntary or involuntary? BJOG, 113(3), 268-275.

8. Blanchette, H., Blanchette, M., McCabe, J., & Vincent, S. (2001). Is vaginal birth after cesarean safe? Experience at a community hospital. Am J Obstet Gynecol, 184(7), 1478-1484; discussion 1484-1477.

9. Bo, K. (2009). Does pelvic floor muscle training prevent and treat urinary and fecal incontinence in pregnancy? Nat Clin Pract Urol, 6(3), 122-123.

10. Borello-France, D., Burgio, K. L., Richter, H. E., Zyczynski, H., Fitzgerald, M. P., Whitehead, W., et al. (2006). Fecal and urinary incontinence in primiparous women. Obstet Gynecol, 108(4), 863-872.

11. Cardwell, C. R., Stene, L. C., Joner, G., Cinek, O., Svensson, J., Goldacre, M. J., et al. (2008). Caesarean section is associated with an increased risk of childhood-onset type 1 diabetes mellitus: A meta-analysis of observational studies. Diabetologia, 51(5), 726-735.

12. Childbirth Connection. (2004). Harms of cesarean versus vaginal birth: A systematic review. Retrieved 4/17/2004, from http://childbirthconnection.org/article.asp?ck=10271

13. Chin, H. Y., Chen, M. C., Liu, Y. H., & Wang, K. H. (2006). Postpartum urinary incontinence: A comparison of vaginal delivery, elective, and emergent cesarean section. Int Urogynecol J Pelvic Floor Dysfunct.

14. Coalition for Improving Maternity Services. (2007). Step 2: Provides accurate, descriptive, statistical information about birth care practices. J Perinat Educ, 16(1), 20S-22S.

15. Coalition for Improving Maternity Services. (2009). Breastfeeding is priceless: There is no substitute for human milk, a cims fact sheet. Retrieved 11/12/09, from http://www.motherfriendly.org/pdf/BreastfeedingisPricelessMarch2009.pdf

16. Crenshaw, J. (2009). Healthy birth practices from lamaze international. #6: Keep mother and baby together-it's best for mother, baby, and breastfeeding. Retrieved 2009, from http://www.lamaze.org/Portals/0/carepractices/CarePractice6.pdf

17. Daltveit, A. K., Tollanes, M. C., Pihlstrom, H., & Irgens, L. M. (2008). Cesarean delivery and subsequent pregnancies. Obstet Gynecol, 111(6), 1327-1334.

18. Declercq, E., Barger, M., Cabral, H. J., Evans, S. R., Kotelchuck, M., Simon, C., et al. (2007). Maternal outcomes associated with planned primary cesarean births compared with planned vaginal births. Obstet Gynecol, 109(3), 669-677.

19. Declercq, E., Cunningham, D. K., Johnson, C., & Sakala, C. (2008). Mothers' reports of postpartum pain associated with vaginal and cesarean deliveries: Results of a national survey. Birth, 35(1), 16-24.

20. Declercq, E., Sakala, C., Corry, M. P., & Applebaum, S. (2006). Listening to mothers ii: Report of the second national u.S. Survey of women's childbearing experiences. New York: Childbirth Connection.

21. Declercq, E., Sakala, C., Corry, M. P., & Applebaum, S. (2008). New mothers speak out:. National survey results highlight women's postpartum experiences. . New York: Childbirth Connection.

22. Deneux-Tharaux, C., Carmona, E., Bouvier-Colle, M. H., & Breart, G. (2006). Postpartum maternal mortality and cesarean delivery. Obstet Gynecol, 108(3), 541-548.

23. DiMatteo, M. R., Morton, S. C., Lepper, H. S., Damush, T. M., Carney, M. F., Pearson, M., et al. (1996). Cesarean childbirth and psychosocial outcomes: A meta-analysis. Health Psychol, 15(4), 303-314.

24. Ekstrom, A., Altman, D., Wiklund, I., Larsson, C., & Andolf, E. (2008). Planned cesarean section versus planned vaginal delivery: Comparison of lower urinary tract symptoms. Int Urogynecol J Pelvic Floor Dysfunct, 19(4), 459-465.

25. Engle, W. A., & Kominiarek, M. A. (2008). Late preterm infants, early term infants, and timing of elective deliveries. Clin Perinatol, 35(2), 325-341, vi.

26. Engle, W. A., Tomashek, K. M., & Wallman, C. (2007). "Late-preterm" infants: A population at risk. Pediatrics, 120(6), 1390-1401.

27. Goer, H. (May 11, 2009). Do cesareans cause endometriosis? Why case studies and case series are canaries in the mine. Science and Sensibility, 11/12/2009, from http://www.scienceandsensibility.org/?p=147

28. Goer, H., Sagady Leslie, M., & Romano, A. (2007). Step 6: Does not routinely employ practices, procedures unsupported by scientific evidence. J Perinat Educ, 16(1), 32S-64S.

29. Gray, R., Quigley, M., Hockley, C., Kurinczuk, J., Goldacre, M., & Brocklehurst, P. (2007). Caesarean delivery and risk of stillbirth in subsequent pregnancy: A retrospective cohort study in an english population. BJOG, 114(3), 264-270.

30. Hamilton, B. E., Martin, J. A., & Ventura, S. J. (2009). Births: Preliminary data for 200. Natl Vital Stat Rep, 57(12), 1-23.

31. Hansen, A. K., Wisborg, K., Uldbjerg, N., & Henriksen, T. B. (2007). Elective caesarean section and respiratory morbidity in the term and near-term neonate. Acta Obstet Gynecol Scand, 86(4), 389-394.

32. Hansen, A. K., Wisborg, K., Uldbjerg, N., & Henriksen, T. B. (2008). Risk of respiratory morbidity in term infants delivered by elective caesarean section: Cohort study. BMJ, 336(7635), 85-87.

33. Hicks, T. L., Goodall, S. F., Quattrone, E. M., & Lydon-Rochelle, M. T. (2004). Postpartum sexual functioning and method of delivery: Summary of the evidence. J Midwifery Womens Health, 49(5), 430-436.

34. Hodnett, E., Gates, S., Hofmeyr, G., & Sakala, C. (2007). Continuous support for women during childbirth. Cochrane Database Syst Rev(3), CD003766.

35. International Cesarean Awareness Network. (Feb 20, 2009). New survey shows shrinking options for women with prior cesarean. from http://www.ican-online.org/ican-in-the-news/trouble-repeat-cesareans

36. Ip, S., Chung, M., Raman, G., Chew, P., Magula, N., DeVine, D., et al. (2007). Breastfeeding and maternal and infant health outcomes in developed countries. Evid Rep Technol Assess (Full Rep)(153), 1-186.

37. Jukelevics, N. (2008). Understanding the dangers of cesarean birth. Westport, CT: Praeger Publishers.

38. Kacmar, J., Bhimani, L., Boyd, M., Shah-Hosseini, R., & Peipert, J. (2003). Route of delivery as a risk factor for emergent peripartum hysterectomy: A case-control study. Obstet Gynecol, 102(1), 141-145.

39. Kalish, R. B., McCullough, L., Gupta, M., Thaler, H. T., & Chervenak, F. A. (2004). Intrapartum elective cesarean delivery: A previously unrecognized clinical entity. Obstet Gynecol, 103(6), 1137-1141.

40. Kennare, R., Tucker, G., Heard, A., & Chan, A. (2007). Risks of adverse outcomes in the next birth after a first cesarean delivery. Obstet Gynecol, 109(2 Pt 1), 270-276.

41. Klein, M. C., Kaczorowski, J., Firoz, T., Hubinette, M., Jorgensen, S., & Gauthier, R. (2005). A comparison of urinary and sexual outcomes in women experiencing vaginal and caesarean births. J Obstet Gynaecol Can, 27(4), 332-339.

42. Knight, M., Kurinczuk, J. J., Spark, P., & Brocklehurst, P. (2008). Cesarean delivery and peripartum hysterectomy. Obstet Gynecol, 111(1), 97-105.

43. Koroukian, S. M. (2004). Relative risk of postpartum complications in the ohio medicaid population: Vaginal versus cesarean delivery. Med Care Res Rev, 61(2), 203-224.

44. Labbok M, & Taylor E. (2008). Achieving exclusive breastfeeding in the united states. Washington D.C.: United States Breastfeeding Committee.

45. Larsson, C., Kallen, K., & Andolf, E. (2009). Cesarean section and risk of pelvic organ prolapse: A nested case-control study. Am J Obstet Gynecol, 200(3), 243 e241-244.

46. Lin, S. Y., Hu, C. J., & Lin, H. C. (2008). Increased risk of stroke in patients who undergo cesarean section delivery: A nationwide population-based study. Am J Obstet Gynecol, 198(4), 391 e391-397.

47. Liu, S., Heaman, M., Joseph, K. S., Liston, R. M., Huang, L., Sauve, R., et al. (2005). Risk of maternal postpartum readmission associated with mode of delivery. Obstet Gynecol, 105(4), 836-842.

48. Liu, S., Liston, R. M., Joseph, K. S., Heaman, M., Sauve, R., & Kramer, M. S. (2007). Maternal mortality and severe morbidity associated with low-risk planned cesarean delivery versus planned vaginal delivery at term. CMAJ, 176(4), 455-460.

49. Loebel, G., Zelop, C. M., Egan, J. F., & Wax, J. (2004). Maternal and neonatal morbidity after elective repeat cesarean delivery versus a trial of labor after previous cesarean delivery in a community teaching hospital. J Matern Fetal Neonatal Med, 15(4), 243-246.

50. Lydon-Rochelle, M., Holt, V. L., Martin, D. P., & Easterling, T. R. (2000). Association between method of delivery and maternal rehospitalization. JAMA, 283(18), 2411-2416.

51. MacDorman, M. F., Declercq, E., Menacker, F., & Malloy, M. H. (2008). Neonatal mortality for primary cesarean and vaginal births to low-risk women: Application of an "intention-to-treat" model. Birth, 35(1), 3-8.

52. MacDorman, M. F., Menacker, F., & Declercq, E. (2008). Cesarean birth in the united states: Epidemiology, trends, and outcomes. Clin Perinatol, 35(2), 293-307, v.

53. Makoha, F. W., Felimban, H. M., Fathuddien, M. A., Roomi, F., & Ghabra, T. (2004). Multiple cesarean section morbidity. Int J Gynaecol Obstet, 87(3), 227-232.

54. Martin, J. A., Hamilton, B. E., Sutton, P. D., Ventura, S. J., Menacker, F., Kirmeyer, S., et al. (2007). Births: Final data for 2005. Natl Vital Stat Rep, 56(6), 1-103.

55. McMahon, M. J., Luther, E. R., Bowes, W. A., Jr., & Olshan, A. F. (1996). Comparison of a trial of labor with an elective second cesarean section. N Engl J Med, 335(10), 689-695.

56. Mollison, J., Porter, M., Campbell, D., & Bhattacharya, S. (2005). Primary mode of delivery and subsequent pregnancy. BJOG, 112(8), 1061-1065.

57. Moore, E., Anderson, G., & Bergman, N. (2007). Early skin-to-skin contact for mothers and their healthy newborn infants. Cochrane Database Syst Rev(3), CD003519.

58. National Institute for Clinical Excellence. (April 2004). Caesarean section, clinical guideline. Retrieved 12/18/09, from http://www.nice.org.uk/nicemedia/pdf/CG013fullguideline.pdf

59. Nelson, R. L., Westercamp, M., & Furner, S. E. (2006). A systematic review of the efficacy of cesarean section in the preservation of anal continence. Dis Colon Rectum, 49(10), 1587-1595.

60. Nisenblat, V., Barak, S., Griness, O. B., Degani, S., Ohel, G., & Gonen, R. (2006). Maternal complications associated with multiple cesarean deliveries. Obstet Gynecol, 108(1), 21-26.

61. Pistiner, M., Gold, D. R., Abdulkerim, H., Hoffman, E., & Celedon, J. C. (2008). Birth by cesarean section, allergic rhinitis, and allergic sensitization among children with a parental history of atopy. J Allergy Clin Immunol, 122(2), 274-279.

62. Press, J. Z., Klein, M. C., Kaczorowski, J., Liston, R. M., & von Dadelszen, P. (2007). Does cesarean section reduce postpartum urinary incontinence? A systematic review. Birth, 34(3), 228-237.

63. Raju, T. N., Higgins, R. D., Stark, A. R., & Leveno, K. J. (2006). Optimizing care and outcome for late-preterm (near-term) infants: A summary of the workshop sponsored by the national institute of child health and human development. Pediatrics, 118(3), 1207-1214.

64. Repeat c-sections climb by more than 40 percent in 10 years. . (April 15, 2009). AHRQ News and Numbers Retrieved 11/13/09, from http://ww.ahrq.gov/new/nn/nn041509.htm

65. Richter, R., Bergmann, R. L., & Dudenhausen, J. W. (2006). Previous caesarean or vaginal delivery: Which mode is a greater risk of perinatal death at the second delivery? Eur J Obstet Gynecol Reprod Biol, 132(1), 51-57.

66. Rortveit, G., Brown, J. S., Thom, D. H., Van Den Eeden, S. K., Creasman, J. M., & Subak, L. L. (2007). Symptomatic pelvic organ prolapse: Prevalence and risk factors in a population-based, racially diverse cohort. Obstet Gynecol, 109(6), 1396-1403.

67. Rotas, M. A., Haberman, S., & Levgur, M. (2006). Cesarean scar ectopic pregnancies: Etiology, diagnosis, and management. Obstet Gynecol, 107(6), 1373-1381.

68. Sagady Leslie, M., & Romano, A. (2007). Appendix: Birth can safely take place at home and in birthing centers. J Perinat Educ, 16(1), 81S-88S.

69. Sagady Leslie, M., & Storton, S. (2007). Step 1: Offers all birthing mothers unrestricted access to birth companions, labor support, professional midwifery care. J Perinat Educ 16(1), 10S-19S.

70. Saisto, T., Ylikorkala, O., & Halmesmaki, E. (1999). Factors associated with fear of delivery in second pregnancies. Obstet Gynecol, 94(5 Pt 1), 679-682.

71. Schwarz, E. B., Ray, R. M., Stuebe, A. M., Allison, M. A., Ness, R. B., Freiberg, M. S., et al. (2009). Duration of lactation and risk factors for maternal cardiovascular disease. Obstet Gynecol, 113(5), 974-982.

72. Silver, R. M., Landon, M. B., Rouse, D. J., Leveno, K. J., Spong, C. Y., Thom, E. A., et al. (2006). Maternal morbidity associated with multiple repeat cesarean deliveries. Obstet Gynecol, 107(6), 1226-1232.

73. Smith, G. C., Pell, J. P., & Dobbie, R. (2003). Caesarean section and risk of unexplained stillbirth in subsequent pregnancy. Lancet, 362(9398), 1779-1784.

74. Smith, G. C., Wood, A. M., Pell, J. P., & Dobbie, R. (2006). First cesarean birth and subsequent fertility. Fertil Steril, 85(1), 90-95.

75. Spong, C. Y., Landon, M. B., Gilbert, S., Rouse, D. J., Leveno, K. J., Varner, M. W., et al. (2007). Risk of uterine rupture and adverse perinatal outcome at term after cesarean delivery. Obstet Gynecol, 110(4), 801-807.

76. Taylor, L. K., Simpson, J. M., Roberts, C. L., Olive, E. C., & Henderson-Smart, D. J. (2005). Risk of complications in a second pregnancy following caesarean section in the first pregnancy: A population-based study. Med J Aust, 183(10), 515-519.

77. Tegerstedt, G., Miedel, A., Maehle-Schmidt, M., Nyren, O., & Hammarstrom, M. (2006). Obstetric risk factors for symptomatic prolapse: A population-based approach. Am J Obstet Gynecol, 194(1), 75-81.

78. Thavagnanam, S., Fleming, J., Bromley, A., Shields, M. D., & Cardwell, C. R. (2008). A meta-analysis of the association between caesarean section and childhood asthma. Clin Exp Allergy, 38(4), 629-633.

79. Tollanes, M. C., Melve, K. K., Irgens, L. M., & Skjaerven, R. (2007). Reduced fertility after cesarean delivery: A maternal choice. Obstet Gynecol, 110(6), 1256-1263.

80. Tower, C. L., Strachan, B. K., & Baker, P. N. (2000). Long-term implications of caesarean section. J Obstet Gynaecol, 20(4), 365-367.

81. Uma, R., Libby, G., & Murphy, D. J. (2005). Obstetric management of a woman's first delivery and the implications for pelvic floor surgery in later life. BJOG, 112(8), 1043-1046.

82. van Brummen, H. J., Bruinse, H. W., van de Pol, G., Heintz, A. P., & van der Vaart, C. H. (2007). The effect of vaginal and cesarean delivery on lower urinary tract symptoms: What makes the difference? Int Urogynecol J Pelvic Floor Dysfunct, 18(2), 133-139.

83. Whiteman, M. K., Kuklina, E., Hillis, S. D., Jamieson, D. J., Meikle, S. F., Posner, S. F., et al. (2006). Incidence and determinants of peripartum hysterectomy. Obstet Gynecol, 108(6), 1486-1492.

84. World Health Organization. (2009). Monitoring emergency obstetric care: A handbook. France: World Health Organization.

85. Yang, Q., Wen, S. W., Oppenheimer, L., Chen, X. K., Black, D., Gao, J., et al. (2007). Association of caesarean

APPENDIX E

THE BIRTH DOULA'S CONTRIBUTION TO MODERN MATERNITY CARE

The birth of each baby has a long-lasting impact on the physical and mental health of mother, baby and family. In the twentieth century, we have witnessed vast improvements in the safety of childbirth, and now efforts to improve psychosocial outcomes are receiving greater attention.

The importance of fostering relationships between parents and infants cannot be overemphasized, since these early relationships largely determine the future of each family, and also of society as a whole. The quality of emotional care received by the mother during labor, birth, and immediately afterwards is one vital factor that can strengthen or weaken the emotional ties between mother and child.[1-4] Furthermore, when women receive continuous emotional support and physical comfort throughout childbirth, their obstetric outcomes may improve.[5-10]

Women have complex needs during childbirth. In addition to the safety of modern obstetrical care, and the love and companionship provided by their partners, women need consistent, continuous reassurance, comfort, encouragement, and respect. They need individualized care based on their circumstances and preferences. The role of the birth doula encompasses the non-clinical aspects of care during childbirth.

This paper presents the position of DONA on the desirability of the presence of a birth doula at childbirth, with references to the medical and social sciences literature. It also explains the role of the doula in relation to the woman's partner, the nurse, and medical care providers. This paper does not discuss the postpartum doula, who provides practical help, advice, and support to families in the weeks following childbirth. The postpartum doula is the subject of another DONA position paper.

Role of the Doula

In nearly every culture throughout history, women have been surrounded and cared for by other women during childbirth.[11] Artistic representations of birth throughout the world usually include at least two other women, surrounding and supporting the birthing woman. One of these women is the midwife, who is responsible for the safe passage of the mother and baby; the other woman or women are behind or beside the mother, holding and comforting her. The modern birth doula is a manifestation of the woman beside the mother.

Birth doulas are trained and experienced in childbirth, although they may or may not have given birth themselves. The doula's role is to provide physical and emotional support and assistance in gathering information for women and their partners during labor and birth. The doula offers help and advice on comfort measures such as breathing, relaxation, movement, and positioning. She also assists the woman and her partner to become informed about the course of their labor and their options. Perhaps the most crucial role of the doula is providing continuous emotional reassurance and comfort. Doulas specialize in non-medical skills and do not perform clinical tasks, such as vaginal exams or fetal heart rate monitoring. Doulas do not diagnose medical conditions, offer second opinions, or give medical advice. Most importantly, doulas do not make decisions for their clients; they do not project their own values and goals onto the laboring woman.[12]

The doula's goal is to help the woman have a safe and satisfying childbirth as the woman defines it. When a doula is present, some women feel less need for pain medications, or may postpone them until later in labor; however, many women choose or need pharmacological pain relief. It is not the role of the doula to discourage the mother from her choices. The doula helps her become informed about various options, including the risks, benefits, and accompanying precautions or interventions for safety. Doulas can help maximize the benefits of pain medications while minimizing their undesirable side effects. The comfort and reassurance offered by the doula are beneficial regardless of the use of pain medications.

The Doula and the Partner Work Together

The woman's partner (the baby's father or another loved one) is essential in providing support for the woman. A doula cannot make some of the unique contributions that the partner makes, such as a long-term commitment, intimate knowledge of the woman, and love for her and her child. The doula is there in addition to, not instead of, the partner. Ideally, the doula and the partner make the perfect support team for the woman, complementing each other's strengths.

In the 1960s, the earliest days of fathers' involvement in childbirth, the expectation was that they would be intimately involved as advisors, coaches, and decision makers for the woman. This turned out to be an unrealistic expectation for most men because they had little prior knowledge of birth or medical procedures and little confidence or desire to ask questions of medical staff. In addition, some men felt helpless and distressed over the women's pain and were not able to provide the constant reassurance and nurturing that women need. With a doula present, the pressure on the father is decreased and he can participate at his own comfort level. Fathers often feel relieved when they can rely on a doula for help; they enjoy the experience more. For those fathers who want to play an active support role, the doula assists and guides them in effective ways to help their loved ones in labor. Partners other than fathers (lovers, friends, family members) also appreciate the doula's support, reassurance, and assistance.

Doulas as Members of the Maternity Care Team

Each person involved in the care of the laboring woman contributes to her emotional well-being. However, doctors, nurses, and midwives are primarily responsible for the health and well-being of the mother and baby. Medical care providers must assess the condition of the mother and fetus, diagnose and treat complications as they arise, and focus on a safe delivery of the baby. These priorities rightly take precedence over the non-medical psychosocial needs of laboring women. The doula helps ensure that these needs are met while enhancing communication and understanding between the woman or couple and the staff. Many doctors, midwives and nurses appreciate the extra attention given to their patients and the greater satisfaction expressed by women who were assisted by a doula.[17]

Research Findings

In the late 1970s, when Drs. John Kennell and Marshall Klaus investigated ways to enhance maternal-infant bonding, they found almost accidentally that introducing a doula into the labor room not only improved the bond between mother and infant, but also seemed to decrease the incidence of complications.[6,7] Since their original studies, published in 1980 and 1986, numerous scientific trials have been conducted in many countries, comparing usual care with usual care plus a doula.

The table below summarizes the findings of North American trials and a meta-analysis of all trials of continuous labor support.[12] Obstetric outcomes were most improved and intervention rates most dramatically lowered by doulas in settings where the women had no loved ones present, the intervention rates were routinely high (as indicated by the data for the control groups), and the doulas were not healthcare professionals.

Services and Costs

There are two basic types of doula services: independent doula practices and hospital/agency doula programs. Independent doulas are employed directly by the parents. They usually have telephone contact and one or more prenatal meetings with their clients to establish a relationship. When labor begins, the doula arrives and stays with the woman until after the birth. A postpartum meeting to process the birth is usually included in the doula's service. Most

---

Labor Support Terminology
The terminology describing labor support can be confusing. When a person uses any of the terms below to describe herself, she may need to clarify what she means by the term.
- *doula*: a Greek word meaning "a woman who serves." In labor support terminology, *doula* refers to a specially trained birth companion (not a friend or loved one) who provides labor support. She performs no clinical tasks. *Doula* also refers to lay women who are trained or experienced in providing postpartum care (mother and newborn care, breastfeeding support and advice, cooking, child care, errands, and light cleaning) for the new family. To distinguish between the two types of doulas, the terms *birth doulas* and *postpartum doulas* are used.
- *monitrice*: a French word originally used by Fernand Lamaze to refer to a specially trained nurse or midwife who provides nursing care and assessment in addition to labor support. Today, *monitrice* is often used as a synonym for *birth assistant* or *labor assistant*.
- *labor support professional, labor support specialist, labor companion*: synonyms for *birth doula*.
- *birth assistant, labor assistant*: sometimes these terms are used as synonyms for *doula*, but also may refer to lay women who are trained to assist a midwife (vaginal exams, set up for birth, fetal heart checks, and so on) as well as to provide some labor support.

---

doulas charge a flat fee for their services, and many base their fees on a sliding scale.

Some doula programs are associated with or administered by a hospital or community service agency. The doulas may be volunteers or paid employees of the hospital or agency. These programs vary widely in their design. In some, the hospital or agency contracts with an independent community-based doula group to provide the doulas. Others train and employ their own staff of doulas. Payment of the doula may come from the institution, the client, or it may be shared by the two. Some hospital/agency services are set up as on-call doula services. A rotating call schedule ensures that there are one or more doulas available at all times. They meet the client for the first time and establish their relationship during labor.

Other hospital/agency doula programs make doula services available to expectant mothers or couples, who may meet and choose their doula, or have one assigned to them, along with a backup doula. They may work with their doula in much the same way that private doulas and clients work together.

Over twenty-five insurance companies have provided variable third-party reimbursement for labor support. Grant funding is also occasionally available, and some Medicaid-funded health agencies have contracts with doula organizations to support women in poverty and women with special needs. Although some health insurance and flex pay plans pay for doulas, at present doula care is usually paid for directly by the client.

Training and Certification of Doulas

Doula training focuses on the emotional needs of women in labor, and non-medical physical and emotional comfort measures. The programs require that participants have some prior knowledge, training, and experience relating to childbirth, and consists of an intensive two- or three-day seminar, including hands-on practice of such skills as relaxation, breathing, positioning and movements to reduce pain and enhance labor progress, massage, and other comfort measures.

For certification, the doula must have a background of work and education in the maternity field, or observation of a series of childbirth classes; a doula training course offered by a DONA-Approved Doula Trainer; background reading; and an essay that demonstrates understanding of the integral concepts of labor support. Positive evaluations from clients, doctors or midwives, and nurses are also required along with detailed observations and essays from a minimum of three births.

Summary and Conclusion

In summary, the doula is emerging as a positive contribution to the care of women in labor. By attending to the women's emotional needs, some obstetric outcomes are improved. Just as importantly, early mother-infant relationships and breastfeeding are enhanced. Women's satisfaction with their birth experiences and even their self-esteem appears to improve when a doula has assisted them through childbirth.

Analysis of the numerous scientific trials of labor support led the prestigious scientific group, The Cochrane Collaboration's Pregnancy and Childbirth Group in Oxford, England to state: "Given the clear

---

Questions to Ask a Doula

To discover the specific training, experience, and services offered by a birth doula, potential clients, nursing supervisors, physicians, midwives, and others should ask the following questions of that person.

- What training have you had? (If a doula is certified, you might consider checking with the organization)
- Tell me about your experience with birth, personally and as a doula.
- What is your philosophy about childbirth and supporting women and their partners through labor?
- May we meet to discuss our birth plans and the role you will play in supporting me through childbirth?
- May we call you with questions or concerns before and after the birth?
- When do you try to join women in labor? Do you come to our home or meet us at the hospital?
- Do you meet with us after the birth to review the labor and answer questions?
- Do you work with one or more backup doulas for times when you are not available?
- May we meet them?
- What are your fees and your refund policies?

---

benefits and no known risks associated with intrapartum support, every effort should be made to ensure that all labouring women receive support, not only from those close to them but also from specially trained caregivers. This support should include continuous presence, the provision of hands-on comfort, and encouragement."[15]

Outcomes of Labor Support Studies in North America

Table 1: Results of 7 North American trials of labor support including 2,259 women (comparing continuous labor support by doulas with "usual care")

Author, Year (# Subjects)	Cesarean Rate	Oxytocin Use	Epidural Rate	Narcotic Use	Instrumental Delivery	Maternal Emotional Distress	5 min. Apgar <7 NICU
Cogan13, 1988 (25)	n.a.	no diff.	n.a.	decrease	n.a.	n.a.	decrease
Hodnett14, 1989 (103)	no diff.	increase	n.a.	decrease	no diff.	n.a.	n.a.
Kennell7, 1991 (616)	decrease	decrease	decrease	no diff.	decrease	n.a.	decrease
Kennell8, 1993 (570)	decrease	n.a.	no diff.	n.a.	n.a.	n.a.	n.a.
Gordon15, 1999 (314)	no diff.	no diff.	decrease	no diff.	no diff.	decrease	n.a.
McGrath9, 1999 (531)	decrease	decrease	decrease	decrease	no diff.	n.a.	n.a.
Trueba16, 2000 (100)	decrease	decrease	decrease	n.a.	n.a.	n.a.	n.a.

Key
- no diff.: no statistically significant difference between groups
- n.a.: not assessed
- increase: statistically significant increase in the supported group
- decrease: statistically significant decrease in the supported group

The results of 3 North American trials[3,18,19] including 8,052 women (comparing continuous labor support by NURSES – not doulas – with usual care) showed no differences in any outcomes listed in Table 1.

Findings of Hodnett's et al meta-analysis of 15 trials of continuous labor support from North America, Europe, and Africa10 Women cared for during labor by a birth doula, compared to those receiving "usual care" were:
- 26% less likely to give birth by cesarean section
- 41% less likely to give birth with a vacuum extractor of forceps
- 28% less likely to use any analgesia or anesthesia
- 33% less likely to be dissatisfied or to negatively rate their birth experience

References

1. Hofmeyr J, Nikodem VC, Wolman WL, Chalmers BE, Kramer T. "Companionship to modify the clinical birth environment: effects on progress and perceptions of labour, and breastfeeding," Br J Obstet Gynaecol, 98:756–764, 1991.
2. Wolman WL, Chalmers B, Hofmeyr J. Nikodem VC. "Postpartum depression and companionship in the clinical birth environment: a randomized, controlled study," Am J Obstet Gynecol, 168:1388–1393, 1993.
3. Langer A, Campero L, Garcia C, Reynoso S. "Effects of psychosocial support during labour and childbirth on breast feeding, medical interventions, and mothers' well-being in a Mexican public hospital: a randomised clinical trial." Br J Obstet Gynaecol, 105:1056–1063, 1998.

4. Martin S, Landry S, Steelman L, Kennell JH, McGrath S. "The effect of doula support during labor on mother-infant interaction at 2 months," Infant Behav Devel, 21:556, 1998.

5. Sosa R, Kennell JH, Klaus MH, Robertson S, Urrutia J. "The effect of a supportive companion on perinatal problems, length of labor, and mother-infant interaction," N Engl J Med, 303:597–600, 1980.

6. Klaus MH, Kennell JH, Robertson SS, Sosa R. "Effects of social support during parturition on maternal and infant morbidity," Br Med J, 293:585–587, 1986.

7. Kennell JH, Klaus MH, McGrath SK, Robertson S, Hinkley C. "Continuous emotional support during labor in a US hospital: a randomized controlled trial," JAMA, 265:2197–2201, 1991.

8. Kennell JH, McGrath SK "Labor support by a doula for middle-income couples; the effect on cesarean rates," Pediatric Res, 32:12A, 1993.

9. McGrath SK, Kennell JH, "Induction of labor and doula support," Pediatric Res, 43(4):Part II, 14A, 1998.

10. Hodnett E, Gates S, Hofmeyr G, Sakala C. Continuous support for women during childbirth. The Cochrane Database of Systematic Reviews 2003. Issue 3, Art. No. CD003766. DOI: 10.1002/14651858.CD003766.

11. Ashford JI. George Engelmann and Primitive Birth. Janet Isaacs Ashford, Solana Beach, CA, 1988.

12. Doulas of North America, Code of Ethics and Standards of Practice, DONA, Jasper, IN, 1992.

13. Cogan R, Spinnato JA. "Social support during premature labor: effects on labor and the newborn," J Psychosom Obstet Gynaecol, 8:209–216, 1988.

14. Hodnett ED, Osborn RW. "Effects of continuous intrapartum professional support on childbirth outcomes," Res Nurs Health, 12:289–297, 1989.

15. Gordon NP, Walton D, McAdam E, Derman J, Gallitero G, Garrett L. "Effects of providing hospital-based doulas in health maintenance organization hospitals." Obstet Gynecol, 93(3):422–426, 1999.

16. Trueba G, Contreras C, Velazco M, Lara E, Martinez H. Alternative strategy to decrease cesarean section: support by doulas during labor. J Perinat Educ, 9:1–6, 2000.

17. Gilliland AL. "Commentary: nurses, doulas, and childbirth educators," J Perinatal Ed, 7:18–24, 1998.

18. GagnonA, Waghorn K, Covell C. A randomized trail of one-to-one nurse support of women in labor. birth, 24:7180. 1997.

19. Hodnett E, Lowe N, Hannah M, Willan A, Stevens B, Weston J et al. Effectiveness of nurses as providers of labor support in North American hospitals: A randomized controlled trial. JAMA 288:1474–81, 2002.

This paper was written by Penny Simkin and Kelli Way, and reviewed and edited by Connie Livingston, Director of Publications, and the 1998 DONA Board of Directors. The second edition was revised and updated by Penny Simkin, Debbie Young, Director of Publications, and the 2005 DONA Board of Directors.

For more information about doulas, contact:
DONA International
888-788-DONA
http://www.DONA.org

To purchase copies of this paper, contact DONA at the number above or order them on-line in the Doula Boutique on the DONA website at http://www.DONA.org.

NOTES

Preface

1. Sakala, C. and M. Corry. (2008). *Evidence-Based Maternity Care: What It Is and What It Can Achieve*. New York: Milbank Memorial Fund.

Chapter 1: Having a Safe, Healthy Birth

1. World Health Organization Department of Reproductive Health and Research. (1999) "Care in Normal Birth: A Practical Guide." Geneva: World Health Organization, 3.2.

2. Sakala, C. and M. Corry. (2008). *Evidence-Based Maternity Care: What It Is and What It Can Achieve*. New York: Milbank Memorial Fund.

3. Declercq, E., andet al. (2006) *Listening to Mothers II: Report of the Second National U.S. Survey of Women's Childbearing Experiences*. New York: Childbirth Connection.

4. National Center for Health Statistics, Centers for Disease Control and Prevention, Hyattsville, Md 20782; 301-458-4000, http://www.cdc.gov/nchs.

5. Enkin, M., et al. (2000) *A Guide to Effective Care in Pregnancy and Childbirth*. New York: Oxford University Press; Goer, H., Leslie, M. and A. Romano. (2007). "The Coalition for Improving Maternity Services' evidence basis for the Ten Steps of Mother-Friendly Care: Step 6: Does not routinely employ practices, procedures unsupported by scientific evidence." *Journal of Perinatal Education* 16(1): 48S–56S.

6. National Vital Statistics (2010).

7. See note 1 above.

8. Childbirth Connection. (2007) *What Every Pregnant Woman Needs to Know About Cesarean Section*. New York: Childbirth Connection (Full text available at www.childbirthconnection.org.); Goer, H., Leslie, M. and A. Romano. (2007). "The Coalition for Improving Maternity Services' evidence basis for the Ten Steps of Mother-Friendly Care: Step 6: Does not routinely employ practices, procedures unsupported by scientific evidence." *Journal of Perinatal Education* 16(1): 48S–56S; Appendix D.

9. Ad Council and U.S. Department of Health and Human Services. (2004) Breastfeeding Awareness Ad Campaign, www.adcouncil.org.

10. American Academy of Pediatrics. (2005) "Breastfeeding and the use of human milk." *Pediatrics*. 115, no. 2: 496–506.

11. See note 3 above.

12. Simkin, P. (1992) "Just another day in a woman's life? Nature and consistency of women's long term memories of their first birth experience." *Birth* 19:64–81.

13. Hodnett, E. (2002) "Pain and women's satisfaction with the experience of birth: A systematic review." *American Journal of Obstetrics and Gynecology* 186, no. 5:s160.

14. Knapp, L. (1996) "Childbirth satisfaction: the effect of internality and perceived control." *Journal of Perinatal Education* 5: 7–15.

15. Simkin, P., interview by Jillian Hanson. "Mother-Friendly Trends." *Pregnancy Today: The Journal for Parents-To-Be*.

Chapter 2: The History of Birth: Back to the Future

1. Rooks, J. (1997) *Midwifery and Childbirth in America*. Philadelphia: Temple University Press, chapter 2.

2. Ibid., chapter 1.

3. Ibid., 29–32.

4. White House Conference on Child Health and Protection (1932).

5. See note 1 above.

6. Olsen, O. and D. Jewell. "Home versus hospital birth." *Cochrane Database of Systematic Reviews* 1998, Issue 3. Art. No.: CD000352. DOI: 10.1002/14651858.CD000352); Leslie, M. and A. Romano. (2007). "The Coalition for Improving Maternity Services' evidence basis for the Ten Steps of Mother-Friendly Care: Birth can safely take place at home and in birthing centers." *Journal of Perinatal Education* 16(1): 81S–84S.

7. Sullivan, N. (March 6, 2002) midwifeinfo.com.

8. Gaskin, I. M. (2003) *Ina May's Guide to Childbirth*. New York: Bantam, 131

9. Enkin, M., et al. (2000) *A Guide to Effective Care in Pregnancy and Childbirth*. New York: Oxford University Press.

10. Bing, E. (1996) "Lamaze Childbirth: Then and Now." *Lamaze Parents' Magazine*.

11. Jordan, B. (1975) *American Journal of Obstetrics and Gynecology* 80, no. 2:284–90.

12. Odent, M. (1984) *Birth Reborn*. New York: Pantheon Books, 50.

13. Rooks, J. (1997) *Midwifery and Childbirth in America*. Philadelphia: Temple University Press, 246–47.

14. House of Commons Health Committee. (1992) *Second Report, Maternity Services* 1. London: HMSO, xciv.

15. See www.cia.gov/cia/publications/factbook for a rank ordering of world's nations on infant mortality rates.

16. *The Cochrane Library*. Oxford: Update Software. (www.cochrane.org)

17. See note and9 above.

18. Ibid.

19. Sakala, C. and M. Corry. (2008). *Evidence-Based Maternity Care: What It Is and What It Can Achieve*. New York: Milbank Memorial Fund.

20. Goer, H., M. Leslie, and A. Romano. (2007). "The Coalition for Improving Maternity Services'

evidence basis for the Ten Steps of Mother-Friendly Care: Step 6: Does not routinely employ practices, procedures unsupported by scientific evidence." and *Journal of Perinatal Education* 16(1): 48S–56S.; Enkin, M., et al. (2000) *A Guide to Effective Care in Pregnancy and Childbirth.* New York: Oxford University Press, chapter 30.

21. Ryan, K. J. (1988) "Giving Birth in America." *Family Planning Perspectives.* 20:298–301.

22. See note 15 above.

23. Rooks, J. (1997) *Midwifery and Childbirth in America.* Philadelphia: Temple University Press.

24. See note 9 above.

25. Luce, B. (March 2004) "A Natural Choice." *Swarthmore.*

26. American College of Nurse-Midwives, www.midwife.org; Midwives Alliance of North America, www.mana.org.

27. See note 25 above.

28. Lamaze International, www.lamaze.org.

29. Coalition for the Improvement of Maternity Services, www.motherfriendly.org.

30. McGhee, C. "The Value and Purpose of Labor Support." *International Doula* 11, no. 3.

31. Childbirth Connection, www.childbirth connection.org.

32. See note 18 above.

33. Choices in Childbirth, www.choicesinchildbirth.org.

34. The Birth Survey, www.thebirthsurvey.com.

35. International Cesarean Awareness Network,www.ican-online.org.

36. Birthing Project USA, 1900 T. Street, Sacramento, Ca 95814; 888-657-9790, www.birthingprojectusa.com.

37. Rogers, F. (1998) Lifetime Achievement Award acceptance speech given at the Daytime Emmy Awards ceremony.

Chapter 3: You're Pregnant!

1. Flaxman, S. and P. W. Sherman. (June 2000) *The Quarterly Review of Biology* 75, no. 2:113–48.

2. England, P. and R. Horowitz. (1998) *Birthing from Within.* Albuquerque, New Mexico: Partera Press, 256.

3. Harding, R. and A. Bocking, ed. (2001) *Fetal Growth and Development.* New York: Cambridge University Press.

4. Gaskin, I. M. (2003) *Ina May's Guide to Childbirth.* New York: Bantam, 303.

5. Fernandes, O., et al. (1998) "Moderate to heavy caffeine consumption and relationship to spontaneous abortion and abnormal fetal growth: a meta-analysis." *Reproductive Toxicology* 12:435–44.

6. Jahanfar, S. and H. Sharifah. "Effects of restricted caffeine intake by mother on fetal, neonatal and pregnancy outcome." *Cochrane Database of Systematic Reviews* 2009, Issue 2. Art. No.: CD006965. DOI: 10.1002/14651858.CD006965.pub2.

7. Enkin, M., et al. (2000) *A Guide to Effective Care in Pregnancy and Childbirth.* New York: Oxford University Press, chapter 5.

Chapter 4: Choosing a Caregiver and Birth Site

1. *Rights of Childbearing Women.* New York. Childbirth Connection. (See Appendix C.)

2. World Health Organization. (1999) "Care in normal birth: Report of a technical work group." Geneva: World Health Organization.

3. Rooks, J. (1997) *Midwifery and Childbirth in America.* Philadelphia: Temple University Press, chapter 1.

4. Devitt, N. (1979) "The statistical case for the elimination of the midwife: fact versus prejudice, 1890–1935 (Parts 1 and 2)." *Women and Health* 4:(part 1) 81–96 (part 2) 169–83.

5. Enkin, M., et al. (2000) *A Guide to Effective Care in Pregnancy and Childbirth.* New York: Oxford University Press.

6. Childbirth Connection. (2007) *What Every Woman Needs to Know About Cesarean Section.* New York: Childbirth Connection; Appendix D.

7. Olsen, O. and D. Jewell. "Home versus hospital birth." *Cochrane Database of Systematic Reviews* 1998, Issue 3. Art. No.: CD000352. DOI: 10.1002/14651858.CD000352);

8. de Jonge, A., B. Y. van der Goes, et al. (2009) "Perinatal mortality and morbidity in a nation-wide cohort of 529,688 low risk planned home and hospital births." *BJOG* 2009; DOI: 10.1111/j.1471-0528.2009.02175.x.

9. Johnson, K and B. Daviss. (2005) "Outcomes of planned home births with certified professional midwives: Large prospective study in North America." *British Medical Journal* 330:14–16.

10. Janssen, P., K. Shoo, L. Ryan, et al . (2002) "Outcomes of planned home births versus planned hospital births after regulation of midwifery in British Columbia." *Can. Med. Assoc. Journal:* 166(3).

11. Janssen, P, L. Saxell, et al. (2009) "Outcomes of planned home birth with registered midwife versus planned hospital birth with midwife or physician." *Can. Med. Assoc. Journal* 181(6–7):377–83.

12. Ibid.

13. Mayberry, L., D. Clemmens, and A. De. (2002) "Epidural analgesia side effects, co-interventions, and care of women during childbirth: A systematic review." *Supplement to American Journal of Obstetrics and Gynecology.* 186, no. 5:s81–s93.

14. Enkin, M., et al. (2000) *A Guide to Effective Care in Pregnancy and Childbirth.* New York: Oxford University Press; Leslie, M. and S. Storton. (2007). "Evidence basis for the ten steps of mother-friendly care: Offers all birthing mothers unrestricted access to birth companions, labor

support, professional midwifery care." *Journal of Perinatal Education* 16(1): 10S–20S.

15. Enkin, M., et al. (2000) *A Guide to Effective Care in Pregnancy and Childbirth*. New York: Oxford University Press, 21; Leslie, M. and A. Romano. (2007). "The Coalition for Improving Maternity Services' evidence basis for the Ten Steps of Mother-Friendly Care: Birth can safely take place at home and in birthing centers." and *Journal of Perinatal Education* 16(1): 81S–84S.

16. Goer, H., M. Leslie, and A. Romano. (2007). "The Coalition for Improving Maternity Services' evidence basis for the Ten Steps of Mother-Friendly Care: Step 6: Does not routinely employ practices, procedures unsupported by scientific evidence." *Journal of Perinatal Education* 16(1): 32S–64S.

17. Leslie, M. and S. Storton. (2007). "Evidence basis for the ten steps of mother-friendly care: Offers all birthing mothers unrestricted access to birth companions, labor support, professional midwifery care." *Journal of Perinatal Education* 16(1):10S–20S.

18. Enkin, M., et al. (2000) *A Guide to Effective Care in Pregnancy and Childbirth*. New York: Oxford University Press, 21.

19. Declercq, E., et al. (2006) *Listening to Mothers II: Report of the Second National U.S. Survey of Women's Childbearing Experiences*. New York: Childbirth Connection.

20. Rooks, J. (1997) *Midwifery and Childbirth in America*. Philadelphia: Temple University Press, 448.

21. See note 18 above.

22. Rooks, J. (1997) *Midwifery and Childbirth in America*. Philadelphia: Temple University Press, 458.

23. See note 18 above.

24. Gaskin, I. M. (2003) *Ina May's Guide to Childbirth*. New York: Bantam, 310.

25. Fein, E., CNM. Personal communication with authors.

26. Rooks, J. (1997) *Midwifery and Childbirth in America*. Philadelphia: Temple University Press, 106.

27. Rosenblatt, R. (1988) "The future of obstetrics in family practice." *Journal of Family Practice* 26:127–29.

28. Coalition for Improving Maternity Services. (2000) *Having a Baby? Ten Questions to Ask*. www.motherfriendly.org.

29. Tumblin, A. and P. Simkin. (2001) "Pregnant women's perceptions of their nurse's role during labor and birth." *Birth* 28, no. 1:52–56.

30. Hodnett, E., S. Gates, G. Hofmeyrand C. Sakala. (2007) "Continuous support for women during childbirth." *Cochrane Database of Systematic Reviews*. Issue 3. Art No.: CD 003766. DOI:

10.1002/14651858.CD003766 pub 2. (Full text available at www.childbirthconnection.org.)

31. Knapp, L. (1996) "Childbirth satisfaction: the effect of internality and perceived control." *Journal of Perinatal Education* 5: 7–14.

32. Enkin, M., et al. (2000) *A Guide to Effective Care in Pregnancy and Childbirth*. New York: Oxford University Press, 250–51.

33. Ibid.

34. Enkin, M., et al. (2000) *A Guide to Effective Care in Pregnancy and Childbirth*. New York: Oxford University Press, 248–49.

35. American College of Nurse Midwives. (2003) "Criteria for Provision of Home Birth Services." *Clinical Bulletin* 7. (www.acnm.org)

36. Kitzinger, S. (2002) *Birth Your Way*. London: DK Publishers.

Chapter 5: Moving through Pregnancy

1. Enkin, M., et al. (2000) *A Guide to Effective Care in Pregnancy and Childbirth*. New York: Oxford University Press, chapter 6.

2. Ibid.

3. Eskenazi, B. (1999) "Caffeine-filtering the facts." *New England Journal of Medicine* 341, no. 22:1688–89.

4. Jahanfar, S. and H. Sharifah. "Effects of restricted caffeine intake by mother on fetal, neonatal and pregnancy outcome." *Cochrane Database of Systematic Reviews* 2009, Issue 2. Art. No.: CD006965. DOI: 10.1002/14651858.CD006965.pub2.

5. Raikkonen, K. (2005) "Sweet babies: Chocolate consumption during pregnancy and infant temperament at 6 months." Early Human Development 76:139.

6. American Academy of Pediatrics. (2005) "Policy Statement: Breastfeeding and the Use of Human Milk." *Pediatrics* 115, no. 2:496–506.

7. American Academy of Pediatrics, www.aap.org.

8. *OBGYN Headline News*. (April 15, 2004) www.obgyn.net.

9. Torloni, N., et al. (2009) "Safety of ultrasonography in pregnancy: WHO systematic review of the literature and meta-analysis." *Ultrasound Obstet Gynecol* 33: 599–608.

10. Enkin, M., et al. (2000) *A Guide to Effective Care in Pregnancy and Childbirth*. New York: Oxford University Press, 58.

11. Wagner, M. (1994) *Pursuing the Birth Machine: The Search for Appropriate Birth Technology*. Sevenoaks, Kent, UK: ACE Graphics.

12. *USA Today*. (February 3, 2004) "Long-held prenatal beliefs challenged." 1D.

13. Enkin, M. et al. (2000) *A Guide to Effective Care in Pregnancy and Childbirth*. New York. Oxford University Press, 77.

14. Schrag, S., R. Gorwitz, K. Fultz-Butts, A. Schuchat. "Prevention of perinatal group B streptococcal disease. Revised guidelines from CDC." *MMWR Recomm Rep* 2002;51(RR–11): 1–22

15. Illuzzi, J. L. and M. B. Bracken. "Duration of intrapartum prophylaxis for neonatal group B streptococcal disease: a systematic review." *Obstet Gynecol* 2006;108(5): 1254–65

16. Rothman, B. K., et al. (2001) *Birth by Design.* New York: Routledge, 180–98.

17. Ibid.

18. Engle, W. A., et al, and the Committee on Fetus and Newborn. (2007)."Late-Preterm" Infants: A Population at Risk." *Pediatrics* 120 (6)r 2007: 1390–1401.

19. Kamath, B., J. Todd, J. Glazner, D. Lexotte and A. Lynch. (2009) "Neonatal outcomes after elective cesarean delivery." *Obstetrics and Gynecology* 113:6, 1231–38.

20. Hall, K, (September 24, 2000) "Whispers, Dreams, and Blessings: Ancient Rituals for a New Millennium." Talk given at Lamaze International Conference, Memphis, Tenn.

Chapter 7: The Simple Story of Birth

1. Odent, M. (2003) *Birth and Breastfeeding: Discovering the needs of women during pregnancy and breastfeeding.* East Sussex, UK: Clarview Books.

2. Righard, L. and M. Alade. (1990) "Effect of delivery room routines on success of first breastfeed." *Lancet* 336, no. 8723:1105–107. (See also Delivery Self Attachment and The Amazing Talents of the Newborn in Recommended Resources.)

3. Kitzinger, S. (2000) *Rediscovering Birth.* New York: Pocket Books, 142.

Chapter 8: Keeping Your Birth Safe and Healthy

1. Kitzinger, S. (2002) *Birth Your Way.* London: Dorling Kindersley Limited, 151.

2. Kramer, M., et al. (2000) "The contribution of mild and moderate preterm birth to infant mortality." *Journal of the American Medical Association* 284, no. 7:843–49.

3. Goer, H., M. Leslie, and A. Romano. (2007). "The Coalition for Improving Maternity Services' evidence basis for the Ten Steps of Mother-Friendly Care: Step 6: Does not routinely employ practices, procedures unsupported by scientific evidence." *Journal of Perinatal Education* 16(1): 42S–45S.

4. American Congress of Obstetricians and Gynecologists. (2000) *Planning your pregnancy and birth.* Washington, DC: ACOG.

5. American Congress of Obstetricians and Gynecologists. (2002) "ACOG news release: Cesarean delivery more likely with labor induc-
tion of a large baby." Washington, DC: ACOG; Sanchez-Ramos, et al. (2002) "Expectant management versus labor induction for suspected fetal macrosomia: A systematic review." *Obstetrics and Gynecology* 100, no. 5: 997–1002.

6. Alexander, J., et al. (2000) "Forty weeks and beyond: Pregnancy outcome by week of gestation." *Obstetrics and Gynecology* 96, no. 2:291–94; Enkin, M., et al. (2000) *A Guide to Effective Care in Pregnancy and Childbirth.* New York: Oxford University Press.

7. Roberts, J., et al. (1983) "The effects of maternal position on uterine contractility and efficiency." *Birth* 10:243–49.

8. Kroger, M. (2004) *Maternal positions in labor, birth, and breastfeeding. Impact of birthing practices on breastfeeding: Protecting the mother and baby continuum.* Sudbury, Ma.: Jones and Bartlett Publishers, 70.

9. Carlson, J., et al. (1986) "Maternal positions during parturition in normal labor." *Obstetrics and Gynecology* 68, no. 4:443–47.

10. Storton, S. (2007). "The Coalition for Improving Maternity Services' evidence basis for the Ten Steps of Mother-Friendly Care: Step 4: Provides the birthing woman with freedom of movement to walk, move, assume positions of her choice." *Journal of Perinatal Education* 16(1): 25S–28S.

11. Lawrence, A., L. Lewis, G. J. Hofmeyr, T. Dowswell, and C. Styles. "Maternal positions and mobility during first stage labour." *Cochrane Database of Systematic Reviews* 2009, Issue 2. Art. No.: CD003934. DOI: 10.1002/14651858.CD003934.pub2.

12. Declercq, E., et al. (2006) *Listening to Mothers II: Report of the Second National U.S. Survey of Women's Childbearing Experiences.* New York: Childbirth Connection.

13. Adachi, K., M. Shimada, and A. Usai. (2003) "The relationship between parturient's positions and perceptions of labor pain intensity." *Nursing Research* 52, no. 1:47–51.

14. Kitzinger, S. (2000) *Rediscovering Birth.* New York: Pocket Books, 99.

15. Hodnett, E., S. Gates, G. Hofmeyrand C. Sakala. (2007) "Continuous support for women during childbirth." *Cochrane Database of Systematic Reviews.* Issue 3. Art No.: CD 003766. DOI: 10.1002/14651858.CD003766 pub 2. (Full text available at www.childbirthconntection.org).

16. Leslie, M. and S. Storton. (2007). "The Coalition for Improving Maternity Services' evidence basis for the Ten Steps of Mother-Friendly Care: Step 1: Offers all birthing mothers unrestricted access to birth companions, labor support, professional midwifery care." *Journal of Perinatal Education* 16(1): 10S–20S.

17. Tumlin, A. and P. Simkin. (2001) "Pregnant women's perceptions of their nurse's role during labor and birth." *Birth* 28, no. 1:52–56.

18. Hodnett, E. (1996) "Nursing support of the laboring woman." *Journal of Obstetric, Gynecologic, and Neonatal Nursing* 25:257–64.

19. Kennell, J. Personal communication.

20. Enkin, M., et al. (2000) *A Guide to Effective Care in Pregnancy and Childbirth*. New York: Oxford University Press, chapter 50.

21. Declercq, E., et al. (2006) *Listening to Mothers II: Report of the Second National U.S. Survey of Women's Childbearing Experiences*. New York: Childbirth Connection.

22. O'Sullivan, G. (1994) "The stomach—fact and fantasy: eating and drinking during labour." *International Anesthesiology Clinics* 32:31–44.

23. American Society of Anesthesiologists Task Force on Obstetric Anesthesia. (2007). "Practice guidelines for obstetric anesthesia: An updated report by the American Society of Anesthesiologists Task Force on Obstetric Anesthesia." *Anesthesiology* 104(4). 843–63.

24. Ibid.; American Congress of Obstetricians and Gynecologists. (2002) "ACOG practice bulletin: Obstetric analgesia and anesthesia." *Obstetrics and Gynecology* 100, no. 1:177–91.

25. American College of Nurse-Midwives. (2008). "Providing oral nutrition for women in labor." *Journal of Midwifery and Women's Health*. 53(3), 276–83.

26. Singata, M., J. Tranmer, G. M. L. Gyte. "Restricting oral fluid and food intake during labour." *Cochrane Database of Systematic Reviews* 2010, Issue 1. Art. No.: CD003930. DOI: 10.1002/14651858 .CD003930.pub2.

27. Begum, M., et al., ed. (1999) *Obstetrics for Postgraduates and Practitioners*. New Delhi: BI Churchill Livingstone.

28. Simkin, P. (1986a) "Stress, pain and catecholamines in labor: Part 1. A Review." *Birth* 13:227–33

29. See note 20 above.

30. Goer, H., M. Leslie, and A. Romano. (2007). "The Coalition for Improving Maternity Services' evidence basis for the Ten Steps of Mother-Friendly Care: Step 6: Does not routinely employ practices, procedures unsupported by scientific evidence." *Journal of Perinatal Education* 16(1): 35S–36S.

31. Enkin, M., et al. (2000) *A Guide to Effective Care in Pregnancy and Childbirth*. New York: Oxford University Press, chapter 30.

32. Goer, H., M. Leslie, and A. Romano. (2007). "The Coalition for Improving Maternity Services' evidence basis for the Ten Steps of Mother-Friendly Care: Step 6: Does not routinely employ practices, procedures unsupported by scientific evidence." *Journal of Perinatal Education* 16(1): 39S–42S.

33. American Congress of Obstetricians and Gynecologists. (2005) "ACOG practice bulletin: Intrapartum fetal heart rate monitoring." *Obstetrics and Gynecology* 105, no. 5:1161–1168.

34. American College of Nurse-Midwives. (2007) "Intermittent auscultation for intrapartum fetal heart rate surveillance." *Journal of Midwifery and Women's Health* 52(3), 314–19.

35. See note 20 above.

36. Fraser, W., et al. (2003) "Amniotomy for shortening spontaneous labour." *The Cochrane Library* 2. Oxford: Update Software.

37. Enkin, M., et al. (2000) *A Guide to Effective Care in Pregnancy and Childbirth*. New York: Oxford University Press, chapter 35.

38. See note 36 above.

39. Enkin, M., et al. (2000) *A Guide to Effective Care in Pregnancy and Childbirth*. New York: Oxford University Press, 337.

40. Declercq, E., et al. (2006) *Listening to Mothers II: Report of the Second National U.S. Survey of Women's Childbearing Experiences*. New York: Childbirth Connection.

41. Mayberry, L., D. Clemmens, and A. De. (2002) "Epidural analgesia side effects, co-interventions, and care of women during childbirth: A systematic review." *Supplement to American Journal of Obstetrics and Gynecology*. 186, no. 5:s81–s93.

42. Lieberman, E. and C. O'Donoghue. (2002) "Unintended effects of epidural analgesia during labor: a systematic review." *Supplement to American Journal of Obstetrics and Gynecology* 186, no. 5:s31–s68.

43. Howell, C. J. (2003) "Epidural versus non-epidural analgesia for pain relief in labor." *The Cochrane Library* 3. Oxford: Update Software; . Leslie, M., A. Romano, and D. Woolley. (2007) "The Coalition for Improving Maternity Services' evidence basis for the Ten Steps of Mother-Friendly Care: Step 7: Educates staff in non-drug methods of pain relief and does not promote use of analgesic, anesthetic drugs." *Journal of Perinatal Education* 16(1): 69s-73s.

44. Righard, L. and M. Alade. (1990) "Effect of delivery room routines on success of first breastfeed." Lancet 336, no. 8723: 1105–107.

45. Matthiesen, A., et al. (2001) "Maternal analgesia during labor disturbs newborn behavior: Effects on breastfeeding, temperature, and crying." Birth 28, no. 1:5–12.

46. Schaffer, J., S. Bloom, , B. Casey, D. McIntire, M. Nihira, and K. Leveno. (2006. "A randomized trial of the effects of coached vs. uncoached maternal pushing during the second stage of labor on postpartum pelvic floor structure and function." *American Journal of Obstetrics and Gynecology* 192(5): 1692–96.

47. See note 20 above.

48. See note 40 above.
49. See note 20 above.
50. Gupta, J. and C. Nickoderm. (2000) "Maternal posture in labour." *European Journal of Obstetrics and Gynecology and Reproductive Biology* 92, no. 2:273–77; see note 20 above.
51. Gupta, J. K., G. J. Hofmeyr, and R. Smyth. (2004) "Position in the second stage of labour for women without epidural anaesthesia." *Cochrane Database of Systematic Reviews*, Issue 4. Art. No.: CD002006.
52. Johnson, N., V. Johnson, and J. Gupta. (1991) "Maternal positions during labor." *Obstetrical and Gynecological Survey* 46, no. 7:428–34.
53. See note 20 above.
54. Anderson, G., et al. (2003) "Early skin-to-skin contact for mothers and their healthy newborn infants." *The Cochrane Library* 3. Oxford: Update Software.
55. Uvnas-Moberg, K. (1998) "Oxytocin may mediate the benefits of positive social interactions and emotions." *Psychoneuroendocrinology* 23, no. 8:819–38.
56. American Academy of Pediatrics (AAP) and American Congress of Obstetricians and Gynecologists (ACOG). (2002) *Guidelines for Perinatal Care*. Elk Grove, Il. and Washington, DC: AAP and ACOG; American Academy of Breastfeeding Medicine Protocol and Committee. (2003) "Clinical protocol #5: Peripartum breastfeeding management for the healthy mother and infant at term." *Academy of Breastfeeding Medicine News and Views* 9, no. 1; Association of Women's Health, Obstetric and Neonatal Nurses. (2000) *Evidence-based clinical practice guideline: Breastfeeding support: Prenatal care through the first year*. Washington, DC: AWHONN; World Health Organization (WHO). (1998) *Evidence for the 10 steps to successful breastfeeding*. Geneva, Switzerland: WHO.
57. Mikiel-Kostyra, K., J. Mazur, and I. Boltruszko. (2002) "Effect of skin-to-skin contact after delivery on duration of breastfeeding: a prospective study." *Acta Paediatrica* 91, no. 12;1301–306.
58. Christenssen, K., et al. (1992) "Temperature, metabolic adaptation and crying in healthy full-term newborns cared for skin-to-skin or in a cot." *Acta Paediatrica* 81, no. 6–7:488–93; ——— (1998) "Randomised study of skin-to-skin versus incubator care for rewarming low-risk hypothermic neonates." *Lancet* 352, no. 9134:1115; Bystrova, K., et al. (2003) "Skin-to-skin contact may reduce negative consequences of 'the stress of being born': A study on temperature in newborn infants subjected to different ward routines in St. Petersburg." *Acta Paediatrica* 92, no. 3:320–26.
59. Washington, DC: AWHONN; World Health Organization (WHO). (1998) *Evidence for the 10 steps to successful breastfeeding*. Geneva, Switzerland: WHO.
60. Christenssen, K., C. Siles, Moreno, L. Belaustequi, A., De La Fuente, et al. (1992); Christenssen, K., et al. (1995). "Separation distress call in the human neonate in the absence of maternal body contact." *Acta Paediatrica* 84, no. 5:468–73; Johanson, R., et al. (1992) "Effect of post-delivery care on neonatal body temperature." *Acta Paediatrica* 81, no. 11:859–63.
61. Righard, L. and M. Alade. (1990) "Effect of delivery room routines on success of first breastfeed." *Lancet* 336, no. 8723:1105–107.
62. Gaskin, I. M. (2003) *Ina May's Guide to Childbirth*. New York: Bantam.

Chapter 9: Finding Comfort in Labor

1. Simkin, P. (2001) *The Birth Partner*. Cambridge, Ma.: Harvard Common Press.
2. Kitzinger, S. (2000) *Rediscovering Birth*. New York: Pocket Books, chapter 7.
3. Trolle, B., et al. (1991) "The effect of sterile water blocks on low back labor pain." *American Journal of Obstetrics and Gynecology* 164, no. 5:1277–281.

Chapter 10: Birth Plans and Baby Plans

1. Hodnett, E., S. Gates, G. Hofmeyr, and C. Sakala. (2007) "Continuous support for women during childbirth." *Cochrane Database of Systematic Reviews* Issue 3. Art No.: CD 003766. DOI: 10.1002/14651858.CD003766 pub 2. (Full text available at www.childbirthconntection.org.)
2. Enkin, M., et al. (2000) *A Guide to Effective Care in Pregnancy and Childbirth*. New York: Oxford University Press, chapter 30.
3. Ibid., chapter 29.
4. American Society of Anesthesiologists Task Force on Obstetric Anesthesia. (2007) "Practice guidelines for obstetric anesthesia: An updated report by the American Society of Anesthesiologists Task Force on Obstetric Anesthesia." *Anesthesiology* 104(4): 843–63; American Congress of Obstetricians and Gynecologists Committee on Obstetric Practice, "ACOG Committee Opinion No. 441: Oral Intake During Labor," *Obstet Gynecol* 2009, 114(3): 714.
5. Enkin, M., et al. (2000) *A Guide to Effective Care in Pregnancy and Childbirth*. New York: Oxford University Press, chapter 29.
6. Ibid., chapter 35.
7. Ibid., chapter 32.
8. Lieberman, E. and C. O'Donoghue. (2002) "Unintended effects of epidural analgesia during labor: A systematic review." *Supplement to Journal of Obstetrics and Gynecology* 186, no. 5:s31–s68.

9. Leslie,M., A. Romanoand D. Woolley. (2007) "The Coalition for Improving Maternity Services' evidence basis for the Ten Steps of Mother-Friendly Care: Step 7:Educates staff in nondrug methods of pain relief and does not promote use of analgesic, anesthetic drugs" *Journal of Perinatal Education*16(1): 68S–73S.

10. Ibid.

11. See note 7 above.

12. Sakala, C., M. Corry, and H. Goer. (2007) *Vaginal Birth and Cesarean Birth: How Do the Risks Compare?* New York: Maternity Center Association. (Full report available at www.maternitywise.org.); Goer, H., M. Leslie, and A. Romano. (2007). "The Coalition for Improving Maternity Services Evidence basis for the Ten Steps of Mother Friendly Care: Step 6: Does not routinely employ practices, procedures unsupported by scientific evidence." *Journal of Perinatal Education* 16(1): 48S–56S.

13. Klaus, M., J. Kennell, and P. Klaus. (1998) *Your Amazing Newborn*. Reading, Ma: Perseus Books.

14. ———. (1998) *The Amazing Talents of the Newborn*. Johnson and Johnson Pediatric Institute.

15. American Academy of Pediatrics. (February 2005) "Policy Statement: Breastfeeding and the Use of Human Milk." *Pediatrics* 115, no. 2:496–506. (http://aappolicy.aappublications.org/cgi/content/full/pediatrics;115/2/496)

Chapter 12: Greeting Your Newborn

1. Kitzinger, S. (2002) *Birth Your Way*. London: DK Publishers, 177.

2. Knoki-Wilson, U. (2003) "Keeping the Sacred in Childbirth Practices: Navajo Perspective." Lamaze International Annual Conference, Albuquerque, New Mexico.

3. Klaus, M. and J. Kennell. (1983) *Bonding: The Beginning of Parenting*. New American Library.

4. Gaskin, I. M. (2003) *Ina May's Guide to Childbirth*. New York: Bantam, 259.

5. Righard, L. and M. Alade. (1990) "Effect of delivery room routines on success of first breast-feed." *Lancet* 336, no. 8723:1105–107.

6. Matthiesen, A., et al. (2001) "Postpartum maternal oxytocin release by newborns: Effects of infant hand massage and suckling." *Birth* 28, no. 1:13–19.

7. Waldenstrom, U. and A. Swenson. (1991) "Rooming-in in the postpartum ward." *Midwifery* 7, no. 2:82–89; Keefe, M. (1987) "Comparison of neonatal nighttime sleep-wake patterns in nursery versus rooming-in environments." *Nursing Research* 36, no. 3:140–44; ——— (1988) "The impact of infant rooming-in on maternal sleep at night." *Journal of Obstetric, Gynecologic, and Neonatal Nursing* 17, no. 2:122–26.

8. Kushner, H. (2003) *The Lord Is My Shepherd: Healing Wisdom of the Twenty-Third Psalm*. New York: Knopf.

9. Crenshaw, J. (2009). "Lamaze Healthy Birth Practice # 6: Keep mother and baby together: It's best for mother, baby, and breastfeeding." Washington, DC: Lamaze International.

10. Yamauchi, Y. and I. Yamanouchi. (1990) "The relationship between rooming-in/not rooming-in and breastfeeding variables." *Acta Pediatrica* 79, no. 11:1017–1022.

11. Syafruddin, M., et al. (1988) "A study comparing rooming-in with separate nursing." *Paediatrica Indonesiana* 79, no. 11:116–23.

12. Keefe, M. (1987) "Comparison of neonatal nighttime sleep-wake patterns in nursery versus rooming-in environments." *Nursing Research* 36, no. 3:140–44; ——— (1988) "The impact of infant rooming-in on maternal sleep at night." *Journal of Obstetric, Gynecologic, and Neonatal Nursing* 17, no. 2:122–26.

13. Prodomidis, M., et al. (1995) "Mothers touching newborns: A comparison of rooming-in versus minimal contact." *Birth* 22, no. 4:196–200; Klaus, M., et al. (1972) "Maternal attachment: Importance of the first postpartum days." *The New England Journal of Medicine* 286, no. 9:460–63; Norr, K., et al. (1989) "Early postpartum rooming-in and maternal attachment behaviors in a group of medically indigent primiparas." *Journal of Nurse Midwifery* 34, no. 2:85–91.

14. Hutton, E. and E. Hassan. (2007) "Late vs. early clamping of the umbilical cord in full-term neonates: Systematic review and met-analysis of controlled trials." *JAMA* 297(11): 1241–252 ; Chaparro, C., R. Fornes, L. Neufeld, G. Alavez, et al. (2007) "Early umbilical cord clamping contributes to elevated blood lead levels among infants with higher lead exposure." *Journal of Pediatrics* 151:505–12.

15. Mercer, J. and R. Skovgaard, R. (2002) "Neonatal transitional physiology: A new paradigm." *Journal of Perinatal and Neonatal Nursing* 15(4): 56–75.

16. American Academy of Pediatrics. (1999). "Cord blood banking." *Pediatrics* 104, no. 1: 116–18.

17. Dick-Reed, G. (2004 edition) *Childbirth without Fear: The Principles and Practice of Natural Childbirth*.

18. Enkin, M., et al. (2000) *A Guide to Effective Care in Pregnancy and Childbirth*. New York: Oxford University Press, chapters 44 and 46.

19. Gray, L., et al. (2002). "Breastfeeding is analgesic in healthy newborns." *Pediatrics* 4: 590–95.

20. Academy of Breastfeeding Medicine. (1999) "Guidelines for Glucose Monitoring and Treatment of Hypoglycemia in Term Infants." (Available at www.bfmed.org/protocol/protocol.html.)

21. American Academy of Pediatrics. (1999) "Circumcision Policy Statement." (Available at www.aap.org.)

22. Ibid.
23. Gartner, M. and M. Herschel. (2000) "Jaundice and breastfeeding." *Pediatric Clinics of North America* 48, no. 2: 389–97.
24. Klaus, M., J. Kennell, and P. Klaus. (2001) *Your Amazing Newborn*. Cambridge, Ma: Perseus, 52.
25. Ibid., 32–41.
26. Ibid., chapter 5.
27. Ibid., chapter 6.
28. Ibid., chapter 3.
29. Bell, S. and M. Ainsworth. (1973) "Infant crying and maternal responsiveness." *Child Development* 43: 1171.
30. See note 24 above, 31.

Chapter 13: Early Parenting

1. Bergman, N. (2000) "Kangaroo mother care: Restoring the original paradigm for infant care and breastfeeding." (http://www.kangaroo mothercare.com/)
2. McKenna, J. "Cultural Influences on Infant Sleep." (www.attachmentparenting.org/cosleepmckenna.shtml)
3. McKenna, J., et al. (1997) "Bedsharing promotes breastfeeding." *Pediatrics* 100: 214–19; McKenna, J. (1991) "Sleep and arousal patterns among co-sleeping mother-infant pairs: Implications for SIDS." *American Journal of Physical Anthropology* 83: 331–37.
4. Academy of Breastfeeding Medicine. (2008) "Guidelines for Co-Sleeping and Breastfeeding." (www.bfmed.org/)
5. McKenna, J. and S. Mosko. (1994) "Sleep and arousal, synchrony and independence: Nursing infants and mothers sleeping apart and together." *Acta Paediatrica[* 397: 94–102.
6. McKenna, J. (1991) "Sleep and arousal patterns among co-sleeping mother-infant pairs: Implications for SIDS." *American Journal of Physical Anthropology* 83: 331–37.
7. Coburn, Jennifer, "The benefits of co-sleeping: Lower your baby's risk of stress disorders, SIDS and more," *The Compleat Mother* (www.breast-feeding.com)
8. Fox, M. "Stressed Babies May Be Prone to Trouble Later." www.atlc.org (Alliance for Transforming the Lives of Children.)
9. Consumer Product Safety Commission. (October 1999) "Hazards for Babies on Adult Beds." Position paper in *The Archives of Pediatrics and Consumer Medicine*.
10. Sears, William, "Safe Co-Sleeping." (iparenting.com)
11. Newman, J. and T. Pitman. (2000) *The Ultimate Breastfeeding Book of Answers*. New York: Prena Publications.
12. American Academy of Pediatrics. (February 2005) "Policy Statement: Breastfeeding and the Use of Human Milk." *Pediatrics* 115, no. 2: 496–506. (http://aappolicy.aappublications.org/cgi/content/ full/pediatrics;115/2/496)
13. Ibid.
14. http://www.who.int/child-adolescent-health/NUTRITION/infant_exclusive.htm
15. Beck, K. (March/April 2004) "Baby fat: The new mom's struggle with body image" *Mothering* 123.
16. Rogers, F. (2003) *The World According to Mister Rogers: Important Things to Remember*. New York: Hyperion, 168.

RECOMMENDED RESOURCES

Books, Booklets, Blogs, and Articles

Block, J. (2008) *Pushed: The Painful Truth about Childbirth and Modern Maternity Care*. New York: Da Capo Press.

The Boston Women's Health Book Collective. (2008) *Our Bodies: Ourselves: Pregnancy and Birth*. New York: Touchstone/Fireside.

Childbirth Connection. (2006) *What Every Pregnant Woman Needs to Know About Cesarean Section*. (available at http://www.childbirthconnection.org and http://www.lamaze.org)

Coalition for Improving Maternity Services. (2007) *Coalition for Improving Maternity Services: Evidence Basis for the Ten Steps of Mother-Friendly Care*. (available at http://www.motherfriendly.org/downloads.php; a summary of the evidence fact sheet also available at this website)

Davis, E. and Pascali-Bonaro, D. (2010) *Orgasmic Birth: Your Guide to a Safe, Satisfying, and Pleasurable Birth Experience*. New York: Rodale Books.

Declercq, E., Sakala, C., Corry, M., et al. (2006) *Listening to Mothers II: Report of the Second National U.S. Survey of Women's Childbirth Experiences*. New York: Childbirth Connection. (available at http://www.childbirthconnection.org)

DeVries, R. (2005) *A Pleasing Birth*. Philadelphia: Temple University Press.

England, P. and Horowitz, R. (1998) *Birthing from Within: An Extra-Ordinary Guide for Childbirth Preparation*. Partera Press.

Enkin, M., Keirse, M., Neilson, J. et al (2000) *A Guide to Effective Care in Pregnancy and Childbirth*. New York: Oxford University Press. (Full text of this book is available at http://www.maternitywise.org, or visit the Cochrane Library at http://www.cochrane.org.)

Gaskin, I. M. (2003) *Ina May's Guide to Childbirth*. New York: Bantam Books.

Gaskin, I. M. (2009) *Ina May's Guide to Breastfeeding*. New York: Bantam Books.

Goer, H. and Romano, A. (2010) *Obstetric Myths versus Research Realities*. Ann Arbor, Michigan: University of Michigan Press.

Goer, H. and Wheeler, R. (1999) *The Thinking Woman's Guide to a Better Birth*. Perigee Books.

Jukelevics, N. (2008) *Understanding the Dangers of Cesarean Birth: Making Informed Decisions*. Praeger.

Kitzinger, S. (2002) *Birth Your Way*. DK Publishing.

Kitzinger, S. (2003). *The Complete Book of Pregnancy and Childbirth*. New York: Knopf.

Kitzinger, S. (2000) *Rediscovering Birth*. New York: Pocket Books

Klaus, M., Kennell, J., Klaus, P. (1998) *Your Amazing Newborn*. Perseus Books.

Klaus, M., Kennell, J., Klaus, P. (2002) *The Doula Book*. Cambridge, Ma.: Perseus Books.

Lake, R. and Epstein, A. (2009) *Your Best Birth: Know All Your Options, Discover the Natural Choices, and Take Back the Birth Experience*. Wellness Central.

La Leche League. (2004) *The Womanly Art of Breastfeeding*. Seventh Edition. La Leche League Publishing.

Lamaze International. (2009) Healthy Birth Practice papers. (available at http://www.lamaze.org)

————. Giving Birth with Confidence blog, http://givingbirthwithconfidence.org.

————. Science & Sensibility blog, http://scienceandsensibility.org.

Mohrbacher, N. and Kendall-Tackett, K. (2005) *Breastfeeding Made Simple: Seven Natural Laws for Nursing Mothers*. Oakland, CA: New Harbinger Publications.

Newman, J. and Pitman, T. (2000) *The Ultimate Breastfeeding Book of Answers*. New York: Prima Publishing.

O'Mara, P. (2003) *Mothering Magazine's Having a Baby Naturally*. Atria Books.

Rooks, J. (1997) *Midwifery and Childbirth in America*. Philadelphia: Temple University Press.

Simkin, P., et al. (2010) *Pregnancy, Childbirth, and the Newborn*. Minnetonka, Mn.: Meadowbrook Press.

DVDs and Videos

Many of these DVDs and videos are used in Lamaze classes; ask your childbirth educator about them. Those marked with an asterisk are reasonably priced and valuable to view early in your pregnancy.

* *Amazing Talents of the Newborn*. (1998) with Marshall Klaus. phyllisklaus@gmail.com.

Celebrate Birth. Injoy Videos with Lamaze International. 800-326-2082. http://www.lamaze.org

* *Everyday Miracles*. Injoy Videos with Lamaze International. View in its entirety on http://www.lamaze.org.

* *The First Hour of Life* with Marshall Klaus. phyllisklaus@gmail.com.

* *Healthy Birth Your Way*. Injoy Videos with Lamaze International. View in its entirety on http://www.lamaze.org.

Open Minds to Birth. (2002) Vida Health Communications. Available from http://www.vidahealth.com

* *Orgasmic Birth: The Best Kept Secret*. (2009) with Debra Pascali-Bonaro. Available from http://www.orgasmicbirth.com or http://www.amazon.com.

Pregnant in America: A Nation's Miscarriage. (2008) with Steve Buonaugurio. Available from http://www.pregnantinamerica.com or http://www.amazon.com.

* *The Business of Being Born*. (2007) with Ricki Lake and Abby Epstein. Available from http://www.thebusinessofbeingborn.com or http://www.amazon.com.

*Timeless Way: A History of Birth from Ancient to
   Modern Times.* Injoy Videos. 800-326-2082
Gentle Birth Choices. (1996) 800-641-baby
Follow Me Mum: The Key to Successful Breastfeeding.
   (2003). Available from reblact@iinet.net.au or
   Hale Publishing (http://ibreastfeeding.com).
The Real Deal on Breastfeeding. Available from
   www.realdealvideos.com
Penny Simkin's Comfort Measures for Childbirth.
   (2009) with Penny Simkin. Available from
   http://www.pennysimkin.com
* *Birth Day.* (2003) with Naoli Vinaver Lopez.
   Sage Femme productions. Available from
   http://www.homebirthvideos.com/birthday_
   dvd.asp and http://www.amazon.com.

Organizations

American Academy of Pediatrics (AAP)
141 Northwest Point Boulevard
Elk Grove Village, IL 60007-1098
Phone: 847-434-4000
Fax: 847-434-8000
http://www.aap.org

American College of Nurse-Midwives (ACNM)
8403 Colesville Road, Suite 1550
Silver Spring, MD 20910-6374
Phone: 240-485-1800
Fax: 240-485-1818
http://www.midwife.org

Canadian Association of Midwives
http://www.canadianmidwives.org

Canadian Doula Association
4 Lamplight Bay
Spruce Grove, Alberta T7X 4N2
Phone: 780-962-1846
http://www.canadiandoulas.com

Canadian Paediatric Society
2305 St. Laurent Boulevard
Ottawa, Ontario K1G 4J8
Phone: 613-526-9397
Fax: 613-526-3332
http://www.cps.ca

Childbirth Connection
281 Park Avenue South, 5th Floor
New York, NY 10010
Phone: 212-777-5000
Fax: 212-777-9320
http://www.childbirthconnection.org

Citizens for Midwifery
P.O. Box 82227
Athens, GA 30608
http://www.cfmidwifery.org

The Coalition for Improving Maternity Services (CIMS)
1500 Sunday Drive, Suite 102
Raleigh, NC 27607
Phone: 919-863-9482
Fax: 919-787-4916
http://www.motherfriendly.org

The Cochrane Library
http://www.cochrane.org

DONA International
P.O. Box 626
Jasper, IN 47547
Phone: 888-788-DONA
Fax: 812-634-1491
http://www.dona.org

International Cesarean Awareness Network (ICAN)
1304 Kingsdale Avenue
Redondo Beach, CA 90278
Phone: 800-686-ICAN or 310-542-6400
Fax: 310-542-5368
http://www.ican-online.org

International Lactation Consultant Association (ILCA)
2501 Aerial Center Parkway, Suite 103
Morrisville, NC 27560
Phone: 888-ILCA-IS-U (452-2478) or 919-861-5577
Fax: 919 459-2075
http://www.ilca.org

La Leche League International (LLLI)
P.O. Box 4079
Schaumburg, IL 60168-4079
Phone: 847-519-7730
Fax: 847-519-0035
http://www.lalecheleague.org

Lamaze International
2025 M Street NW, Suite 300
Washington, DC 20036
800-368-4404
http://www.lamaze.org

Midwives Alliance of North America (MANA)
4805 Lawrenceville Highway, Suite 116-279
Lilburn, GA 30047
Phone: 888-923-MANA (6262)
Fax: 417-777-6181
http://www.mana.org

Vaginal Birth After Cesarean (VBAC)
Nicette Jukelevics, MA, ICCE
Center For Family
24050 Madison Street, Suite 200
Torrance, CA 90505
310-375-3141
http://www.vbac.com

INDEX

Real women sharing stories,
finding answers and
supporting each other.

Giving Birth
with Confidence Blog

GivingBirthwithConfidence.org

Pregnancy, Childbirth, and the Newborn, 4th Edition

This book covers all aspects of childbearing, from conception through early infancy.
It offers detailed information, suggestions, and advice to help make pregnancy, childbirth, and new parenthood an enjoyable, healthy experience. It presents the latest
research-based information, including new information on complementary medicine
approaches, updated information on interventions during childbirth, and new advice
to help you make informed decisions about your care. It's the most authoritative,
yet easy to use.

Extra information, resources, and worksheets are located on PCNGuide.com.

100,000+ Baby Names

This is the #1 baby name book and is the most complete guide for helping you name
your baby. It contains more than 100,000 popular and unusual names from around the
world, complete with origins, meanings, variations, and famous namesakes. It also
includes the most recently available top 100 names for girls and boys, as well as over
300 helpful lists of names to consider and avoid.

First-Year Baby Care

This recently updated, time-tested book provides new parents with essential information
about baby care basics including bathing, diapering, and feeding; help with choices
about circumcision, cloth or disposable diapers, childcare, and more; plus the latest
information about newborn screening tests, SIDS, vaccinations, treatments for common
illnesses, and healthy sleep patterns. It's a quick and easy way for parents to find the
information they need, when they need it.

We offer many more titles written to delight, inform, and entertain.
To order books or browse our full selection of titles, visit our web site at:

www.meadowbrookpress.com

For quantity discounts, please call: 1-800-338-2232